Clinical
Leadership
in Nursing

Clinical Leadership in Nursing

Judith T. Rocchiccioli, PhD, RN

Visiting Professor in Nursing Administration
Louisiana State University
New Orleans, Louisiana
Faculty
Medical College of Virginia
Virginia Commonwealth University
Richmond, Virginia

Mary S. Tilbury, EdD, RN, CNAA

Formerly Visiting Professor in Nursing
  Administration
Louisiana State University
New Orleans, Louisiana
Faculty, University of Maryland School of Nursing
Baltimore, Maryland
Consultant to the Magnet Nursing Services
  Recognition Program
American Nurses Credentialing Center
Washington, D.C.

W.B. SAUNDERS COMPANY
A Division of Harcourt Brace & Company

Philadelphia London Toronto Montreal Sydney Tokyo

W.B. SAUNDERS COMPANY

A Division of Harcourt Brace & Company

The Curtis Center
Independence Square West
Philadelphia, Pennsylvania 19106

Library of Congress Cataloging-in-Publication Data

Clinical leadership in nursing / Judith T. Rocchiccioli, Mary S. Tilbury.—1st ed.

p.   cm.

ISBN 0–7216–5442–8

1. Nursing services—Administration.   2. Leadership.   I. Tilbury,
Mary Sayre.   II. Title.
[DNLM: 1. Nurse Administrators.   2. Nursing, Supervisory.
3. Leadership.   WY 105 R671c 1998]

RT89.R63   1998   362.1′73′068—dc21

DNLM/DLC   97-34010

CLINICAL LEADERSHIP IN NURSING   ISBN 0–7216–5442–8

Printed in the United States of America.

Last digit is the print number: 9   8   7   6   5   4   3   2   1

Contributors

Faye Anderson, RN, MS, CNAA
Doctoral Student, Nursing Administration Program, Louisiana State University Medical Center School of Nursing, New Orleans, Louisiana.
Chief Nursing Officer, Gulf Coast Medical Center, Biloxi, Mississippi.
Performance Management

Christine R. Curran, MSN, RN
Doctoral Candidate in Informatics, University of Maryland School of Nursing, Baltimore, Maryland.
Associate Director, Care Provider Applications, Information Technology Department, Penn State Geisinger Health System, The Milton S. Hershey Medical Center, Hershey, Pennsylvania.
Information Management in a Changing Nursing Environment

Sarah S. Detmer, RN, MS
CEO Rivers Healthcare Resources
Aylett, Virginia
Clinical Leadership in Nursing: The RN as Integrator

Jacqueline A. Dienemann, PhD, RN, CNAA, FAAN
Associate Professor, School of Nursing, and Nursing Systems Expert, Johns Hopkins University, Baltimore, Maryland.
Quality Management

Anne Fortenberry, DNS, RN
Chairperson, Division of Nursing, Louisiana College, Pineville, Louisiana.
Communication, Conflict Management, and Negotiation

Betsy Frank, RN, PhD
Associate Professor and Chair, Department of Health Restoration, Indiana State University, School of Nursing, Terre Haute, Indiana.
Time Management

Carole A. Gassert, PhD, RN
Nurse Consultant, Informatics, Division of Nursing, Department of Health and Human Services, Rockville, Maryland.
Information Management in a Changing Nursing Environment

Mary Etta C. Mills, ScD, RN
Associate Professor and Chair, Department of Education, Administration, Health Policy and Informatics, University of Maryland School of Nursing, Baltimore, Maryland.
Motivation and Motivational Leadership

Ruth November, RN, JD
Attorney in Private Practice
Roanoke, Virginia
Legal Considerations in Clinical Nursing Practice

Dorothy M. Nyberg, MS, RN
Coordinator, Nursing Clinical Quality, Department of Nursing, Johns Hopkins Hospital, Baltimore, Maryland.
Quality Management

J. Anne O'Neil, PhD, RN
Independent Consultant, Ethics, Education, and Research, Baltimore, Maryland.
Ethical Leadership in Nursing

Virginia Kay Rogers, MS, MEd, RNC
Graduate Student, Louisiana State University Medical Center, Nursing Doctoral Program, New Orleans, Louisiana.
Nurse Educator, Department of Veterans Affairs, Biloxi, Mississippi.
   Group Dynamics and Cultural Diversity

Enrica Singleton, DrPH, MBA, RN
Chair and Professor, Division of Nursing, Dillard University, New Orleans, Louisiana.
   Supervision and Delegation

William J. Ward, Jr., MBA
Associate Scientist and Director, MHS Degree Program in Health Finance and Management, Johns Hopkins School of Hygiene and Public Health; and Adjunct Faculty, University of Maryland School of Nursing, Baltimore, Maryland.
Principal, Healthcare Management Resources, Inc., Bel Air, Maryland.
   Fiscal Considerations in Clinical Leadership

Kathleen M. White, PhD, RN
Director for Case Management, Helix Health, Harbor Hospital Center, Baltimore, Maryland.
   Planned Change

Preface

The health care system is undergoing change at an unprecedented rate, and the impact of this process is profound. Reduction, retrenchment, and re-engineering of the hospital industry are all but accomplished. Newspapers and trade journals report hospital closures, mergers, and acquisitions and the formation of regional integrated health care delivery networks. Traditional health care insurance has essentially been replaced by a myriad of managed care structures that look like alphabet soup—HMO, PPO, POS, IPA, MSO—and headlines speak of drive-through deliveries and denial of care. The values, attitudes, and beliefs of a not-for-profit orientation are challenged by an environment characterized by for-profit motives. Against this backdrop, educators are challenged to respond and react, so as to prepare nurses who can provide leadership in this brave new world. This text was prepared with these thoughts in mind.

The registered nurse's role is shaped primarily by environmental factors. Today more than ever before, nurses are focused on the management of patient care, not only in the traditional acute-care setting but increasingly in community-based practice. The emergence of case management is only one reflection of this evolutionary process. On a daily basis, nurses must confront the impact of economic factors on the nursing process. The utilization of assistive personnel, the analysis of supply consumption patterns, the development of tools to map interdisciplinary clinical activities, the acquisition of electronic information systems, and the introduction of quality management methodologies represent only a few initiatives developed and designed to respond to the changing environment.

The need for effective nursing leadership has never been greater. In this text, leadership is used in a generic sense and incorporates the knowledge, skills, and competencies that might, in a theoretical sense, be associated with management. While the authors recognize that leadership and manage-

ment are different, the fundamental principles and concepts associated with these areas of content and those required for practice in today's health care system are inexorably intertwined.

In keeping with this perspective, this text is divided into three sections. The first focuses on the knowledge, concepts, and principles that are fundamental to leadership in the evolving environment. It includes a brief exploration of our health care system in transition, an examination of common organizational structures and their operating principles, a review of nursing care delivery systems, and an introduction to nursing case management. The incorporation of substantive fiscal content and a focus on information management is a direct reflection of the changing environment. Nurses must develop the skills and competencies necessary to include fiscal analytical tools and information management skills in decision-making activities.

The second section highlights concepts that are critical to the achievement of predetermined organizational outcomes. The ability to motivate subordinates in a challenging environment and to manage time wisely; the acquisition of leadership, supervision, and delegation skills are essential. The vital nature of effective communication and conflict management; the need for planned change; and the essentials of multicultural group process are requisite skills and competencies in a managed care environment.

The text concludes by focusing on systems that serve as integrating functions across the organization. Legal and ethical factors must receive the leader's consideration not only in the management of patient care but also in the management of personnel. Finally, the management of quality and of employee performance is at the heart of organizational effectiveness.

Although professional nursing leadership principles and concepts have always been an integral part of the nursing education process, their importance is increased and broadened in the evolving health care system. We must now be concerned with the "business" of nursing. This text is designed to provide the student with the knowledge, skills, and competencies to effectively engage the challenges and opportunities presented by the changing environment.

MARY S. TILBURY, EdD, RN, CNAA
JUDITH T. ROCCHICCIOLI, PhD, RN

Contents

Unit II
Critical Concepts in Contemporary Nursing Leadership 81

Foundations of Contemporary Nursing Leadership

Introduction: A Health Care System in Transition

Mary S. Tilbury, EdD, RN, CNAA

. . . .

LEARNING OBJECTIVES

This chapter will enable the learner to:
1. Analyze how the changing health care environment is being shaped by cost, access, and quality.
2. Describe the primary differences between the traditional and evolving health care systems.
3. Compare and contrast common characteristics of basic managed health care organizations.
4. Identify nursing implications and opportunities generated by this transformational process.

. . . .

INTRODUCTION

Change, challenge, and opportunity are the order of the day in the health care system. A fundamental process designed to restructure health care continues to unfold. As the provision of care moves from illness and acute care to one of wellness and community focus, the nursing profession must react and retool to meet the needs of society. To respond, the acquisition of relevant knowledge, skills, and competencies is essential. The purpose of this introductory chapter is to describe this powerful transformation, identify and explore factors fundamental to its evolution, and examine nursing opportunities created by the process.

THE COST OF HEALTH CARE

The primary factor driving changes in the health care system is cost. The principal actors are consumers, employers, insurance companies, and the federal government. In 1995, 13.6% of the gross domestic product, 988.5 billion dollars, was spent on health care. Since Congress enacted Medicare and Medicaid legislation in 1965, the cost of these programs, which are designed to care for the elderly and the economically disadvantaged, as well as health care costs in general, has risen steadily. As costs rose, insurance companies, such as Blue Cross and Blue Shield, passed increases on to employers. It was, therefore, inevitable that the premiums paid by employees for coverage would increase, affecting take-home pay. In addition, it is essential to recognize that not only did employers find company profits negatively affected by employee health care costs, but their stockholders continued to demand favorable returns on their investments. It became clearer and clearer that major change was inevitable (Table 1-1).

The Social Security Amendments of 1983 (PL 98-21) represents a key event in the process of health care reform. This legislation included provisions that dictated a fundamental shift in the way hospitals are paid for services. Prior to 1983, hospitals were reimbursed on the basis of *reasonable costs*. For example, shortly after discharge, a request would be submitted to the payer (insurance company) requesting reimbursement for services received by the patient. The longer the patient remained in the hospital, the more payment the

Table 1–1.
Changes in the Health Care Environment

OLD ENVIRONMENT	NEW ENVIRONMENT
Emphasis on hospital-based, acute care services	Emphasis on community-based practice in ambulatory settings
Emphasis on illness and treatment	Emphasis on health promotion and disease prevention
Retrospective reimbursement based on resource utilization and length of stay	Prospective reimbursement creates financial risk related to length of stay and resource utilization

hospital received. As the volume of laboratory tests and radiology studies increased, the hospital could request and expect more reimbursement. In financial terms, more was better (see Table 1–1).

The PL 98-21 legislation established a Medicare payment system based on 467 *diagnosis-related* groups, or DRGs. Reimbursement rates were prospectively established for each DRG prior to admission. For example, if DRG #209, total hip replacement, carried a reimbursement of $8000 and it cost the hospital $10,000 to provide the care, the hospital lost $2000. On the other hand, if the cost of caring for the patient was $6500, the hospital kept the $1500 difference. The Medicare DRG payment rate was determined primarily by data on the average length of stay for each DRG. This reimbursement model established a powerful incentive to reduce length of stay. For the first time, increasing the length of stay and doing more procedures did not represent increased revenues. It represented loss. This change in policy signifies a major shift in power among the principal players. Previously, the payer responded to requests for reimbursement, the amount of which was essentially determined by the provider's use of resources. With the advent of a prospective methodology, the payer, not the provider, established payment, irrespective of the resources utilized. The prospective philosophy and methodology of the Medicare system quickly spread to other insurers, such as commercial payers, and

efficiency, cost-containment, and productivity became driving management goals. Length of stay became the major focus of cost reduction activities as hospitals competed for patients.

As trends in admissions and occupancy rates declined, excess capacity was created. In response to the organizational pressures created by fiscal imperatives, each member of the hospital community was called on to find creative and innovative ways to contain costs. The restructuring of nursing service delivery systems, for example, with the goal of reducing costs while maintaining quality, was undertaken by many facilities. As length of stay dropped, inpatient beds were taken out of service and in some cases facilities either closed, merged, or were acquired by other hospital systems in an effort to reduce costs associated with the duplication of services. As a result, some nurses were laid off and the hospital job market was compromised.

ACCESS TO CARE

As the public policy debate regarding the cost of health care and how it would be delivered continued, the Clinton administration offered a plan to maintain quality, contain costs, and guarantee primary and preventive care to children and adults. This national health insurance plan addressed fiscal imperatives, but was also designed to meet the needs of the approximately 37 million citizens who were either uninsured or underinsured. Resistance to the Clinton plan was formidable, and the legislation was not passed. Insurance through employment continued as the primary means of securing coverage. Unparalleled consumer, provider, and payer forces in the marketplace filled the void left by the failed government initiative. Health care now operated in a business-oriented environment characterized by a marketplace centered on competition, cost, and revenue.

QUALITY OF CARE

The "new" health care environment challenged providers to deliver high-quality, low-cost care. Whereas organizational resources focused on analyzing costs, providers emphasized the need to oper-

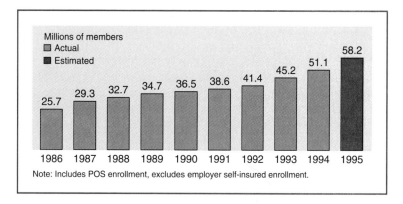

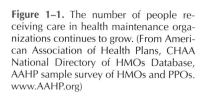

Figure 1–1. The number of people receiving care in health maintenance organizations continues to grow. (From American Association of Health Plans, CHAA National Directory of HMOs Database, AAHP sample survey of HMOs and PPOs. www.AAHP.org)

ationally define the exact nature of quality. Quality is an illusive concept, easily influenced by a variety of factors. Although a comprehensive discussion of quality and issues surrounding it are beyond the scope of this introductory chapter (see Chap. 16), it should be acknowledged that hospitals and health care providers recognized the need to more aggressively manage the process and outcomes of client care. Total quality management and the tools developed to support its implementation were adopted, not only as a means of managing cost, but also as a means of developing standards against which performance might be measured. The goal was to manage quality so as to benefit from experience, enhance the process of care, and achieve established outcomes.

The change process spawned by alterations in reimbursement practices and the failure of national health insurance opened the door to substantial reform. While the environment continues to develop, *managed care* dominates the marketplace as the primary approach designed to control the cost of health services and promote a continuum of care through the development and use of integrated services. The objectives, characteristics, and structures of this developing system are worthy of review.

MANAGED CARE

Managed care is the practice of prospectively paying predetermined amounts of money to selected providers to maintain the health of a defined population. The growth of managed care is extraordinary (Fox, 1997) (Figs. 1–1 and 1–2). Its success is due

primarily to modest premiums, high levels of consumer satisfaction, and employer support. Health care plans are offered as an employment benefit. As cited earlier, the cost of traditional or indemnity insurance plans has increased over time for both employees and employers. In an attempt to control health care costs, employers have either limited employee choices to the less costly managed care programs or encouraged their employees to elect managed care options. Whatever the dynamics operating, managed care organizations have made substantial gains in membership.

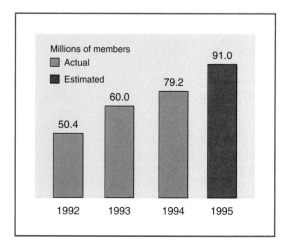

Figure 1–2. The number of people receiving care through preferred provider organizations is growing rapidly. (From American Association of Health Plans, AMCRA Census Database, AAHP sample survey of HMOs and PPOs. www.AAHP.org)

Methods and Structure of Managed Care

It is important to separate the methods that managed care organizations use to achieve organizational goals and objectives from the structures they employ to administer their organizations. Population-based care, for example, emphasizes the promotion of health, patient education, early identification of disease, and self-care. It responds to the fact that it is far less costly to provide this type of care than that associated with acute care and hospitalization. Through the development of contractual arrangements, managed care organizations enter into a variety of relationships with providers, such as hospitals and physicians, to meet the needs of its members. Relationships with primary care physicians are of paramount importance in meeting the needs of participating members and the fiscal goals of the managed care organization. Physicians typically receive a set sum, or capitated rate, for patient care. In this financial arrangement, the physician is paid a specified amount per member per month to provide care, irrespective of services rendered. Thus, the physician is provided with an incentive to keep the patient healthy. The managed care organization monitors the frequency of services such as pap smears, mammograms, and routine physical examinations to ensure that care goals are met through wellness promotion and early detection. In addition, primary care physicians also serve as gatekeepers. This utilization management technique requires that they prospectively authorize specialty care and limit the use of hospital-based services to promote efficient, cost-effective, and appropriate use of resources.

Patient education and responsible self-care are encouraged by managed care organizations, practices that have long been endorsed and practiced by professional nursing. Indeed, the member is expected to accept responsibility for his or her own health and actively participate as a partner in managing his or her health. Members are furnished with educational materials covering a variety of subjects, such as the benefits of a low-fat diet, the health risks of smoking, and the advantages of regular exercise. Diabetic members, for example, are provided with classes designed to enhance their knowledge and improve their health status. Members are also encouraged to use health care resources appropriately, and resources are allocated to assist beneficiaries in meeting this expectation. For example, managed care organizations often utilize professional nurse advice lines to assist in problem-solving. The emphasis is on prevention, health promotion, and early detection. These initiatives contribute not only to quality care but also to the organization's financial goals.

Managed care organizations structure their services in a variety of ways. Over the last few years, the distinction between these various configurations has diminished, but a description of the more common structures and the acronyms used to symbolize them is useful (Wagner, 1997). Three factors—premiums, provider choice, and the manner in which relationships are structured between the managed care organization and physicians—provide a basis for the examination of managed care structures.

Health Maintenance Organizations

The health maintenance organization (HMO) is one of the oldest and most familiar managed care structures. It offers comprehensive coverage for hospital and physician services in exchange for a fixed, prepaid fee. It is both an insurance company and a health care delivery system. When this type of organization is selected by employees for health care coverage, costs and premiums are characteristically low for employer and beneficiary alike. Provider choice runs along a continuum from restricted to permissive (see Fig. 1–3).

Staff models, also known as closed panel HMOs, employ a group of physicians in areas such as family practice, obstetrics and gynecology, internal medicine, and pediatrics to provide member services. The physicians are usually salaried but may also be eligible for bonus or incentive pay, depending on their performance and productivity. Highly specialized care is provided by physicians through contracted services. Member choice in this model is limited.

In the *group* model, the HMO contracts with a physician group to provide member services. The financial arrangement between the parties varies from capitation to reimbursement on the basis of prospectively established fees. In some cases, the physician group may be allowed to see non-HMO patients, and in others, practice is restricted to

HMO members. For the beneficiary, choice in this type of HMO is limited and premiums are low. It should be noted that the primary difference between the staff and group models hinges on the way in which the physician–organization relationship is structured.

The *network* HMO contracts with more than one group of physicians for medical services. Physicians are usually compensated on a capitated basis. Specialist referral is managed by the primary group and the specialists are compensated for their services by the group, not the HMO. Consumer choice varies in this type of HMO. In some cases, the HMO will contract with a limited number of groups, and in others, establish relationships with any physician who meets their participation specifications. Although the element of choice in this arrangement varies for the HMO member, it is usually more liberal than the staff and group models. In accordance, employer costs and beneficiary premiums are typically somewhat higher.

Independent practice association and *direct contract* model HMOs are similar. The independent practice association is a legal entity composed of physician members from a broad range of specialties and subspecialties. It contracts with the HMO to provide medical care. The contract between the HMO and independent practice association typically features a capitated reimbursement arrangement. The reimbursement relationship between the independent practice association and member physicians varies.

In the direct contract model, the HMO enters into contractual arrangements with a variety of individual physicians to provide services. Physician compensation varies from a predetermined fee structure to capitation. Consumer choice is high in these arrangements; thus, the employer's contribution and the employee's premiums are somewhat higher than those of other arrangements.

Preferred Provider Organizations

Preferred provider organizations represent an arrangement between employers and insurance companies that provide member services from a selected group of providers. Physicians, who agree to accept discounted reimbursement rates, can participate in the arrangement. The choice of physicians is typically comprehensive and members can commonly elect to see any participating physician without prior authorization. Preferred provider organizations also permit members to see non-participating physicians, although significant deductibles and co-payments are usually required. Since choice in these arrangements is liberal, the premiums may be the highest of the managed care organization arrangements offered to consumers.

Exclusive Provider Organizations

The exclusive provider organization model parallels the preferred provider organization, with one major exception. Beneficiaries are limited to those providers that are participating physicians for any required health care services. In this plan primary care physicians serve as gatekeepers. If members elect to see physicians outside the exclusive provider organization, services may not be covered. This arrangement is highly attractive to employers because of the degree of regulation, utilization management, and cost savings, but limited provider selection may dissatisfy potential members. It follows, however, that employee premiums are among the lowest in the managed care arena (Fig. 1–3).

Managed care and the structures that reflect this movement will continue to evolve. The models described represent only a fundamental review of the

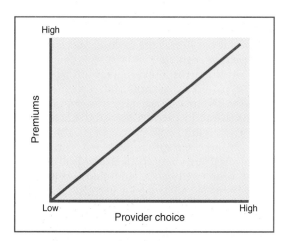

Figure 1–3. Provider choice is a significant factor in determining beneficiary premium levels.

basic factors that shape structures. They will continue to evolve as they respond to changes in the health care marketplace. In a little more than a decade, the system has progressed from one highlighting illness and acute care services to one featuring health promotion, disease prevention, and early detection in an efficient, effective, and fiscally responsible manner. The implications for nursing practice are profound.

NURSING IMPLICATIONS AND OPPORTUNITIES

Today's health care environment offers an opportunity for nurses to gain in professional status by proactively responding to the changing needs and expectations of society. As the single largest provider group, the nursing profession is positioned to influence not only the development of the system but also how practice will be shaped by the changing landscape. This exchange process will affect every aspect of professional practice.

First, nursing has the opportunity to fill the vacuum left by the growth of specialty medical practice and the increased demand for primary care services that emphasize early detection, health promotion, and disease prevention. Advanced practice nurses (APNs)—nurse practitioners, clinical nurse specialists, certified nurse midwives, and certified registered nurse anesthetists—are prepared to provide a wide range of high-quality health care services. These specialties characteristically require education beyond the baccalaureate level and emphasize subspecialty preparation.

Advanced practice opportunities are particularly favorable in today's environment. Although many types of APN educational programs are available, the majority are focused on preparing family, adult, pediatric, geriatric, and women's health practitioners. These clinicians are prepared to take complete medical histories, conduct physical examinations, furnish well-baby and child health care, provide prenatal and routine gynecological services, and diagnose and treat common acute and chronic health care problems. They are particularly skilled in patient teaching, health promotion, and disease prevention.

These practitioners, through their knowledge, skill, and competency, offer the health care system high-quality, cost-effective care, but the opportunity to practice is frequently limited by state regulations. As noted earlier, not only must nursing respond to the opportunities presented by a health care system in transition, but it must also engage in activities designed to change state and federal regulations and the scope of practice limitations. A definitive review of issues such as certified nurse midwives' practicing under the supervision of physicians and APNs' being granted prescriptive authority are beyond the scope of this introductory chapter, but they represent barriers to advanced practice in its fullest sense. Suffice it to say that the nursing community must engage in the politics of health care as one means of advancing the profession and meeting the needs of society.

Case management represents a second opportunity in the new environment. (Refer to Chapter 4 for a thorough review of this topic.) This developing role focuses on the needs and problems of individuals and families across the health care system and strives to direct the attainment of established patient outcomes while meeting consumer expectations in a cost-effective manner. The case manager reduces care fragmentation by working closely with other disciplines; acts as a patient advocate; and coordinates all aspects of the patient's care through the complex health care system. The role of case managers is valued by managed care organizations and acute care agencies alike because of their broad knowledge base and quality of care. Nurses are uniquely qualified to fill this role (Bower, 1992).

The roles described require, however, knowledge, skill, and competencies beyond those of the traditional or advanced clinician. An understanding and appreciation for organizational concepts and principles is required to influence decision-making. Communication skills are paramount in roles emphasizing coordination and transdisciplinary contact. In addition, as population demographics change and cultural diversity among clients and coworkers is evidenced, professionals must be sensitive to the impact of differing attitudes, values, and beliefs, as they affect not only patient care but also organizational policy. Concepts traditionally emphasized in health services administration education, such as motivation, performance management, and supervision and delegation, now provide a functional foundation for practice in the new environment.

Managed care organizations will also develop information systems that can track patients and provide data on practice patterns and trends, costs, and utilization of services across organizational units and boundaries. Specialization in nursing informatics provides many opportunities for nurses to augment the development of sophisticated patient care systems in the acute care arena and managed care settings, but the practice environment will require that all nurses develop computer competency and recognize the potential that this technology offers.

The development of complex legal and ethical health care issues is inevitable. The allocation of scarce resources, particularly fiscal ones, frequently raises utilization questions. Practices such as drive-through deliveries and same-day mastectomies are examples of the continuing struggle that exists between the use of organizational resources and the formulation of practice standards. The patient advocacy role is informed and expanded by knowledge in these fields.

Of paramount importance is the need for professional nurses to acquire fiscal competencies and skills. The cost of health care is the central factor driving system reform. Change creates opportunity. Nursing's potential to play a major role in the evolution of the health care system may well depend on the ability of each nurse to grasp the importance of financial management and contribute to the achievement of patient care outcomes through the development of creative and innovative, cost-effective practices. The fundamental concepts and principles of budgeting, revenue generation, cost accounting, variance analysis, return on investment, and benefit-cost analysis are critical to decision-making in health care organizations. These represent analytical tools that the nursing profession can use to promote its health care agenda. The opportunities are limitless and their potential exciting.

SUMMARY

The health care landscape is replete with change. The need for skilled nurse leaders and managers has never been greater. This chapter focused on factors driving change in the health care system, explored the basic elements of managed care, and described the structures that managed care employs to provide health care. The implications and nursing practice opportunities spawned by this transformation are profound and will require the nursing profession to retool and react to meet the needs of those it seeks to serve. Clinical proficiency must be informed by management and leadership theory and the skills and competencies that flow from and are supported by this knowledge base.

■ DISCUSSION QUESTIONS ■

1. Identify mechanisms that you might use to reduce the cost of care in the acute care setting, in the home health care setting, and in the community nursing center.
2. How might the role of the nurse case manager differ in a community setting as opposed to a hospital?
3. Why is the measurement of patient outcomes essential in the evolving health care system? Identify three mechanisms that might be used to evaluate nursing's contribution to patient outcomes.
4. What marketplace factors might receive primary consideration in designing types of managed care organizations?
5. How might a health maintenance organization manage the patient care evaluation; how might a preferred provider organization? What are the differences and similarities? Which type of managed care organization is best structured to manage quality? Why?
6. Identify and discuss factors that are driving the restructuring of acute care nursing service delivery systems.
7. Do advanced practice nurses have prescriptive authority in your state? If so, explore how it was obtained. If not, is it under consideration and what issues are operating in the environment?

■ LEARNING ACTIVITIES ■

1. You have been asked by a young, newly married couple what factors they should consider in selecting a managed care organization. How would you respond? How would you go about investigating this area of inquiry? What factors might be important to this young couple as opposed to a middle-aged one?

2. Collaboration and cooperation among health care providers is essential in achieving efficient and cost-effective care. Maintain a log describing your observations of mechanisms established to facilitate communication between the members of different health care disciplines. How did the mechanisms affect patient care? Were the mechanisms effective?

3. On a weekly basis, review current events in newspapers, magazines, newsletters, and other media reports regarding the health care system. Analyze one during each week of the semester. Specify the nursing implications and opportunities generated by the report.

■ REFERENCES ■

Bower R (1992). *Case management by nurses.* Washington, DC: American Nurses Publishing.

Brock R (1996). *The business of nursing.* Chicago: American Hospital Publishing.

Fagin CM (1992). Collaboration between nurses and physicians: No longer a choice. *Nursing and Health Care* 13(7):354–363.

Fottler M, Smith H, Muller H (1986). Retrenchment in health care organizations: Theory and practice. *Hospitals and Health Services Administration* Sept/Oct:30–43.

Fox PD (1997). An overview of managed care. In Kongstvedt PR (ed). *Essentials of Managed Health Care.* Gaithersburg, MD: Aspen Publishers, pp 3–16.

Heenan DO (1991). The right way to downsize. *The Journal of Business Strategy* 12(5):4–7.

Jones KR (1989). Evolution of the prospective payment system: Implications for nursing. *Nursing Economics* 7(6):299–304.

Keith JM (1996). Flattening the hierarchy. *Health Progress* 77(4):60–62.

Kongstvedt PR (ed) (1996). *The Managed Health Care Handbook,* 3rd ed. Gaithersburg, MD: Aspen Publishers.

Lamm RD (1996). The coming dislocation in the health professions. *Healthcare Forum Journal* 39(1):58–62.

Mckinley W (1992). Decreasing organizational size: To untangle or not to tangle? *Academy of Management Review* 17:112–123.

Pew Health Professions Commission (1995). *Critical Challenges: Revitalizing the Health Care Professions for the Twenty-First Century.* San Francisco, CA: UCSF Center for the Health Professions.

Sovie MD (1995). Tailoring hospitals for managed care and integrated healthcare systems. *Nursing Economics* 13(2):72–77.

Wagner ER (1997). Types of managed care organizations. In Kongstvedt PR (ed). *Essentials of Managed Health Care.* Gaithersburg, MD: Aspen Publishers, pp 36–48.

Weber LJ (1994). Ethical downsizing. *Health Progress* 75(6):24–26.

Zimmerman P (1994). Handling inevitable layoffs. *Journal of Emergency Medicine* 20(6):475–477.

2

Structural Foundations for Health Care Delivery

Mary S. Tilbury, EdD, RN, CNAA

LEARNING OBJECTIVES

This chapter will enable the learner to:
1. Analyze the development of a mission statement and the formulation of goals and objectives in shaping organizational function.
2. Identify and discuss concepts and principles central to organizational structures and their potential impact on nursing services.
3. Describe fundamental principles that have an impact on organizational relationships.
4. Identify key structural factors shaping decision-making and problem-solving activities.

We were trained hard . . . but it seemed that every time we were beginning to form up into teams, we would be reorganized. I was to learn later in life that we tend to meet any new situation by reorganizing and a wonderful method it can be for creating the illusion of progress while producing confusion, inefficiency and demoralization.

Petronius Arbiter, Roman Satirist, 1 AD

INTRODUCTION

There are those who would argue that things have not changed much since the 1st century AD. Re-structuring, resizing, right-sizing, and re-engineering of health care agencies is the order of the day. Acquisitions, mergers, takeovers, and joint ventures are common responses to a changing health care environment. Within each organization, administrators and managers strive to arrange or configure services so as to create a structure that will effectively and efficiently promote the achievement of quality patient outcomes. Organizational structure can be thought of as a coat rack. It provides the means by which the activities of an organization are "hung" together. Structures outline how business is conducted. Individuals interact with organizations from birth to death. It is, therefore, vital that nurse leaders appreciate the concepts and principles fundamental to organizational structure and how structure can influence nursing practice. This chapter is devoted to the achievement of these goals.

DEFINING ORGANIZATIONAL FUNCTION

Organizations exist for specific reasons. Restaurants, for example, provide consumers with food in a variety of ways, and schools serve the educational needs of individuals and groups across a wide spectrum. Hospitals provide acute care services; home health care agencies focus on serving needs outside the acute care setting; and hospices exist to care for the dying. These and other health care organizations function on a continuing basis to achieve a designated purpose, and the relationships established with them vary accordingly.

Mission Statement

Organizations specify and communicate their service intent primarily through two means. First, they develop a mission statement, which communicates in broad terms the reason for the organization's existence, the geographical area it serves, and the attitudes and beliefs within which the organization functions.

An example is Riverside Hospital's mission statement, shown in Figure 2–1. It declares that the organization provides acute care services and appropriate hospital-based services and specifies that all services are of high quality and are personalized. The statement limits the service area to Riverside and nearby counties and communities. Mission statements serve as an anchor in the development and delivery of products and services. Nurse leaders refer to mission statements in the design and execution of client care services. The use of the word *personalized* commits Riverside Hospital to a high level of service and influences how its human and financial resources are allocated. Nurse leaders recognize the characteristics valued in their organization and strive to provide services that are consistent with established values.

Although mission statements usually specify purpose, service area, and values, they may also speak to missions other than those directed at patients. Note, for example, that Riverside's statement does not include a teaching or research mission. Agencies whose purpose includes the training and education of health care providers or clinical research reference such activities in their mission statement. Indeed, the education of health care providers may be the primary mission of the organization and a principal focus of the mission statement.

It is the mission of the Riverside Hospital to provide high quality, personalized, acute patient care, and appropriate hospital-based services for the city of Riverside and areas of nearby counties and municipalities

Figure 2–1. Organizations use mission statements as one means of communicating service intent to their public.

Goals and Objectives

Once organizations have developed a mission statement, they turn to the ongoing formation of programs and services that address the attainment of their mission. The generation of goals and objectives (G&O) specific to the development of designated programs and services is the second means by which an organization specifies and communicates service intent. *Goals* are aspirations, and *objectives* are measurable activities. A home health care agency may establish a goal to implement an oncology chemotherapy administration program. The agency's objectives delineate how and what must occur for the program to function, such as staff training and equipment acquisition.

Goals and objectives are formulated to address planned change in any aspect of organizational life, such as the creation or development of new or existing services, the renovation of a clinical unit, or the introduction of case management as a care delivery role. The process by which G&O are formulated can take many forms. Typically, however, different groups or departments develop G&O in response to those established for the institution. For example, the organization's top executives, in concert with the board of directors, formulate G&O through a planning process designed to maintain and advance the organization's mission. Thereafter, the nursing department is expected to generate G&O at the department and unit level that support the attainment of those developed at the institutional level. Additionally, the nursing department formulates G&O that address needs specific to the department, unit, or team. Nurse leaders participate in and recognize the process of G&O development as critical to building commitment and cohesion in an organization.

It is essential that employees have a clear understanding of where the organization is going and how work activities contribute to its success. The mission statement and the formulation of G&O throughout the organization serve to facilitate and coordinate a team-oriented effort.

ORGANIZATIONAL STRUCTURE

As stated earlier, organizations arrange their activities so as to efficiently and effectively control work directed at achieving predetermined outcomes. Max Weber (1864–1920), a German sociologist, is commonly acknowledged as a key figure in the development of organizational theory. Weber conceived of an organizational structure called *bureaucracy* as a type of hierarchical arrangement designed to coordinate employee activities. Aspects of Weber's work continue to influence contemporary organizational design. An understanding of fundamental bureaucratic principles and concepts is essential to the analysis of organizational structure.

The Bureaucratic Model

Weber proposed a structure that featured a clear-cut division of labor that is hierarchical in nature and features several layers of management. Positions within the structure are typically filled on the basis of technical qualifications. The recruitment and employment process designed to fill positions frequently involves competency-verifying procedures such as examinations; however, once someone is employed, the dominant expectation is for a long-term or lifetime association with the organization.

The bureaucratic setting featured employee activities governed by defined rules and established procedures that typically provided little or no opportunity for managerial discretion or employee innovation. Problems were frequently categorized on the basis of designated criteria and acted upon using previously established courses of action. Such practices were designed to promote equity, objectivity, and fairness in organizational life. The working environment consequently was highly impersonal, precluding variation in the application of regulations or the exercise of partiality by managers. In addition, work life and private life were rigidly separated. Personal or family-related needs on the part of the employee were seen as beyond organizational consideration. The organization was the priority and employees were expected to accede to this expectation.

The dominant mode of bureaucratic communication was written, reflecting the impersonal nature of the environment. Memoranda and letters were preferred over personal contact of a verbal nature, reflecting the value placed on formality. Technical efficiency was the hallmark of Weber's bureaucracy, with a premium placed on quickness, control, continuity, and high returns on inputs. The resulting structures and practices proved beneficial in the life of organizations caught up in the production-oriented focus of the industrial revolution.

Although the environment in which organizations conduct their activities has changed significantly since Weber developed the bureaucratic model, many of the characteristics of that model continue in today's organizations. People still complain about the "red tape" of formal written communication and the inflexibility of an organization in dealing with a problem. Social reactions to reductions in workforce or layoffs are directly influenced by the bureaucratic practice that places value in long-term or lifetime employment, whereas highly competitive environments, such as those we find today, favor companies that can frequently reconfigure themselves to react to changes in the marketplace. Although the times have changed, many bureaucratic concepts and principles are evident in today's organizations and must be understood by nurse leaders to effectively engage organizational life.

THE FORMAL ORGANIZATION

Organizations arrange or structure themselves to coordinate activities and manage the performance of their employees. Departmentation is one of the primary ways in which this is achieved, whereby working relationships are specified and responsibilities systematically defined. Hospitals are commonly divided into major units or divisions such as finance, medical affairs, nursing, and marketing, among others. These large structural units are composed of departments such as materials management, medical records, food service, and advertising (Fig. 2–2). This type of organizational arrangement reflects fundamental bureaucratic principles.

The departments cited in the figure are organized on the basis of function, but some organizations elect to configure units around products, such as cardiac services, oncology, or maternal and child health services. In these structures, functions such as cardiac rehabilitation, electrocardiography, cardiac catheterization, and the nursing units that care for cardiac patients may be placed in the same division or organizational unit. The individual with organizational responsibility for this department

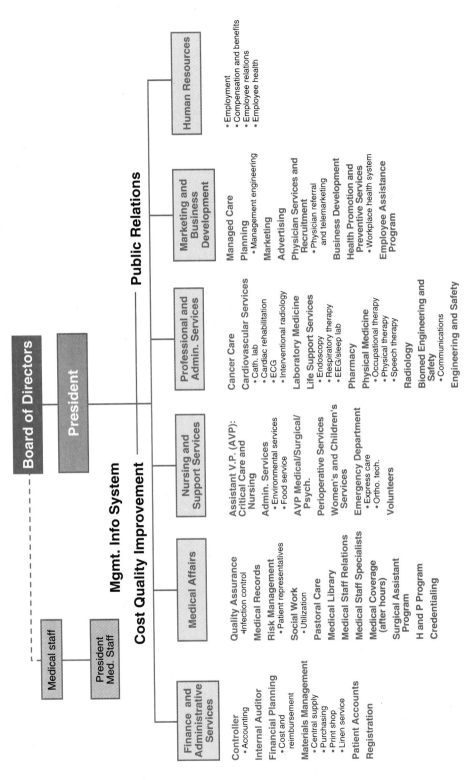

Board of Directors

President

President Med. Staff

Mgmt. Info System

Cost Quality Improvement

Public Relations

| Finance and Administrative Services | Medical Affairs | Nursing and Support Services | Professional and Admin. Services | Marketing and Business Development | Human Resources |

Finance and Administrative Services

Controller
• Accounting

Internal Auditor

Financial Planning
• Cost and reimbursement

Materials Management
• Central supply
• Purchasing
• Print shop
• Linen service

Patient Accounts

Registration

Medical Affairs

Quality Assurance
• Infection control

Medical Records

Risk Management
• Patient representatives

Social Work
• Utilization

Pastoral Care

Medical Library

Medical Staff Relations

Medical Staff Specialists

Medical Coverage (after hours)

Surgical Assistant Program

H and P Program

Credentialing

Nursing and Support Services

Assistant V.P. (AVP): Critical Care and Nursing

Admin. Services
• Environmental services
• Food service

AVP Medical/Surgical/ Psych.

Perioperative Services

Women's and Children's Services

Emergency Department
• Express care
• Ortho. tech.

Volunteers

Professional and Admin. Services

Cancer Care

Cardiovascular Services
• Cath. lab
• Cardiac rehabilitation
• ECG
• Interventional radiology

Laboratory Medicine

Life Support Services
• Endoscopy
• Respiratory therapy
• EEG/sleep lab

Pharmacy

Physical Medicine
• Occupational therapy
• Physical therapy
• Speech therapy

Radiology

Biomed Engineering and Safety
• Communications

Engineering and Safety

Marketing and Business Development

Managed Care

Planning
• Management engineering

Marketing

Advertising

Physician Services and Recruitment
• Physician referral and telemarketing

Business Development

Health Promotion and Preventive Services
• Workplace health system

Employee Assistance Program

Human Resources

• Employment
• Compensation and benefits
• Employee relations
• Employee health

Figure 2–2. An organizational chart is a graphic representation of the organization's structure and provides information regarding formal relationships, lines of communication, unity of command, span of control, and levels of management.

14

may or may not be a registered nurse. The consequences of how an organization elects to structure itself are significant in that the structure identifies authority and control relationships that have a profound impact on the nurse leader and the provision of care.

The organizational chart depicts and thereby communicates to all parties how activities are arranged, how authority relationships are defined, and how communication channels are established (see Fig. 2–2). The formal organization is communicated to employees and interested parties through the organizational chart. At the top of the chart is the Board of Directors, a group that has overall responsibility for the functioning of the organization. This group is commonly composed of community leaders, and its membership typically reflects community racial, ethnic, and gender demographics. Members usually serve in a voluntary capacity and thus receive no monetary compensation for their services. The board of directors is responsible for hiring and evaluating the chief executive officer (CEO) or president; frames organizational policies that define activities, such as whether the hospital will offer pediatric services; participates in setting the organization's agenda; and retains responsibility for financial performance. Obligation for the overall operation of the organization on a day-to-day basis is delegated by the board to the CEO.

The Chief Executive Officer

The CEO, in conjunction with members of the executive group, determines how the organization's structural hierarchy is organized. The executive group, or top-level management, represents the first of three management levels characteristically seen in organizations. The executive group's composition varies according to how the organization is structured. In the chart depicted in Figure 2–2, the president and those responsible for the major divisions (human resources, marketing and business development, professional and administrative services, nursing and support services, medical affairs, and finance and administrative services) make up top-level management. Their activities are focused on providing direction in the formulation of goals and objectives, achievement of fiscal performance targets, and defining and controlling operational policy.

In assessing how the practice of nursing is valued in the organization, it is important to determine if the chief nursing officer is a member of this executive group. The position of the chief nursing officer may be designated by a number of different titles, such as vice president for nursing, nursing administrator, or vice president for patient care, and may vary in its structural location. The presence or absence of a nursing perspective in upper level management decision-making has significant implications for nursing and patient care.

Middle-Level Managers

Middle-level managers serve primarily to coordinate activities between the upper and lower levels of the hierarchy and represent the main channel of communication between levels. These managers, who may include assistant vice presidents, department heads, shift supervisors, case managers, and nurse managers, are focused on the day-to-day operation of the nursing function and frequently play a major role in developing the policies and procedures that guide nursing and organizational activities. Furthermore, the participation of these individuals in the development of institutional, divisional, and departmental goals and objectives is key because of their proximity to the clinical operation. In the organizational chart depicted in Figure 2–2, for example, middle-level managers include the individuals responsible for materials management, medical records, perioperative services, laboratory medicine, advertising, and employee health, among others.

First-Level Managers

First-level managers, on the other hand, are focused primarily on the activities of their own work units. Within the nursing function, individuals such as assistant nurse managers, primary nurses, unit-based case managers, team leaders, and charge nurses are examples of those who act as first-level managers and have a major impact on delivery of care.

Unlicensed Assistive Personnel

As the health care system responds to increasing economic pressures, many organizations, particularly hospitals, elect to restructure nursing care delivery systems with the introduction of unlicensed assistive personnel. The use of these personnel places additional management responsibilities and leadership expectations on registered nurses, who must work through them to achieve patient and unit or organizational G&O. Therefore, the management and leadership skills required of registered nurses in such structures are fundamentally different than those required in units that, for example, might use only registered nurses, such as intensive care units. (See Chaps. 3, 8, and 10 for a more comprehensive discussion of relevant factors.)

The organizational chart also defines lines of communication within the organization and how authority is allocated. Solid vertical lines between positions define the organization's formal chain of command and communication. Positions that have been granted greater authority are located in the upper levels of the chart, whereas those at the lower levels have less authority. Vertical lines also indicate how communication should travel up and down the organization, whereas solid horizontal lines depict how departments with different functions, but similar levels of responsibility, conduct communication.

For example, in the organizational chart depicted in Figure 2–2, the manager with responsibility for medical-surgical and psychiatric nursing services can independently communicate up and down the vertical line of the nursing and support services division. If, however, he or she needs to communicate with the head of materials management in the finance and administrative services division, the nursing division administrator should also be advised regarding the communication. This can be accomplished verbally in a regular meeting, or by a duplicate of written communication or memoranda between the individuals that is sent to the division director. Although communication in modern organizational life is seldom this rigid, professionals should be mindful of formal communication standards and channels, as expectations can vary within the organizational setting. The basic idea is to keep everyone apprised who needs to be informed. The achievement of this objective is a challenge. A comprehensive review of effective communication principles and techniques is found in Chapter 11.

The organizational chart also provides information regarding line and staff positions. Line positions are directly concerned with achieving organizational objectives and are indicated by either vertical or horizontal solid lines on the chart. Staff positions, on the other hand, are focused on supporting, assisting, or advising the line in moving forward and typically provide expertise in areas deemed vital to the organization. Staff positions or relationships are represented by broken or dotted lines on the chart. The staff relationship of the medical staff to the board of directors is indicated by a dotted line on the chart in Figure 2–2. The medical staff assists the board in its decision-making activities, primarily through the exercise of influence, but does not have legitimate organizationally based authority.

Staff or advisory positions in nursing, such as clinical specialist, nurse researcher, or staffing coordinator, also lack legitimate authority in the organization and primarily influence the organization through building relationships and through demonstration of professional expertise. Consider the example of the clinical specialist who consults with nurses on skin integrity issues. Typically, this specialist recommends modifications in nursing interventions, but the unit nurse who is responsible for the patient's care makes the final decision as to how the plan of care will be altered. It is rare that the nurse would ignore the assistance of such a valuable resource, but within the context of structural relationships, line position authority dominates.

The lack of formal authority in staff positions can lead to the development of conflict between individuals in line and staff positions. Nurse managers, for example, can effectively block or otherwise thwart the suggestions or recommendations of the staffing coordinator or staff development instructor, based on their positional authority and responsibility. The concept of staff and line positions is sometimes difficult for registered nurses to understand, since the majority of health care organizations refer to clinical positions as "staff nurses." Staff nurses are actually in line positions, because they are instrumental in achieving the organization's primary quality care goal. *Line* and *staff* are organizational concepts that refer to an element or option in bureaucratic design, not position title.

UNITY OF COMMAND AND SPAN OF CONTROL

Unity of command and *span of control* are concepts that can also be evaluated using the organizational chart. Unity of command is depicted on the chart by vertical solid lines between individuals, specifying that each employee has one manager to whom he or she is responsible. The staff nurse is organizationally responsible to the nurse manager, and in the sample chart (see Fig. 2–2), the controller, for example, is responsible to the vice president for finance and administrative services. Although unity of command simplifies organizational relationships, it is difficult to maintain in complex health care organizations, which emphasize a team or multidisciplinary approach to patient care. Nurses frequently express concern that they have several bosses—nurse managers, physicians, and case managers, for example. Conflict and confusion are natural by-products of an intense and sometimes chaotic environment. The nurse leader is challenged by this complexity and should clarify responsibility relationships whenever doubt exists.

Span of control refers to the number of employees reporting to a manager. Until very recently, an optimal span of control was six to eight individuals. As health care organizations confront financial constraints, traditional standards, such as span of control, that increase the number of managers and divert fiscal resources from patient care are questioned, and factors such as manager skill, employee competence, and functional complexity are considered in the determination of manager-to-employee ratios. In the final analysis, a manager's span of control is established after careful consideration of relevant factors, such as those mentioned earlier, recognizing that arrangements that optimize performance and satisfy managers, leaders, and employees alike are ideal.

INTEGRATING ORGANIZATIONAL CONCEPTS

Comprehensive patient care requires the skill of many professionals who are located in different departments and who occupy different positions in the organization. The formal organization uses integrating mechanisms to allow linkage and coordination across various departments. Norms or expected methods of managing are frequently established through the development of structure standards such as policies and procedures. Critical pathways

are examples of integrating standards, in that they establish expected behaviors of professionals, on behalf of the patient, across the organization. Staff roles frequently serve to meet the integrational needs of the formal organization. The case manager and the clinical specialist, for example, work across departments and up and down the hierarchy to facilitate the achievement of patient care objectives.

Organizations also develop departments whose primary function is focused on integrating activities. Functions such as quality management, strategic planning, and information systems are typically housed in their own departments and work across the organization as a means of bringing the organization together. Finally, committees, task forces, and teams are structures often used as a means of responding to the need for integration across the formal organization. Groups who develop critical pathways or propose solutions to identified problems are examples of those that integrate activities.

COMMUNITY AND MATRIX STRUCTURES

Although bureaucratic structures tend to dominate organizational life, two other arrangements for organizing work are routinely seen: community and matrix structures.

Community Structures

The community structure is, in many respects, the opposite of bureaucracy. It is usually seen in small organizations composed of highly educated, skilled, and competent individuals. Extensive or complex hierarchy is precluded in community structures and the roles of its members are seldom formally articulated, although they may be well defined. Leadership is diffuse and transient and decisions are normally made by consensus. The special expertise of any member is only indirectly acknowledged and does not result in special status or privileges. The focus of organizational life is the group. Relationships are close, and communication is intimate and informal. People and their needs are a primary focus and there is far less division of labor than that found in a bureaucracy. Tradition plays a major role in this type of organization, and sanctions and social pressures are applied to and by all members in concert.

Organizations referred to as "think tanks" commonly use this structure to organize their activities. It has been suggested that the Supreme Court of the United States reflects community structure characteristics. In nursing, the staff development department, although housed in a large bureaucratic organization, may operate much like a community structure. A rural home health care agency, with a small staffing component, might elect to operate in the "community" manner. Otherwise, these structures are not frequently seen in the health care arena.

Matrix Structures

Matrix structures generate a high degree of complexity. In this arrangement, a second bureaucratic-like structure overlies the primary one, thus establishing two levels of authority, communication, and responsibility for those involved. Matrix structures are typically focused on production as opposed to the functional orientation of the underlying bureaucratic structure. It creates multiple reporting relationships, yielding an increased potential for conflict, uncertainty, and ambiguity.

For example, the organization may elect to create a product-focused structure responsible for managing its cardiac services. The nurse manager of the coronary care unit must not only respond to this management structure, but also to that of the nursing function. Matrix structures are commonly used in unstable environments subject to frequent changes and varying pressures, such as that in which health care currently exists. Through these types of structures, the nurse leader has an opportunity to influence how services are delivered to patients. Matrix structures can produce quality outcomes through the focus of experts on the development and management of service opportunities, but they require productive levels of communication, effective relationship-building skills, and a high degree of employee understanding, commitment, and competence.

Structures, as noted earlier, are designed to promote the achievement of organizational goals and objectives and they are frequently altered so as to better organize activities and improve communication and decision-making. It is important for nurse leaders to develop a basic understanding of how organizations are structured so that they can evaluate what structural changes might mean to the nursing function and analyze how they can use structure to better meet client needs. Organizations, however, do not live by structure alone. The analysis of organizational structure takes on an added dimension when the individuals occupying the positions are taken into consideration and their impact on function is evaluated.

THE INFORMAL ORGANIZATION

In every enterprise, an informal social organization exists in addition to the formal one defined and communicated in the organizational chart (Fig. 2–3). The informal organization serves as an indispensable communication system and establishes attitudes, customs, and habits at the work unit and organizational level. This system serves to meet the social needs of employees by supporting a sense of belonging in the frequently impersonal bureaucratic environment. The informal organization is not found on the organizational chart or in the employee handbook. It must be assessed and analyzed

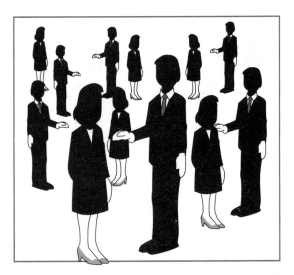

Figure 2–3. The informal system serves as an indispensable communication mechanism and establishes attitudes, customs, and habits at the unit and organizational level.

through experience. It can be hostile or friendly, it can facilitate or impede organizational goals, and it can change the experience, knowledge, attitudes, and emotions of those who are affected by it.

Grapevine Communication

The most obvious reflection of the informal system is the "grapevine," whereby information flows and rumors flourish. The grapevine is a vital aspect of any organization's communication network and can be effectively used to address the needs of employees. The grapevine picks up on issues that employees feel are important, such as those that generate anxiety and concern. It acts, therefore, as both a feedback mechanism and a filter. Situations involving appointments to vacant positions, declining volumes, changes in organizational structure, concerns regarding restructuring nursing delivery systems, and layoffs are only a few examples of situations that are subjects for the grapevine. Leaders engage in a continuing assessment of the grapevine and take steps to minimize the negative impact of rumors, whenever possible. This is accomplished by clarifying events that may seem inconsistent, establishing timetables for announcements about important decisions, and openly discussing best- and worst-case scenarios.

Outcomes of Informal Communication

The informal organization also establishes behavioral norms or expected behaviors. Consider the nurse who knows that only one radiological procedure stands in the way of a patient's discharge. The formal system calls for transcription of the order and notification of the radiology department. The nurse using the established formal system waits for notification by the radiology department that the procedure has been scheduled. Then consider the nurse leader who also uses the informal system. This nurse supervises the transcription and notification processes, but also calls a fellow member of the hospital bowling team, who happens to work in the radiology department. The patient's test is worked into the schedule within hours.

Another example is the nursing home employee who finds that recently installed water savers are causing dissatisfaction among the residents. The formal system calls for the nurse leader to notify the nurse manager, who in turn advises the nursing supervisor, who notifies the chief nurse executive, who calls the maintenance manager. Consider the nurse leader who also, or instead, approaches and briefs the chief nurse executive in the hallway, facilitates the inclusion of residents in the exchange, and demonstrates how the water savers have restricted water flow. The outcomes of informal communication enhance resolution of the problem, because the impact is real to those who have the authority to resolve employee and patient care issues. The ability of employees to utilize the informal system is enhanced as length of service with the organization increases and relationships are established and nourished. Through participation, nurse leaders can influence the values, attitudes, and beliefs of the informal system and thus how it responds and reacts to the activities of organizational life.

Some informal systems may include expectation of social functions. Such expectations may be reflected in unit-level parties for departing employees or celebrations related to marriages, impending births, engagements, and holidays. Other activities may involve staff members' meeting at a local restaurant or lounge on a regular basis. These activities meet employee socialization needs and support adjustment. On the other hand, some employees prefer to keep their personal and professional lives separated. Depending on the emphasis placed on socializing by the informal system the employee's integration into the organization is facilitated or impeded.

Informal Leadership

Informal systems also have informal leaders. These individuals influence organizational behavior and decision-making. The extent of the influence of an informal leader is frequently related to tenure, expertise, and close associations with those occupying key positions in the organization. Although the norms and functions of the informal organization may seem contrary to and even destructive to the formal organization, the system should be regarded as a mechanism for maintaining and supporting the individual against the effects of formal organization which, as identified earlier, tend to create a rigid and inflexible environment. Attempts to block or eliminate the informal organization are ill-advised, primarily because of the rapidity with which it can effect communication and because it serves as a means of alerting managers to employee concerns. A balance between the formal and informal organizations is generally productive in meeting the needs of the organization as a whole and those of the employee specifically.

PROFESSIONAL–BUREAUCRATIC CONFLICT

The potential for conflict is present between people in line positions and those in staff positions and between the formal and informal organizations. The other factor that frequently generates organizational conflict occurs when the values and attitudes of professionals are at odds with those of the organization. This dilemma is referred to as the *professional–bureaucratic conflict*. Professionals share similar characteristics or attributes and are bound by a code of ethics. The code calls for the professional to give priority to client needs. Individuals occupying positions of responsibility and authority in the organization are asked to represent and promote the interests of the organization. A professional's source of power is based on his or her knowledge and expertise. Bureaucratic authority is based on an employment relationship with the organization. Professional decisions are frequently governed by professional standards, and bureaucratic decisions are governed by compliance with policies, procedures, and directives from superiors. Professional actions are evaluated and sanctioned by peer groups with similar expertise. Bureaucratic actions are evaluated and sanctioned by superiors whose knowledge and skills may differ from those of the subordinate. The ability of the nurse leader to recognize and respond to these inherently conflicting factors is vital in maintaining a productive organizational environment.

The adjustment and adaptation of nurses to potential sources of conflict is critical. Some organizational expectations are pivotal and require cooperation, whereas others are subject to varying degrees of flexibility. Personal and professional adjustments to organizational life depend on the nurse leader's

skills and competencies. A theoretical understanding of organizational structures, principles, and concepts offers an opportunity to evaluate the organization's activities and to shape responses accordingly.

FOUNDATIONS FOR ORGANIZATIONAL DECISION-MAKING

The organizational chart is an invaluable management tool that discloses how activities are structured, communication conducted, and superior and subordinate relationships defined. The organizational chart, however, does not detail how decisions are made and who has the authority to make them.

Authority, Responsibility, and Accountability

Authority, or legitimate power, is defined as the official right to act. For example, a nurse manager has the authority to discipline and counsel an employee who is frequently absent from work. A registered nurse has the authority to defer the administration of a medication based on clinical assessment data, and the shift supervisor has the right to reassign employees from one unit to another. Authority is closely tied to the concept of responsibility. *Responsibility* is commonly defined as the duty to act. The nurse manager of an employee who is frequently absent is expected to act when the standards of the organization are breached. The shift supervisor who is authorized to reassign personnel has a duty to appropriately use staff to achieve patient care goals, and the nurse who withholds a medication does so because of his or her responsibility for safe and effective patient care.

The terms *responsibility* and *accountability* are often used interchangeably. Accountability, however, is a moral concept and involves acceptance, by the professional nurse, of the consequences of a decision or action. For example, the nurse manager has responsibility and authority for developing the unit's work schedule. The nurse manager, after careful consideration, elects to approve a request for a day off that will place the number of scheduled staff just below minimum levels. On the day in question the census and acuity are high and one of the registered nurses scheduled to work is involved in an accident on the way to work. Personnel from other floors are reassigned to help out, but the regular staff feel overwhelmed and express concerns regarding the quality of patient care. Does the nurse manager feel both responsible and accountable for the staffing decision? While it is clear that the organization has assigned this staffing decision responsibility to the nurse manager, only the nurse manager, through word and deed, can demonstrate the moral internalization of the decision, which is accountability.

The organization possesses a number of other mechanisms that further structure decision-making activities. Policies, procedures, and protocols are frequently used as guides in defining appropriate courses of action. Policies carry a high expectation of compliance and are sometimes referred to as *rules*. Some policies are formulated because external accrediting agencies such as the Joint Commission on the Accreditation of Healthcare Organizations (JCAHO) or the National Committee on Quality Assurance (NCQA) require them, whereas others are developed by the organization, department, or unit to shape employee behavior.

Procedures and Protocols

Procedures and protocols outline an accepted course of action, step by step, for achieving a specific outcome. The term *procedure* is used when defining a task, whereas *protocol* signifies the definition of a clinical process. For example, when a patient is required to undergo a diagnostic procedure that requires transportation to another facility, a procedure outlines step by step how arrangements are made for the patient's safe transportation. On the other hand, consider the patient who arrives in the emergency department with the classic signs and symptoms of a stroke. The physician may elect to use a clot-breaking drug such as streptokinase or tissue plasminogen activator. The emergency department uses a protocol detailing the process by which the drug will be administered and the role that nurses and representatives of other disciplines are expected to play in the process.

Centralization and Decentralization

Earlier in this chapter it was recognized that the CEO plays a major role in how an organization is structured. Top-level management also plays a major role in determining how responsibility and authority are delegated or distributed throughout the organization. When decisions are made by a limited number of individuals at the top of the organization or by the managers of a department or unit, and thereafter communicated to the employees, the decision-making is termed *centralized*.

When, on the other hand, authority is distributed throughout the organization, to allow for increased responsibility and delegation in decision-making, the organization is referred to as *decentralized*. In a health care environment emphasizing the need for efficient and effective operations, it is essential that managers, leaders, and clinicians have the authority necessary to make decisions that, for example, might affect the patient's length of stay or referral to an extended care facility. Over-centralization of decision-making and problem-solving activities creates an atmosphere characterized by apprehension and intimidation. Such an environment tends to be rigid and inflexible and employees are reluctant to act unilaterally, even when the outcome is clearly positive.

The organizational chart can provide important but not complete information regarding the decentralization of authority within the organization. Taller structures communicate multiple levels of management, with decision-making and problem-solving responsibilities that are cumbersome and time-consuming and do not involve those who are affected by these processes. Flatter structures, with fewer layers of management, are typical of organizations that have delegated authority for decision-making and problem-solving activities down the organization, involving those who are most directly affected by these activities. Each of these structures is illustrated in Figure 2–4.

The process of organizational decentralization has been accelerated by the changing environment and economic factors in the health care arena. In some situations, managers and staff have assumed new responsibilities, such as those focusing on reducing the length of stay. To adapt, the authority and responsibility for selected functions are decentralized. Consider the nurse manager who has accepted increased responsibilities for the fiscal management of his or her unit. In this case, the employees may be expected to assume staffing responsibilities that were once included in the nurse

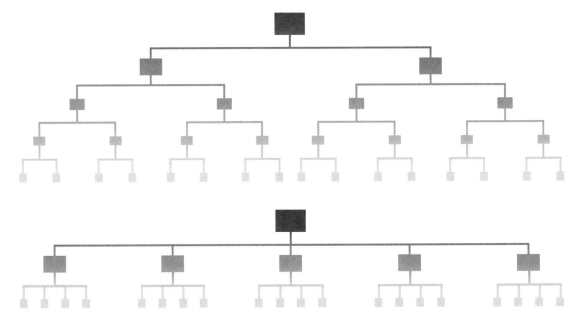

Figure 2–4. Tall centralized structures with multiple layers of management (top) are being replaced with flat decentralized structures (bottom) as economic resources diminish.

manager's duties. Thus, although the levels of management may remain the same, the nature of the positions within the organization may change substantially. Over time, however, and as reimbursement and revenues decrease, priorities dictate that finite resources be focused on patient care. In these organizations, the levels of management are decreased, the knowledge and skill required of those working in the organization are increased, and employee expectations are expanded.

Decentralization, however, is a qualitative concept and one that requires additional information by which to evaluate how the organization has designated responsibility and authority. The organizational chart does not communicate whether the nurse manager makes 24-hour staffing decisions or whether a registered nurse can call a physician regarding the patient's condition without first checking in with the charge nurse. Both of these situations provide information regarding the degree to which the department is decentralized. If decisions regarding staffing must be made or reviewed by the nurse manager's superior, the decision-making process is lengthened and the nurse manager's authority is limited. If a nurse is required to clear physician calls with the charge nurse, responsibility and authority are more centralized than they are when such a requirement is not in effect. It is essential to evaluate many factors to conduct an informed and accurate assessment regarding the decentralization of any organization.

STRUCTURE AND OUTCOMES

Organizational culture and climate are two different but vital outcomes of the principles and concepts related to structural foundations. Organizational climate involves how employees feel about their organization and can, for many reasons, change rapidly. Employee surveys, for example, are one means of capturing data related to the organization's climate on a variety of issues.

Organizational culture is much more lasting than climate and not as easily influenced by environmental factors. Culture may be defined as values, attitudes, and beliefs. Just as individuals vary in relation to these elements, so do organizations. Some organizations value the expertise of clinical nurse specialists and others do not; some organizations are paternalistic and some are empowering; some organizations focus on internal competition and others on cooperation; some organizations value employee participation in decision-making, others do not; and some organizations believe in and practice planned change, while others drift amid chaos.

Numerous factors are inherent in shaping an organization's culture, but none is more important than the leader's values, attitudes, and beliefs. Thus, it is vital that leaders are cognizant of their own viewpoints and those of the organization. In the evolving health care environment, nurse leaders may be required to dismantle aspects of the culture to enhance the organization's ability to respond efficiently and effectively. The more entrenched a pattern of organizational behavior, the more difficult the transition and change process. Consider the importance of health care economics in today's environment and the challenge of incorporating cost in the decision-making processes concerning patient care. Decisions regarding the organization's mission, structures, decision-making, and problem-solving styles all ultimately have an impact on culture. Furthermore, an understanding of the organization's culture is not readily achieved by employees. It is transmitted by leaders and through encounters and interpersonal relationships over time. The skill and competency of leaders profoundly affects these outcomes.

SUMMARY

This chapter focused on concepts and principles fundamental to organizational design. Structures are formulated to arrange the organization's activities in such a manner that efficient and effective operations are achieved. Administrative decisions regarding unity of command, span of control, integrating mechanisms, allocation of authority, and how line and staff positions are used to influence the organization's ultimate effectiveness were explored. Structures may be labeled bureaucratic, community, or matrix and described as tall, flat, centralized, or decentralized. The organizational chart defines the formal organization and its employees define the informal organization. A working knowledge of these concepts and principles, among others, prepares the nurse employee to proactively engage organizational life.

■ DISCUSSION QUESTIONS ■

1. What information might be gathered to make a judgment regarding the centralization versus decentralization of an organization? A unit?
2. Discuss the relationship between authority and responsibility. What are the implications of delegating responsibility without the appropriate levels of authority?
3. What factors must be identified, analyzed, and acted on before a manager's span of control can be altered?
4. What factors increase an individual's ability to informally influence the organization's climate? The culture?
5. What are the professional attributes that may interfere with the establishment of a positive working relationship between the individual (group) and the organization?

■ LEARNING ACTIVITIES ■

1. Collect organizational charts and mission statements from a variety of health care organizations, such as a home health care agency, hospital, nursing home, and ambulatory surgery center. What are the similarities and differences between the documents? What factors account for the differences?
2. Collect organizational charts and mission statements from hospitals of different bed sizes (ie, 500, 300, <100). Identify their similarities and differences. What factors might account for identified differences?
3. In analyzing the organizational charts in Activity 2, identify line and staff positions. What positions are staff in more than one facility? What factors influence decisions to structure positions as staff or line?
4. Interview nurse managers and ask that they respond to the following scenario. You are a nurse manager in a 300-bed community hospital. Your unit is 32 beds and primarily serves the needs of cardiac patients. A short distance away from your unit is another 32-bed unit that admits respiratory, endocrine, and neurology patients. The

Nurse Manager of this floor has just resigned to return to school and you have been asked to accept administrative responsibility for this unit, in addition to your own. First, identify factors you believe should be taken into consideration in making this important decision and then ask each manager what factors he or she would analyze in making a decision to increase his or her span of control.

5. The informal organization is a powerful force. Compare and contrast the formal organization and the informal in a home health care agency and in a hospital. What are the differences? Who are the informal leaders? Does the nurse manager use the informal organization in analyzing employee needs? If so, how?

■ REFERENCES ■

Acorn S, Crawford M (1995). Consider this . . . Decentralized organizational structures and first-line nurse managers. *Journal of Nursing Administration* 25(10):5, 27.

Banner DK, Gagne ET (1994). *Designing Effective Organizations: Traditional and Transformational Views*. Newbury Park, CA: Sage.

Barnard CI (1938). *The Functions of the Executive*. Cambridge, MA: Harvard University Press.

Davis AA (1992). Project management: New approaches. *Nursing Management* 23(9):62–65.

Dirschel KM (1994). Decentralization or centralization: Striking a balance. *Nursing Management* 25(9):49–51.

Doerge J, Hagenow N (1995). Management restructuring: Toward a leaner organization. *Nursing Management* 26(12):32–38.

Drucker P (1992). *Managing for the Future: The 1990s and Beyond*. New York: Truman Tally Books/Dutton.

Dutton JE, Diekerich JM, Harquail CV (1994). Organizational images and member identification. *Administrative Science Quarterly* 39(June):239–263.

Ellefsen B (1995). Bureaucratization of professionals: Conflict and resolution. *Nursing Leadership Forum* 1(3):100–106.

Flarey DL (1991). The social climate scale: A tool for organizational change and development. *Journal of Nursing Administration* 21(4):37–44.

Fleeger ME (1993). Assessing organizational culture: A planning strategy. *Nursing Management* 24(2):39–41.

Gessner T (1996). Organizations as work flow systems. *In* Dienemann J (ed). *Nursing Administration: Strategic Perspectives and Application*. Norwalk, CT: Appleton & Lange.

Hesselbein F, Goldsmith M, Beckhard R (eds) (1997). *The Organization of the Future*, San Francisco: Jossey-Bass Publishers.

Kelduff M (1993). Deconstructing organizations. *Academy of Management Review* 18:13–31.

McDaniel C, Stumpf L (1993). The organizational culture. *Journal of Nursing Administration* 23(4):54–60.

McGill ME, Slocum JW (1994). *The Smarter Organization: How to Build a Business that Learns and Adapts to the Marketplace Needs*. New York: Wiley.

Mintzberg H (1989). *Mintzberg on Management: Inside Our Strange World of Organizations*. New York: Free Press.

Murray-Groher ME, Dicroce HA (1992). *Leadership and Management in Nursing*. San Mateo, CA: Appleton & Lange.

Pabst MK (1993). Span of control on nursing inpatient units. *Nursing Economics* 11(2):87–90.

Peters T (1988). *Thriving on Chaos*. New York: Alfred A. Knopf.

Porter-O'Grady T (ed) (1992). *Implementing Shared Governance*. New York: Mosby Publishers.

Weber M (1958). *In* Gerth H, Mills CW (eds). *From Max Weber: Essays in Sociology*. New York: Oxford University Press.

3

Professional Practice Models: Developing Empowering Delivery Systems

Judith Rocchiccioli, PhD, RN

LEARNING OBJECTIVES

This chapter will enable the learner to:
1. Relate the evolution of nursing science to current nursing practice.
2. Identify the components of professional practice systems.
3. Differentiate a professional practice system from a patient care delivery system.
4. Examine the merits of patient care delivery systems based on professionalism and research.

INTRODUCTION

The model of professional nursing practice is the most important organizational structure in the delivery of patient care. A well-defined delivery system supports the practicing professional nurse in a manner that is knowledge-based rather than task-based and provides an empowering environment for the professional growth of the nursing staff.

As the health care system continues to reform, the way in which patient care is delivered will become more and more important in the cost-constrained health care environment. Consequently, the efficiency of nursing practice patterns in the delivery of patient care is a critical indicator in the

success, and sometimes survival, of health care organizations

Professional practice models (PPMs) are uniquely different from patient care delivery systems. Professional practice models address the organization's vision and strategic plan while allowing for the unique needs and characteristics of the individual patient care unit and the collective vision of the staff on the unit. If the model is indeed a professional one, it will provide for the growth, autonomy, education, and collaboration of the nurse working in a complex organization.

For the purposes of this chapter, the term *patient care delivery system* encompasses the former language noted in the nursing literature that refers to "models of patient care" and "nursing care delivery systems." PPMs suggest that framework for continual professional growth and development of nursing staff.

The purpose of this chapter is threefold. The chapter (1) draws a parallel between the evolution of nursing practice and its effect on patient care delivery models; (2) differentiates between professional practice models and models of patient care delivery; and (3) examines the components of professional practice systems with current patient care delivery systems and explores the research and merits of these models by examining them in a changing health care environment as health delivery systems. Future patient care delivery must foster quality and efficiency at lower costs. An underpinning of the chapter is the knowledge that reform and changes in the health care system have facilitated significant changes in the manner in which nurses have traditionally practiced their profession.

HISTORICAL PERSPECTIVES OF PATIENT CARE DELIVERY

A goal of nursing practice has always been to offer efficient and cost-effective care without compromising quality. Patient care delivery systems facilitated this goal. A number of factors have influenced the development of nursing practice and patient care delivery systems.

Delivery systems generally reflected the current development and state of knowledge in nursing practice. Patient care practices were influenced by the degree of professionalism and development tasks. Social, political, and economic trends, advancing technology, and other environmental factors in health care continue to affect how nursing is practiced and how patient care is delivered. For instance, the economic feasibility of early discharge from hospitals has significantly decreased inpatient admissions days and dramatically increased the number of nurses providing care outside of hospitals. Laser technology has changed traditional surgical procedures, making them available on an outpatient basis, which places an even greater importance on patient education. Other variables that influence nursing care and patient care delivery systems are patient populations, acuity, technology, skill mix, clinical expertise, and education of staff nurses and nursing managers.

The Evolution of Professionalism

The work of registered nurses is professional, although many opponents of nursing would disagree. In fact, as the health care environment becomes more competitive and as nurses are laid off and as the work of nursing is given to lesser qualified caregivers, it is likely that more and more people will question the need for and the professionalism of registered nurses.

Professionalism denotes prestige and status and suggests autonomy, collaboration, responsibility, and accountability for practice. Professionalism suggests maturity within a profession as evidenced by the way it meets and serves the needs of its clients.

Flexner's (1915) classic definition of a profession is often used to enumerate the components of a profession. Flexner identified six criteria that a work group must possess to acquire professional status. They are as follows: (1) the activities of the work group must be intellectual; (2) the activities, because they are based on knowledge, can be learned; (3) the work activities must be practical as opposed to academic or theoretical; (4) the profession must have teachable techniques, which are the work of professional education; (5) there must be a strong internal organization of members of the work group; and (6) the professional worker's motivation must be a desire to provide for the good of society (Flexner, 1915).

Other writers have enlarged upon the work of Flexner to further define the components of a profession. A composite list includes the following: (1) a continually growing body of practice-oriented knowledge established through research and analysis unique to the work group; (2) collaboration with all service groups and individuals for the benefit of the patient; (3) strong peer colleagueship demonstrated by licensing and practice laws designed to protect clients; (4) autonomy, with direct lines of access to clients; and (5) a cohesive, clear, well-articulated code of ethics voluntarily adhered to by members and designed to protect the client (Flexner, 1915; Baldridge, 1969; Caplow, 1954; Goode, 1969).

Although these criteria can be described as idealistic, it is important that professional nurses embrace these components in the reformed health care environment.

Nursing History

A cursory look at the history of nursing helps us understand the evolution of patient care delivery systems. The development and progression of nursing as a profession and the evolutionary development of work tasks and practice models are clearly delineated in nursing history.

Prior to the Civil War, there was no recognized nursing profession in the United States. Nursing care was unskilled and patient-focused, with nurses assuming total responsibility for patients in the home. Much of the work of nursing was household chores. This individualized, patient-focused approach to care is similar to home health care today.

The hospital boom that occurred between 1900 and 1910 allowed nurses to move into the hospitals working under physicians (Zander, 1980). After World War I, most patients were treated in hospitals where one registered nurse supervised care for a ward of patients. Practice moved from an individualized focus to one that was task-based and centered on caring for many patients using large numbers of less skilled health care workers. *Functional nursing* emerged at this time and became the delivery system after World War II, reflecting the popularity of current industrial engineering concepts. LPNs, nursing assistants, and orderlies became the main source of hospital labor while RNs were removed from patient care to perform management functions (Zander, 1980). Much of this practice is being repeated today as hospitals across the country substitute lesser paid labor for professional nurses.

Team nursing evolved when there were too few registered nurses to manage the supervision of task-trained personnel. The team leader was responsible for assigning tasks to team members and for the supervision of patient care. Different caregivers were assigned functional tasks depending on their skill level. This practice was criticized as fragmented and confusing. Team tasks was work that needed to be done during a given shift as opposed to care directly based on patient needs. Team nursing remains a popular patient delivery model today.

In the late 1950s and 1960s, university-based nursing education provided the profession with significant growth, expansion, and prestige. Nurses began to blend their natural science and liberal arts educations to search for holistic ways of offering basic care. Research into developing a theory of nursing began at this time, and this research reflected a growing need for professional autonomy and accountability in meeting patient needs. This led to the development of primary nursing (Zander, 1980).

Primary nursing represented a philosophical basis for patient care delivery. Central to primary nursing is a group of concepts that includes continuity, accountability, autonomy, authority, and other basic beliefs about the role of the nurse in the nurse-patient relationship (Marram et al, 1979; Zander, 1980). Primary nursing reflected the professions' conscious move toward independence

in practice and highlighted an important milestone in the evolution of professional practice. Table 3–1 presents the evolution of nursing practice models.

PROFESSIONAL PRACTICE SYSTEMS AND PATIENT CARE DELIVERY

Professional practice models are different from patient care delivery systems. PPMs provide an empowering and viable alternative to traditional patient practice models and advocate for the continual growth of the professional nurse.

Patient care delivery models describe how nursing care is actually carried out. These models include work tasks, work roles, and work flow systems.

Professional practice models are different and greater in scope in that they provide a professional framework for unit-based practice and self-management. Philosophically, PPMs empower nurses to have authority, control, and accountability for all aspects of their practice. Consequently, traditional nursing practice models are "nested" in the PPMs. A conceptual framework integrating PPMs and patient care delivery systems is shown in Figure 3–1.

This conceptual framework examines traditional patient care delivery systems as being a part of PPMs. The patient care delivery systems describe how nursing care occurs on a nursing unit whereas

Table 3–1.
Evolution of Nursing Practice Models

Dates	Model
1900s	Individualized Care in Home
1920s–1940s	Functional Nursing
1950s–1960s	Team Nursing
1970s–1980s	Primary Nursing Primary Team Total Patient Care Modular Nursing
Late 1980s–1990s	Differentiated Practice Case Management

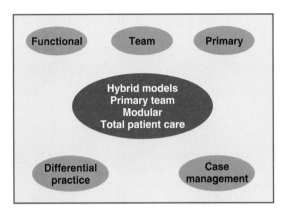

Figure 3–1. Conceptual framework for professional practice model.

the PPM provides for the continual growth and development of the professional nurse.

Professional practice models represent a paradigm shift in nursing practice and within the health care system. PPMs require macro and micro changes in the way nurses do their work. Components of PPMs include decentralized decision-making, peer review, an enhanced salary structure, and gain-sharing for registered nurses. PPMs employ such concepts as decentralization of nursing operations to the unit level, flexible scheduling, established clinical standards, authority, and continual accountability for patient care. Table 3–2 shows the concepts of professional practice models.

Professional practice models also require that nurses have direct control over their human and fiscal resources, work-flow systems, and communication systems as well as built-in reward incentives for committed nurses.

Professional practice models are best noted in the literature when shared governance and case management models are discussed. Shared governance promotes professionalism through the establishment of lateral or peer relationships that function in tangent with managerial relationships. The principles of shared governance are closely aligned with the concepts of continuous quality improvement (Research Box 3–1).

Porter-O'Grady (1984) suggested a model of shared governance that effects a system of administrative integration with councils of management, education, and quality assurance overlapping with a coordinating council.

Table 3–2.
Concepts of Professional Practice Models

Concepts of Professional Practice	Elements of Delivery Systems
Decentralized decision-making	Work flow systems
Unit-based nursing operations	Job descriptions
Self-management	Policies/procedures
Practice control	Defined roles
Authority	Assignment-making
Accountability	
Peer-review	
Flexible scheduling	
Clinical standards	
Control of resources	
Personnel	
Fiscal	

Research Box 3–1
Shared Governance Practice Model

Porter-O'Grady and Finnegan (1984) reported shared governance as cost neutral after factoring in planning and implementation costs. Jenkins (1988) analyzed the incremental costs associated with maintaining a shared governance practice model. She noted a 28% increase in meeting hours per year, but suggested that the costs associated with this expense were almost entirely offset by the elimination of one director's position.

Brodbeck (1992) described the implementation and evaluation of shared governance and case management. The study reported improved patient care outcomes after 1 year and a significant reduction in spending after 1 year. The cost savings were accompanied by reduced lengths of stay for selected patient care groups.

Research on Professional Practice Models

Research suggests a relationship between nursing turnover and nurses' dissatisfaction with working conditions, particularly in the degree of control over work processes and content (Dear et al, 1985). Other research suggests that PPMs are designed to improve nurses' retention by increasing their autonomy and authority to make decisions (Hinshaw et al, 1987; Price & Mueller, 1981).

Positive outcomes have been associated with the implementation of shared governance models, but research conclusions that examined the cost of implementing and maintaining professional practice systems are mixed.

Current Models of Patient Care Delivery

Nursing process, the thinking model of clinical practice, describes how one nurse plans and carries out nursing care for a specific patient. A nursing practice model describes how a group of nurses on a specific unit provide care for a group of patients (Rocchiccioli & Colley, 1989). Three frequently recognized models of patient care delivery systems are noted in the literature prior to 1990: functional nursing, team nursing, and primary nursing. These models are discussed in detail in this section. Several other models are identified that represent a splitting off of the best known models. Among these are total patient care, modular nursing and primary-team nursing. More recently, the literature has addressed differentiated practice and case management as current models of delivery. Differentiated practice is discussed in this chapter, and case management is examined in detail in Chapter 4. These two models encompass the attributes and characteristics of a professional practice system.

Each delivery model has specific characteristics occurring in a defined combination, which are usually adopted to meet a specific set of objectives defined by each patient care unit. For the purposes of this chapter, it is important to note that case management methods and shared governance principles can be applied to all current models of patient care delivery. A more complete discussion of case management is given in Chapter 4.

The application of case management and shared governance concepts are especially important because changes in health care focusing on managed care and capitated costs (see Chaps. 1 and 2) make it necessary to examine these models as they affect patient outcomes, costs, staff satisfaction, efficiency, quality, and productivity.

Patient delivery models are work systems in which nursing tasks and responsibilities are organized. Essential components in patient delivery models include job descriptions, designated responsibilities, assignment-making criteria, interdisciplinary rounds and conferences, unit geographics, physician/nurse/patient communication, and work flow systems.

The following definitions of these models are used throughout this chapter (Table 3–3).

Functional Nursing

Functional nursing is a system of care borrowed from industry that concentrates on duties and activities. The concept of functional nursing arose during the 1920s and continued through the 1940s at a time when time, motion, and efficiency studies were thriving in the United States. Functional nursing is predicated on task completion and concentrates on organizing nursing tasks to optimize the technical skills of nursing staff as opposed to the unique needs of individual patients and staff.

The functional design of patient care involves an assembly-line approach to patient care, with major tasks being delegated by the charge nurse to individual members of the team. For instance, one staff member may make beds and bathe patients, while another serves juice and fills water pitchers. A third staff member may administer medications. The goals of functional nursing are concerned with work productivity at the lowest possible cost. Tasks are generally assigned to the lowest-skilled, lowest-paid workers who are available to do the work.

Functional nursing does not provide a professional practice environment for nursing staff, but rather represents a mechanism for merely getting the work done. Functional patient care delivery does not contribute to the continual development and professional growth of nursing staff, nor does it provide for optimal patient outcomes. Consequently, functional nursing does not represent a professional care delivery system but is a model of patient care.

ADVANTAGES OF FUNCTIONAL NURSING. The major advantages of functional nursing are its effi-

Table 3–3.
Definitions of Nursing Models of Practice

Functional nursing	An assembly-line method assigns each nurse to perform a specific task or set of tasks for every patient.
Team nursing	A group of nursing personnel, including LPNs and nursing extenders, are led by an RN team leader in providing care for a group of patients.
Primary nursing	A single RN is responsible and accountable for providing comprehensive nursing care to a group of patients during their entire hospital stay; delegation of tasks to non-RN personnel is reduced but not eliminated. (Rocchiccioli & Colley, 1989)
Total patient care	A single RN is responsible for providing the nursing care to a group of patients for one shift. Nurse accountability does not extend beyond that shift. (Rocchiccioli & Colley, 1989)
Modular nursing	An RN accompanied by one or two nursing personnel provides care for a group of patients located in a particular geographic area. (Rocchiccioli & Colley, 1989)
Differentiated practice	A philosophy that focuses on the structuring of roles and functions of nurses according to education, experience, and competence. (NCNIP, 1989)
Case management	A professional practice system that manages clinical care of patients across a continuum using managed care concepts and tools.

ciency, cost, and clearly articulated expectations. The ease of monitoring task completion is also an advantage because the charge nurse maintains greater control over work activities.

DISADVANTAGES OF FUNCTIONAL NURSING. There are many disadvantages to functional nursing care. Psychological, social, and unique needs of patients are often overlooked, care is fragmented, quality may not be optimal, and nursing care is depersonalized. Functional care delivery is directly opposed to continuous quality improvement and does not support professional practice and optimal patient outcomes.

Team Nursing

Team nursing became popular after World War II as an effort to employ a large number of health care workers who had been specifically trained to fill registered nursing positions left vacant during the war. These workers, trained with varying clinical skills on a wide range of levels, were used by hospitals to ease the nursing shortage created by the war and later to ease the shortage of nurses created by the hospital boom. The use of these lower-paid personnel had specific fiscal benefits. In essence, hospital administrators found vocational nurses, technicians, and nursing assistants a less expensive way to offer care while providing a cheap source of labor (Marram et al, 1979). The quality of patient care suffered from a lack of well-prepared nursing providers to care for increasing numbers of ill patients. Team nursing, in its operational definition, does not support continuous quality improvement and optimal patient outcomes.

Philosophically, team nursing is founded on the

belief that nursing care is patient-centered and that care is best delivered using a team approach where there is trust and an acknowledged value and worth of each team member. Team nursing is characterized by a large degree of respect and maturity of team members and a high degree of communication and collaboration between members. The team is generally led by the most qualified registered nurse who is responsible for the assessing, diagnosing, planning, and evaluating of each patients' plan of care. Team members, who may be registered nurses, licensed practical nurses, and nurse extenders, then implement the plan of care by dividing up various patient care tasks and responsibilities. An effort is made in patient assignments to decrease fragmentation of care in order to provide individualized patient care.

In an *exemplary model* of team nursing, each staff member works fully within the realm of his or her educational and clinical expertise in an effort to provide comprehensive, individualized patient care. Each staff member is accountable for patient care and outcomes of care delivered in accordance with their licensing and practice scope as determined by hospital policy and state law. For instance, a registered nurse team member may plan, diagnose, implement, and evaluate patient care for his or her patients, whereas a licensed practical nurse may administer medications and perform patient care treatments. Exemplary team nursing occurs when the team considers the values, skills, and experiences of each member and works together cohesively to anticipate and solve difficult situations to facilitate quality care and optimal clinical outcomes.

Team nursing is the most widely used model of nursing care today. This is in part due to the economic benefits of substituting lower-paid employees for higher-paid professional nurses. Team nursing also suggests a reduction in the time and expense of training nursing personnel (Brown, 1982). Team nursing represents a step toward decentralization of nursing care and a higher degree of accountability for registered nurses than functional nursing. The model attempts to bring clinical judgment and decision-making, authority, and autonomy to the unit operations level.

Roles in Team Nursing

There are generally three roles in team nursing: charge nurse, team leader, and team members. In an effort to ensure professional practice, the charge nurse and team leader should be registered nurses and assume accountability for patient care. The role of the registered nurse in team nursing, as in all professional practice systems, is concerned with assessing, diagnosing, planning, and evaluating patient care. While other team members may be charged with the direct implementation of the patient care, it is nevertheless the responsibility of the registered nurse to oversee and monitor the care.

Team members, who may be RNs, LPNs, or nurse extenders, are delegated to implement patient care. Team members' responsibilities for patient care should be within the capabilities of their skill level, education and certification. It is important that all nurses and caregivers be familiar with their hospitals' policies, standards of care, and state laws governing nursing care.

ADVANTAGES OF TEAM NURSING. These rest with the ability of team nursing to provide quality nursing care to groups of patients using ancillary nursing staff to fulfill tasks while registered nurses plan, diagnose, and evaluate individualized nursing care (Rocchiccioli & Colley, 1989). Team nursing also suggests that the skills, talents, and abilities of each staff member are recognized and used fully in caring for patients. Team nursing offers less fragmentation in care than functional nursing, but does not address continuity of care over time. Another strength of team nursing is its thrust toward increased cooperation among team members which can improve unit morale and patient outcomes.

DISADVANTAGES OF TEAM NURSING. These are inherent in the duplication of effort of team leaders and team members in monitoring work tasks and work completion. The greatest disadvantage of team nursing is that it is often poorly implemented. Many nurses approach team assignments by simply dividing the staff into equal groups and distributing an equal number of patients to each group. Often no regard or attention is given to the level of expertise of the staff member, the acuity of the patient's condition, or the long-term comprehensive needs of the patient. Some nursing leaders also believe that the method of assignment in team nursing is more costly because the overall efficiency of the nursing unit is reduced by fragmented distribution of personnel (Douglas, 1988).

Duplication of work is inherent in team nursing when there is overlap or lack of clarity in responsibilities. This may occur when several staff members receive and communicate medical orders or changes in patient conditions. A legal risk also exists when poor communication and cooperation present difficulty in actualizing safe patient outcomes. Team nursing does not address overall accountability for patient outcomes over time.

It is also unlikely that team nursing in its present form can survive in a managed care environment that places considerable emphasis on the integration of care and the optimal use of staff and material resources. A lack of attention to fiscal and patient outcomes needed in managed care environments is also a criticism.

Primary Nursing

The concept of primary nursing represented additional movement toward professionalism. The basis of primary nursing is inherent in a philosophical ideology based on a professional commitment made by registered nurses to direct and provide comprehensive nursing care to specifically assigned patients and their families during their contact with the health care agency (Zander, 1980). Twelve core elements of primary nursing have been identified in an effort to formulate an operational definition. These elements prescribe the nursing actions in directing patient care. These elements include accountability, advocacy, assertiveness, authority, autonomy, continuity, commitment, collaboration, contracting, coordination, communication, and decentralization (Zander, 1980). Conceptually, primary nursing describes a system of interrelated values, beliefs, and principles. Consequently, there should be a relationship between the conceptual model and operational design of the practice, particularly in the areas of model design, role descriptions, staffing patterns, communication systems, work tasks, and assignment of patients to primary nurses. The implementation of primary nursing requires a belief in the philosophical principles underlying the model, a commitment of registered nurses to professional accountability, and a careful design that allows for patient continuity and optimal outcomes in the absence of the primary nurse (Research Box 3–2).

Primary nursing is both a philosophy and a pa-

Research Box 3–2
The Cost Effectiveness of Primary Nursing

Because primary nursing requires a higher ratio of registered nurses, it was initially assumed to be more expensive than team nursing. Some studies suggest that this is not the case and report that in terms of salary, actual operating cost, staff development costs, and actual cost per bed, primary nursing has been found to be less expensive (Marram et al, 1979; McClelland et al, 1987).

tient care delivery system that focuses on patient outcomes as opposed to nursing tasks. Primary nursing is concerned with keeping the nurse at the bedside, actively involved in clinical care while planning goal-directed, individualized patient care. The practice of a primary nursing system suggests clinical experiences and a cadre of competent professionals who can deliver optimal care with little direct supervision.

Conceptual components in the practice of primary nursing are accountability and authority for patient care. Accountability requires that nurses have the authority and the autonomy to make patient care decisions. Unfortunately, primary nursing has been difficult to operationalize because many of the model's conceptual and operational tenets do not work in highly bureaucratic hospital environments. Decentralized nursing environments and highly experienced nurses are pivotal to success in the implementation of models.

At its best, primary nursing meets the physician's need for information via the primary nurse who supplies pertinent, comprehensive, and up-to-date information about patient condition and status. Such enhancement facilitates better patient care outcomes as well as collegiality among caregivers.

Roles in Primary Nursing

Four roles are generally noted in a primary patient delivery system. These roles include the primary nurse, the associate nurse, the charge nurse, and the assistant nurse. The primary nurse has the ultimate authority and accountability for patient care from admission to discharge. The primary nurse is also delegated the responsibility of assessing, diagnosing, planning, and evaluating patient care for his or her primary patients.

The associate nurse is responsible for assisting in patient care planning in the absence of the primary nurse and for performing nursing functions delegated by the primary nurse. The associate nurse may set short-term goals and interventions but is not accountable for the overall progression and comprehensive care of the patient. Associate nurses provide direct care in the absence of the primary nurse and work collaboratively with the primary nurse in all patient care efforts.

The charge nurse in a primary practice delivery model, as in other patient delivery models, is responsible and accountable for the overall functioning of the nursing unit on a given shift. Charge nurses maintain a working knowledge of all primary patients and fill in for primary nurses in selected situations.

Assistant nurses in primary delivery settings are generally nonprofessional staff who implement the patient plan of care and report accordingly to the primary nurse.

Research in Primary Nursing

A review of the literature (Zander, 1980; McAdam, 1985) suggests that considerable confusion exists about many of the operational definitions of primary nurses. The confusion stems from a lack of clear understanding of how to operationalize the philosophical elements of the model.

Research into the practice of primary nursing has reported mixed results. Primary nursing has not been clearly established as a cost-effective delivery model.

Differentiated Practice Models

In the late 1980s, differentiated practice models appeared in the nursing literature. The purpose of these models was to preserve the integrity and essence of primary nursing while maintaining the progress toward professionalism made during the acute nursing shortage of the late 1980s and early 1990s.

The term *differentiated nursing practice* has cus-

tomarily referred to practice expectations that are consistent with the expected competencies of graduates from different kinds of education programs. The Governing Board of the National Commission on Nursing Implementation Project (NCNIP, 1989) has issued the following statement regarding differentiated practice: "In order to improve patient care, effectively utilize health care resources and create a more satisfying work environment, roles and functions of nursing personnel should be based on education, experience and competence and nurses should be compensated accordingly" (Research Box 3–3).

Most differentiated practice models are currently integrated into the present system of nursing care delivery, and roles and responsibilities are developed according to the nurse's education and experience. Koerner and Karpiuk (1994) suggest that differentiated practice recognizes the contribution of all nursing personnel in patient care delivery as unique and valuable and suggest that the model of differentiated practice positions nurses well in the changing practice environment that is beneficial to the nurse and to the patient.

The ICON (Integrated Competencies of Nurses) model addresses entry into practice through the creation of differentiated practice roles (Rotkovitch, 1986) and is an education-based differentiated practice model. The baccalaureate nurse assumes the professional role of assessing, planning, and evaluating the care, and the associate degree nurse functions in an associate role with responsibility for implementing the care. The ICON II model was developed as a transitional model in response to the nursing shortage. The ICON II model grandfathers all RNs into the baccalaureate nursing role and

Research Box 3–3
Model of Differentiated Practice

A demonstration three-dimensional model of differentiated practice was developed at New England Deaconess Hospital. The demonstration project suggested that nurses had more opportunities for almost all phases of direct patient care, particularly in the areas of needs assessment and analysis of change in patient status (Harkness et al, 1992).

grandfathers all licensed practice nurses into the associate role (Rotkovitch & Smith, 1987).

Other Patient Care Delivery Systems

Other delivery systems have appeared more recently in the literature. These systems were designed mainly to preserve the integrity of primary nursing and remedy the fragmented care resulting from the nursing shortage of the late 1980s and early 1990s. Often these models paired up a registered nurse with a nonskilled worker in an effort to decrease fragmentation and to allow the professional caregiver the time needed to plan and evaluate professional nursing care. The primary practice partners model proposed by Manthey (1988) suggested a technical assistant as a partner for each registered nurse in an effort to develop a close working relationship to facilitate patient care. The model further insured maximum utilization of scarce RNs, efficient use of ancillary personnel and close control over nursing practice.

The primary-team model overlays primary nursing responsibilities for a primary nurse while allowing for the flexibility of team members to actually administer patient care. The primary-team model provides an effective may to manage patient care.

SUMMARY

The purpose of this chapter was to discuss and distinguish between professional practice models and models of nursing delivery. A review of the literature revealed that the evolution of nursing delivery systems has paralleled the growth and evolution of the nursing profession. Professional practice occurs in decentralized environments, which provide an empowering environment and allow nurses control over financial and clinical resources. Shared governance, empowerment models, differentiated practice, and case management are PPMs, as they encompass the elements of professional practice. Function, team, primary, and variations of these three models represent models of nursing care delivery based on the organization of tasks in each model.

Each model of nursing delivery was reviewed, and the advantages and disadvantages of the model were discussed. Selected research studies were included as they related to the cost of the delivery system and the degree of nursing and patient satisfaction.

In conclusion, it is clear that the changing health environment with its emphasis on cost, quality, and outcomes will require that nurses refine their patient care delivery methods and skills and become proficient in the clinical and fiscal monitoring of patient care.

■ DISCUSSION QUESTIONS ■

1. Differentiate professional practice models from patient care delivery systems.
2. Identify and define the current models of patient care delivery.
3. How has the evolution of nursing been reflected in the way the profession has cared for patients?
4. Compare and contrast the roles in primary nursing and team nursing and ways in which the models can interface.
5. When does the practice of functional nursing work in clinical nursing?
6. Is an exemplary model of primary nursing better than or superior to an exemplary model of team patient care delivery? Why or why not?
7. How has health reform changed the way in which patient care must be practiced?
8. Discuss how research has examined the way in which nurses have delivered patient care.
9. Why is nursing autonomy important to the profession?

■ LEARNING ACTIVITIES ■

1. You are a clinical leader on a 27-bed neurology unit with four ICU beds. Currently a team patient care delivery model is used. Your manager has asked you to head a task force to implement a professional practice model. How would you plan for this considerable organizational change?
2. Your nursing director has insisted that all nursing units in medicine and surgery change from a team patient care delivery system to a primary patient care delivery system. Your professional staff on the unit only represents 25% of the total number of staff. With cutbacks and down-sizing

you know you will not get new staff. How can you redesign your current delivery system to meet the director's mandate? How will tasks be delegated?

3. In addition to the change in the patient care delivery system in Activity 2, how can a professional practice system be created to increase staff motivation, commitment, and autonomy?

■ BIBLIOGRAPHY ■

Baldridge JV (1969). *Professionalism*. Lecture notes from Stanford University, Palo Alto, CA. October 23, 1969.

Brodbeck K (1992). Professional practice actualized through an integrated shared governance and quality assurance model. *Journal of Nursing Care Quality* 6(2):20–23.

Brown BJ (1982). *Perspectives in Primary Nursing: Professional Practice Environments*. Rockville, MD: Aspen Systems Corporation.

Caplow T (1954). *The Sociology of Work*. Minneapolis: University of Minnesota Press.

Dear M, Weisman C, O'Keefe S (1985). Evaluation of a contract model for professional nursing practice. *Health Care Management Review* 6:65–77.

Douglas LM (1988). *The Effective Nurse Leader/Manager*, 3rd ed. St. Louis: CV Mosby.

Flexner A (1915). Is social work a profession? In *Proceedings of the National Conference of Charities and Correction*. Chicago: Hildeman.

Goode WJ (1969). The theoretical limits of professionalization. *In* Etzioni A (ed). *The Semi-Professionals and Their Organization*. New York: The Free Press.

Harkness GA, Miller J, Hill N (1992). Differentiated practice: A three dimensional model. *Nursing Management* (12):26–30.

Hinshaw AS, Smeltzer CH, Atwood JR (1987). Innovative retention strategies for nursing staff. *Journal of Nursing Administration* 17(6):8–16.

Jenkins JA (1988). A nursing governance and practice model: What are the costs? *Nursing Economics* 6(6):302–311.

Koerner JG, Karpiuk KL (1994). *Implementing Differentiated Nursing Practice: Transformation by Design*. Gaithersburg, MD: Aspen Publications.

Manthey M (1988). Primary practice partners (a nurse-extender system). *Nursing Management* 19(3):58–59.

Marram G, Flynn K, Abaravich W, Carey S (1976). Cost-effectiveness of primary and team nursing. Wakefield, MA: Contemporary Publishing.

Marram GG, Barrett MW, Bevis EM (1979). *Primary Nursing*. St. Louis: CV Mosby.

McAdam E (1985). Primary nursing demands change. *Nursing Management* 13(5):50.

McClelland MR, Kolesar MJ, Bailey MA (1987). From team to primary nursing. *Nursing Management* 18(10):69–71.

National Commission on Nursing Implementation Project (1989). *Nursing Practice Patterns (Differentiated Practice)*. Milwaukee, WI: National Commission on Nursing Implementation Project.

Porter-O'Grady T, Finnegan S (1984). *Shared Governance for Nursing*. Rockville, MD: Aspen Publications.

Price JL, Mueller CW (1981). *Professional Turnover: The Case of Nurses*. New York: Spectrum.

Rocchiccioli J, Colley BB (1989). Models of nursing practice: The basis of diagnosis-based nursing practice. *In* Miller E (ed). *How To Make Nursing Diagnosis Work: Administrative and Clinical Strategies*. Norwalk, CT: Appleton & Lange.

Rotkovitch R (1986). ICON: A model of nursing practice for the future. *Nursing Management* 17(6):54–56.

Rotkovitch R, Smith C (1987). ICON I: The future model; ICON II: The transitional model. *Nursing Management* 18(11):91–96.

Zander KS (1980). *Primary Nursing: Development and Management*. Germantown, MD: Aspen Publications.

Managed Care and Nursing Case Management

Judith Rocchiccioli, PhD, RN

• •

LEARNING OBJECTIVES

This chapter will enable the learner to:
1. Differentiate between managed care and nursing case management.
2. Discuss the importance of tracking the fiscal and clinical outcomes of patient care.
3. Describe the tools used in nursing care management including critical paths and variance analysis.
4. Develop a model of nursing case management.

• •

INTRODUCTION

Managed care, a system of health care that provides a generalized structure and focus when managing the use, cost, quality, and effectiveness of health care services (Cohen & Cesta, 1993) has presented hospitals, physicians, and nurses with a paradigm change that has profoundly affected the delivery of traditional medical care. The move to managed care has been fueled by sky-rocketing health care costs and the financial concerns of health care reformers. Managed care demands that hospitals as well as other health care agencies change and develop new practices that focus on quality, cost, and the outcomes of care.

The rapid growth and continued evolution of managed care organizations, better known as Health Maintenance Organizations (HMOs) and Preferred Provider Organizations (PPOs), have added to the environmental uncertainty that providers are currently facing. Physicians and hospitals, long the economic powers in health care, have given way to the purchasers of health care services which include corporations, insurance companies, and individuals. The shift in power has resulted in a focus on cost containment, the control of resources, and a complete restructuring of the health care environment.

Traditionally, health care operated under a fee-for-service system in which a patient received health care services from a provider for a designated fee. More recently, managed care systems have emerged as control shifted from the provider to the purchaser of health care service (Cohen & Cesta, 1993).

In its purest form, managed care organizations focus on wellness education and disease prevention. Many critics of managed care systems disagree, suggesting that many managed care organizations focus only on costs and limitations of choice for patients. Regardless, survival under managed care requires that hospitals and other health care agencies streamline their delivery systems, control their variability in patient outcomes, and establish efficient physician and nurse practice patterns to maximize hospital revenues and decrease costs. Nurses, the providers of almost 90% of all inpatient care, will play a pivotal role in containing cost through the use of nursing case management, a professional practice model that places emphasis on managing the patient's environment by coordinating and monitoring the appropriate use of patient care resources.

CASE MANAGEMENT DEFINED

The terms *managed care* and *nursing case management* have been used interchangeably for years. Although they are distinctly different, managed care and nursing case management share a common ground because both are rooted in cost containment and quality. Nursing case management can be conceptualized as a component of managed care that supports cost-effective patient outcomes for a duration of illness. In essence, nursing case management serves as a linchpin to facilitate managed care concepts.

In the early 1980s, the advent of diagnosis-related groups (DRGs) suggested that hospitals must achieve cost-effective accountability by developing management strategies for both patient mix and service volume. Early nursing case management delivery systems were directed toward this focus, and recent nursing case management systems provide an interdisciplinary process of clinical care and management directed at meeting these challenges via a network of nursing services organized across a continuum of care. The network of nursing services is illustrated in Figure 4–1.

Case management is not a new framework for providing patient care. In fact, social workers, counselors, and public health nurses have been using concepts of case management for years. An important distinction to note in clinical case management is that **not all patients need to be case-managed**. However, patients who are not case-managed must be managed using critical paths to achieve optimal cost and quality outcomes. High-

risk and high-cost patients, patients with complex illness, patients with a high rate of recidivism, and elderly patients represent populations that generally make up the 20% of case-managed patients.

Case management represents an interdisciplinary health care delivery system designed to promote appropriate use of hospital personnel and material resources to maximize hospital revenues while providing for optimal outcome of care. Case management has been described as an alternative care delivery model that expands the concept of primary nursing to include preadmission care, outpatient care, inpatient care, and post-discharge home care. Case management is closely tied to the concept of primary nursing and represents a health care delivery system process aimed at providing quality health care, decreased fragmentation, enhanced quality of life, and contained costs (American Nurses' Association, 1988).

Zander (1988) describes six realistic goals of managed care and nursing case management: (1) the achievement of expected or standardized patient outcomes; (2) early discharge of patients or discharge within appropriate lengths of stay; (3) appropriate or reduced use of resources; (4) collaborative practice and coordination and continuity of care; (5) professional development and personal satisfaction on the job; and (6) encouragement of contributions by all care providers to the achievement of patient outcomes. These goals enable continuity of patient care and affect cost containment.

Bower (1992) defined the key characteristics of case management programs as (1) episode-based, with case managers attentive to the care needs of patients across a continuum of settings which pro-

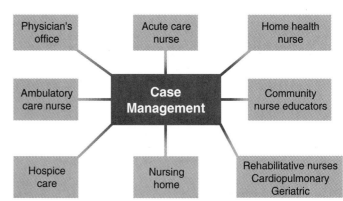

Figure 4–1. Network of nursing services.

motes continuity of a plan of care; (2) longitudinally based, with a case manager following a patient across the continuum of an illness; (3) centrally focused on patients and the entire family unit; (4) interdisciplinary focus, with collaboration among disciplines; (5) concerned with accessibility of services; (6) proactive, preventing problems; and (7) quality- and outcome-driven. Other definitions describe case management as an alternative method of delivery that offers "state-of-the-art" care to patients over a period of time or continuum. At the heart of most of these definitions is the consistent theme of "coordination of care" (Ethridge & Lamb, 1989; Farquhar & Robinson, 1990; Knollmueller, 1989).

The use of case-management professional practice delivery systems is popular today because the systems fit well into the mandates of managed care by assisting hospitals to manage use of resources, costs, productivity, and outcomes. Case management provides a care process that assists hospitals and health care providers to standardize the appropriate use of clinical and material resources to achieve a purposeful and controlled connection between quality of care and cost of care, thereby managing the variability in patient care. Consequently, the main thrust of case management professional practice systems is to manage patient care by managing the patient care environment.

TOOLS OF CASE MANAGEMENT

The accomplishment of goals in the context of case management requires a high degree of collaboration, negotiation, and fiscal monitoring of care. Zander (1988) identified five components of managed care: (1) standard critical paths, which are used as adjuncts to care plans; (2) critical paths, which are used as bases for change-of-shift reports; (3) analysis of positive and negative variance from the critical paths; (4) timely case consultation for the caregiver once a variance occurs; and (5) health care team meetings initiated, conducted, and followed up by nursing staff.

Critical Paths

Critical paths are central to the success of any case-management delivery system and are developed based on appropriate standards of care. Critical paths (Table 4–1) can take the place of the nursing care plan and actually map out the desired clinical progress of a patient during an acute care admission.

Critical paths are developed through the collaborative efforts of physicians, nurses, pharmacists, and other interdisciplinary caregivers with the goal of improving the quality and outcomes of care. Critical paths may be purchased commercially or may be developed by an interdisciplinary committee of health care providers who provide care for a specific group of patients. Critical paths may be organized by diagnosis, DRG, physician, patient age, or body system. For instance, a patient undergoing a coronary artery bypass graft would need, among others, the physician, nurse, pharmacist, and dietitian on the development committee. An elderly patient with complex illness and repeated bouts of pneumonia may need these clinical providers as well as social services, home health services, rehabilitative personnel, and the clinical nurse specialist in gerontology as members of the critical path development committee.

Critical paths offer optimal sequencing and timing of interventions by physicians, nurses, and other caregivers for a particular diagnosis or procedure designed to better use resources, maximize quality, and minimize delays (Coffey et al, 1992). In fact, critical paths provide a road map or blueprint for care during a patient's inpatient stay. Consequently, to be effective, critical paths must be interdisciplinary, so that all disciplines caring for the patient have input into the development of the plan and are vested in using the integrated plan to manage patient progress and care. Ideally, the critical path should represent the interdisciplinary care plan and should replace other care plans currently used by services caring for the patient.

Critical paths provide effective clinical management systems for monitoring care and for reducing or controlling the length of stay. Additionally, management by critical paths assists providers in the early identification and anticipation of additional hospital days and facilitates the negotiation with insurers for securing additional inpatient revenues for extended lengths of stay. Consequently, critical paths are instrumental in monitoring the cost of care. The constant and accurate monitoring of patients against their critical path is pivotal to the

TABLE 4–1.
Critical Path Guideline Pneumonia (DRG 89)

Date	Day 1	Day 2	Day 3	Day 4	Day 5	Day 6	Day 7
Location							
Consultations	Dietitian, if deficit present		Consider pulmonary or infectious disease consult if Pt not improving				
Tests	Sputum CLS/ gram stain Acid fast if indicated EKO (over 55) Theo. level, if on Theo Pulse OK Blood cult CKR, ABGs if indicated CBC, lytes Chem 7, SMA 12	------>	Repeat lab & R. CXR (if normal) ------> Repeat culture if indicated	------>	------>	ABG on room air or within 48 h of DC if home oxygen anticipated CKR if indicated prior to discharge	------>
Activity	SRP with assistance As able ------>	Up in chair bid ------>	Up in chair tid ------>	Ambulate tid, time ------>	------>	------>	------>

40

Treatment	Aerosols q 4-6 hrs with bronchodilator, or HDI with aero chamber Percussion, oxygen per ABG/P. Ox per present policy (If indicated)	-----> Reevaluate need for aerosol	----->	D.C. oxygen ? if P.Ox. 90% Oxygen prn?	----->	-----> D.C. oxygen if not done previously
Diet	OAT, unless otherwise indicated	----->	----->	----->	----->	----->
Medication	IV for hydration Home meds Antibiotic	Antibiotic reevaluated after culture result reported -Evaluation Heplock		Oral antibiotic >	----->	----->
Discharge Planning	Evaluation level of care	Continuing care or refer to S.S. for placement	Eval. & D/C plan MM placement if appropriate Pt/family consult	Request M.D. concurrence & advise	Implement arrs. MM transport home health – DME CRF completed	----->
Teaching	Per teaching plan	----->	----->	----->	----->	----->

41

success of the case-management professional practice system. In the event that a patient "falls off" his or her critical path, the case manager immediately acts on the negative variance that may present and plans accordingly with other caregivers, family, and insurers.

Variance Analysis

Variance analysis occurs continually as the case manager and other caregivers monitor patient outcomes against the critical path. Variances are actual deviations or detours from the critical paths. Variances are either positive or negative, avoidable or unavoidable, and may be caused by a variety of things (Coffey et al, 1992). Positive variance occurs when the patient achieves maximum benefit and is discharged earlier than anticipated on his or her critical path. Negative variance occurs when untoward events preclude a timely discharge and the length of stay is longer than planned for a patient on a specific critical path. The goal of critical paths is to anticipate and recognize negative variance early so that appropriate action can be taken.

Variances may be caused by the patient or the patient's family, a clinical caregiver, an environmental or systems problem within the hospital organization, or a community resource problem. Within many hospital organizations, information systems generate and tabulate variance information. A typical variance analysis form is shown in Figure 4–2.

A patient variance may occur when the patient's family does not attend the discharge planning class, or when the patient simply becomes ill and develops a fever or infection necessitating that the case manager intervene with the insurance company for extra admission days. A staff or clinician problem may be related to caregiver practice. For instance, a physician who always keeps a myocardial infarction patient in the hospital for 4.5 days as opposed to 3.2 days may represent a caregiver problem. A clinician problem may also occur if the case manager does not recognize or immediately act on a deviation from the path and neglects to use timely clinical resources to address the problem. A frequent variance may be concerned with the lack of physical therapy on the weekend, necessitating additional inpatient days. A system or hospital problem may occur when equipment or machinery is broken or

malfunctions, or when laboratory tests or x-rays are delayed or lost. Common systems problems occur when there is no transfer bed for a patient in the intensive care unit. Community problems are usually related to inappropriate knowledge of resources, or the lack of a skilled nursing home bed.

Many hospitals have their own unique variances in patient care and develop variance analysis forms to reflect this uniqueness. Variance should be monitored daily, shift by shift, and should be tabulated weekly and reviewed by the case manager and the nurse manager monthly. In some hospitals, these reports are generated by the hospital information system. The critical care task force should also review variance trends and deviations quarterly and refine critical paths accordingly. It is at this time that organizational change may occur; for instance, the addition of a physical therapist on the weekend or the purchase of new, more reliable equipment. Analysis of variance ensures continual quality monitoring of patient care and outcomes of care and fits well within the guidelines of total quality management.

If variance is noted in a timely fashion and timely case consultation occurs, better patient outcomes can result. Accurate monitoring of critical paths with variance analysis can estimate and track the financial impact of patient care. Consequently, costs are better managed, and, if the variance is predictable, negotiation with insurers for an additional length of stay can maximize patient care revenues. The need for fiscal accountability for patient care is important.

ROLE OF NURSING CASE MANAGERS

The role and responsibility of the nursing case manager in a managed-care environment is comprehensive, complex, and often diverse (Fig. 4–3). Usually, the case manager acts as a coordinator of care and assists the patient and family in making decisions based on need, ability, and available resources (National Council on Aging, 1987).

Case managers also assume accountability for patient outcomes and possess authority that extends across the boundaries of nursing units. Critical tasks for nursing case managers include the coordination, management, and monitoring of patient care via

Day	Initials	Variance and Reason	Code	Action Taken and Response

CODES:

A. Patient/Family
B. Care-Giver
C. Hospital Systems
D. Community Response
E. Other

Critical Pathway Boundaries

A. All Pneumonias
  1. Includes:
    A. Co-Morbidity
  2. Excludes:
    A. Ventilator development

Addressograph

Figure 4–2. Variance analysis form.

Pre-hospital   Acute hospital   Post-hospital

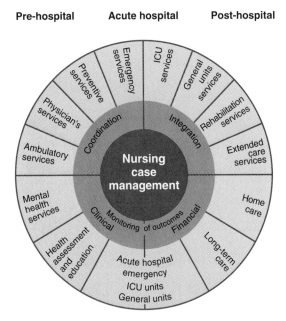

Figure 4–3. Role of nursing care managers: case management services over a continuum.

clinical assessment and variance analysis of assigned patients. The facilitation of care is based on developed standards of care. Nursing case managers are also responsible for the design, implementation, and refinement of critical paths and other case management tools to facilitate care delivery. Variance analysis is a critical part of the case manager's role, as the control of variability is directly linked with the cost, quality, and outcomes of care. Other roles assumed by case managers are similar to RN caregiver roles.

Nursing case managers must have excellent communication and negotiation skills as well as clinical credibility and respect. Hospitals must educate nursing case managers regarding the fiscal aspects of care, the availability of community resources, as well knowledge of quality improvement and utilization management.

An *exemplary model* of case management occurs when the entire hospital has committed to an interdisciplinary professional practice system within a decentralized environment and when case managers are selected based on their education, expertise, and negotiation skills. When these variables occur,

nursing and other professionals have the authority to manage care and accountability for that care. An exemplary model also requires a comprehensive evaluation system for financial, clinical, and perceptual outcomes of the hospital, its patients, and its staff.

ADVANTAGES OF CASE MANAGEMENT

Advantages of case management are numerous in the literature. A considerable advantage of case management is that it can be matrixed over, or used in conjunction with, a primary, team, or functional nursing model with the case manager providing the management and direction of the care. Matrixing this model provides significant cost savings as the entire nursing practice does not have to be changed.

In addition to decreased implementation costs, the literature suggests that case management is associated with cost reductions, a decrease in the fragmentation of patient care, and enhanced job satisfaction for nursing case managers and for patients. Ethridge (1991) noted several key factors that account for how case management can affect cost savings. Ethridge suggests that teaching patients to recognize illness and seek medical care before the illness becomes complex and difficult to treat can provide cost reductions, as can coordinating care with physicians during acute episodes of illness. Also, discussing quality of life issues with chronically ill patients and their families can reduce expensive and unnecessary life support mechanisms prior to an acute crisis. Ethridge and Lamb (1989) noted that the nurse case manager can aid in reducing fragmented care through the development of a long-term relationship with the patient and his or her family. Also, monitoring of a patient response to treatments and services can prevent complications, decrease fragmentation of care, and prevent unnecessary costs. Collaborating with other health care providers, monitoring a patient's response to treatments and services to prevent complications as well as facilitating access to various community-based services and support groups can also reduce fragmentation in patient care.

In addition to reducing the cost of care and the fragmentation of care, the literature suggests an increase in patient satisfaction with case management. Because one case manager coordinates a patient's care, it can be anticipated that enhanced patient outcomes will be realized, as well as patient satisfaction (Lynn-McHale et al, 1993). High patient and family satisfaction has been reported by Ethridge (1988), McElroy and Campbell (1992), and McKenzie et al (1989). Furthermore, McKenzie et al (1989) noted that patients expressed a sense of security by having a familiar individual, such as the nurse case manager, educating and supporting them. Collard and Henderson (1988) reported that patients often improve their behavior simply because they are being closely watched and cared for. High physician satisfaction with case management has been noted by Ethridge (1988) and Loveridge et al (1988).

DISADVANTAGES OF CASE MANAGEMENT

Disadvantages of case management are generally concerned with the difficulties that usually accompany planned change and the perception by administration that the hospital has a lack of qualified staff members to be case managers. Many urban hospitals require the case manager to have a master's degree in nursing, but other hospitals have found that nurses with less education function well within the case manager role. Another disadvantage concerns the interdisciplinary nature of case management. Some hospitals have reported difficulty implementing case management because of this requirement. Frequently, turf and territorial issues arise between representatives of nursing, social work, and the supportive therapy disciplines. To combat this difficulty, hospitals are encouraged to stress the interdisciplinary nature of clinical care management throughout the introduction, planning, implementation, and evaluation of the case-management professional practice system. All interdisciplinary caregivers should be included in the planning and development of critical paths and in the evaluation of case-managed care.

A final difficulty with clinical case-managed care is associated with the lack of physician support for the practice model. Usually the lack of support is directly related to a lack of understanding by the physician. Since physicians are key players in man-

aged care, it is imperative to gain their support and cooperation during the initial phase of planning. Frequently, this can be orchestrated by hospital administration through the medical director via medical staff meetings. This eliminates the perception that the case-management professional practice system is simply "nurses changing things again." It is important to note that case-managed care represents the first attempt at nursing care delivery that has a direct impact on physicians and other interdisciplinary team members.

Case management has also been associated with nurse satisfaction. An increase in nursing satisfaction and a decrease in nursing job stress and turnover under the case-management model was noted by Bower (1992), Lynn-McHale et al (1993), Ahrens (1992), and Ethridge (1987). McKenzie et al (1989) observed that nursing case management is rewarding for nurses because it allows nurses a greater degree of control when caring for patients. Ownership, recognition, and increased involvement in patient care were cited as important consequences of nursing case management.

Case management is a professional practice model because it provides a professional framework for unit-based practice and self-management. A managed-care delivery system in a decentralized nursing environment empowers nurses to have control, authority, and accountability over all aspects of their practice, including the establishment of clinical standards, accountability, and collegiality. Case management can also provide reward incentives, benefits, and gain-sharing for committed case managers. Case management integrates well with continuous quality improvement because of its customer focus. It provides a consistent refinement of care processes through variance analysis and refinement of critical paths.

RESEARCH IN CASE MANAGEMENT

Research suggests that case-management delivery systems can provide an improvement in the length of stay and costs of care (Research Box 4–1). Brooten et al (1986) demonstrated the effects of nurse specialist care on outcomes for low-birthweight infants. Babies cared for by nurse specialists were discharged on an average of more than 11 days earlier than control babies, at a cost savings of approximately $18,560 per family.

Ethridge and Lamb (1989) describe a system of nursing case management staffed by professional nurses and extending from the acute-care hospital into the community. Evaluating case-managed, high-risk patients against lower-acuity standards, the researchers reported a 2-day average reduction in length of stay for patients case-managed by an RN. The New England Medical Center has reduced its average length of stay for patients with myocardial infarction from 9 to 7 days, while the length of stay for cardiac catheterization has been reduced from 5 to 3 days (Ethridge & Lamb, 1989). The New England Medical Center also reports a 29% drop in the average length of stay for ischemic strokes and a 47% drop in the average number of intensive care days (Zander, 1988). Ethridge (1991) provides data on more than 1700 patients in the HMO for senior citizens. The case-managed patients have fewer hospital admissions and an average length of stay of 1.73 days less than a comparison group of Medicare patients. Naylor (1990) examined the impact of discharge planning by nurses on the hospitalization of elderly adults and found that although there was no difference in the initial length of stay between the control group and the experimental group, patients in the control group had significantly higher rehospitalization rates and hence longer lengths of stay.

A study by Mumford et al (1982) demonstrated that clinical management by professional nurses lowered the length of stay and decreased costs. Stillwaggon (1989) examined the costs of nursing care affected when nurses practiced nursing based on patient needs as opposed to institutional policy. The study concluded that the impact of nurse-managed care on the cost of nursing practice and satisfaction resulted in a 20% decrease in nursing costs.

An additional study by McKenzie et al (1989) showed that interventions associated with nursing case management had a significant effect on patient resource consumption and expenditures. Case management plans and critical paths were developed for specific high-volume DRGs associated with diseases and disorders of the circulatory system, coronary artery bypass, and catheterization. This study demonstrated average cost savings per case equivalent to $350 for laboratory charges, $180 per day for radiology charges, and $766 for pharmaceutical charges for nursing case-managed patients. The average length of stay was also reduced by 1.1 days. Within a 1-year period, close to $1 million was saved by using the case-management system of care.

The literature clearly suggests that nursing case-managed care offers better clinical and perceptual outcomes for patients. Financial outcomes are often enhanced because hospitals are able to effect optimal clinical outcomes at a lower cost. Case-managed care also offers enhanced collegiality between providers and prevents the duplication of services. Nursing satisfaction, motivation, and retention is also enhanced when nurses are working in a professional practice system.

Research Box 4–1

Case Management and Length of Stay

Cohen (1991) demonstrates significant difference in length of stay between a traditional unit and one using a nursing case-management system. Nursing case-managed patients stayed an average of 4.86 days whereas patients on traditional nursing units stayed an average of 6.02 days. Furthermore, the nurse-managed patients received significantly more direct care time from RNs and nurse extenders than did the patients on the traditional unit, and yet the cost per patient case was lower for the case-managed patient, with a savings of $930.40 per case reported. McKenzie et al (1989) reported shorter lengths of stay, lower costs, and higher levels of patient, nurse, and physician satisfaction associated with nursing case-managed patients and savings of $960,000 and 430 patient days.

SUMMARY

The purpose of this chapter was to discuss and differentiate between managed care and nursing case management. An overview of a case management professional practice model was presented and a review of the literature validated case management delivery systems as cost-efficient, effective, and satisfying to staff and patients.

The reformed health care environment with its emphasis on cost, quality, and outcomes will continue to require that nurses refine their skills and become proficient in the clinical monitoring and fiscal tracking of care. Delivery systems of the future will foster quality and efficiency at lower costs.

■ DISCUSSION QUESTIONS ■

1. Discuss how health care reform has changed the way in which patients receive care.
2. Distinguish between managed care and nursing case management.
3. Explain why all patients do not have to be case-managed.
4. Discuss the tools of case management and their importance in quality and cost monitoring.
5. Discuss the changing role of the clinical leader in case management.
6. What are the goals of managed care and nursing case management?
7. Discuss how case management is a professional practice model.
8. What has nursing research validated about case management?

■ LEARNING ACTIVITIES ■

1. You are an RN in a breast clinic in a large medical center. Explain how the network of nursing services can be best used to provide quality care and control costs.
2. As a clinical leader in a cardiac unit, you have been assigned the task of establishing a critical path to manage patients after myocardial infarction. Explain how you would do this and who should be included in the process.
3. At the January variance analysis meeting you notice that the length of stay for patients with strokes has increased 1.6 days over the last quarter. How would you and the committee analyze the data, explain the variance, and adjust the critical path?
4. You are an emergency department nurse, and your hospital wants to decrease the number of emergency room visits for certain patient populations. It has been decided that you will be the new emergency department case manager. How would you define and integrate your role?

■ BIBLIOGRAPHY ■

Ahrens T (1992). Nurse clinician model of managed care. *AACN Clinical Issues on Critical Care Nursing* 3:761—768.

American Nurses' Association (1988). *Nursing Case Management.* Kansas City, MO: Author, Publication No. N5-32.

Bower K (1992). *Case Management by Nurses.* Washington, DC: American Nurses Publishing.

Brooten D, Jumar S, Brown L, et al (1986). A randomized clinical treatment of early hospital discharge and home follow-up of very low birth weight infants. *New England Journal of Medicine* 315:934–939.

Coffey RJ, Richards JS, Remmert CS, et al (1992). An introduction to critical paths. *Quality Management in Health Care* 1(1):45–54.

Cohen EL (1991). Nursing case management: Does it pay? *Journal of Nursing Administration* 21(4):20–25.

Cohen S, Arnold L, Brown L, Brooten M (1991). Taxonomic classification of transitional follow-up case nursing interventions with low birthweight infants. *Clinical Nurse Specialist* 5(1):31–36.

Cohen EL, Cesta TG (1993). *Nursing Case Management: From Concept to Evaluation.* St. Louis: Mosby.

Collard A, Henderson M (1988). Measuring quality in medical case management programs. *Case Management: Guiding Patients Through the Health Care Maze*, JACHO.

Cronin CJ, Makelbust JK (1989) Case-managed care: Capitalizing on the CNS. *Nursing Management* 20(3):38–47.

Dear M, Weisman C, O'Keefe S (1985) Evaluation of a contract model for professional nursing practice. *Health Care Management Review* 65–77.

DelTogno-Armanasco V (1989). Developing an integrated nursing case management model. *Nursing Management* 20 (10):26–29.

Douglas LM (1988). *The Effective Nurse Leader/Manager.* St. Louis: CV Mosby.

Ethridge P (1987). Nurse accountability program improves satisfaction turnover. *Health Progress* 68:44–49.

Ethridge P (1988). Professional nurse case management reduces hospital costs. *Arizona Nurse* 41:1, 8

Ethridge PE (1991). A nursing HMO: Carondelet St. Mary's experience. *Nursing Management* 22:22–27.

Ethridge P, Lamb G (1989). Professional nursing case management improves quality, access, and costs. *Nursing Management* 20(3):35–38.

Farquhar S, Robinson J (1990). The geometry of case management. *Michigan Nurse* 63(5):7–8.

Haley-Boyce JA, Dulin J (1996). Actualizing Empowerment. *Nursing Management* 27(1):47–48.

Harkness GA, Miller J, Hill N (1992). Differentiated practice: A three dimensional model. *Nursing Management* (12):26–30.

Hogan A, Rohrer J (1989). The effects of nursing and physician services: Some preliminary results. *Social Science Medicine* 29(4):527–536.

Hurt LW (1995). Care management: Providing a connecting link. *Nursing Management* 24(11):27–33.

Knollmueller R (1989). Case management: What's in a name. *Nursing Management* 20(10):3–40, 42.

Lancero AW, Gerber RM (1995). Comparing work satisfaction in two case management models. *Nursing Management* 26(11):45–48.

Loveridge C, Cummings S, O'Malley J (1988). Development case management in the primary nursing system. *Journal of Nursing Administration* 18:36–39.

Lynn-McHale D, Fitzpatrick E, Shaffer R (1993). Case management: Development of a model. *Clinical Nurse Specialist* 7(6):299–307.

McElroy M, Campbell S (1992). Case management with the nurse manager in the role of case manager in an interventional cardiology unit. *AACN Clinical Issues on Critical Care Nursing* 3:749–760.

McKenzie C, Torkelson N, Holt M (1989). Care and cost: Nursing case management improved both. *Nursing Management* 20:30–34.

Mumford E, Schlesinger H, Glass G (1982). The effects of psychological intervention on recovery from surgery and heart attacks: An analysis of the literature. *American Journal of Public Health* 72:141–51.

National Council on Aging (1987). *Standards for Case Management*. Washington, DC: Author.

Naylor M (1990). Comprehensive discharge planning for hospitalized elderly: A pilot study. *Nursing Research* 39(3):156–161.

Oliver GS, DelTogno-Armanasco V, Ericksosn JR, Harter S (1989). Case management: A bottom-line delivery model. Part I: the concept. *Journal of Nursing Administration* 19(11):16–20.

Stillwaggon CA (1989). The impact of nurse managed care of the cost of nurse practice and nurse satisfaction. *Journal of Nursing Administration* 19(11):21–27.

Zander K (1988). Nursing case management: strategic management of cost and quality outcomes. *Journal of Nursing Administration* 18(5):23–30.

Zander K (1991). Care maps: the core of cost/quality care. *The New Definition* 6(3):1–3.

5

Fiscal Considerations in Clinical Leadership

William J. Ward, Jr., MBA

LEARNING OBJECTIVES

This chapter will enable the learner to:

1. Analyze the content of the balance sheet and income statement.
2. Identify the factors that cause operating costs to rise and fall.
3. Discuss the importance of budgeting in the management of resources.
4. Evaluate the use of analytical tools such as variance analysis, benefit-to-cost ratio analysis, forecasting, and break-even analysis.
5. Appreciate the need for business skills to balance clinical know-how.

INTRODUCTION

The fiscal concerns of providers of health care in the next millennium are such that the only successful approach to clinical leadership will be a balanced one. A successful approach will empower leaders to give appropriate, balanced consideration to both the clinical needs of the patients served and business needs of the health care entity striving to survive to continue to provide the clinical needs of its patients. The days of worrying solely about clinical issues to the exclusion of business reality are long gone.

THE IMPACT OF MANAGED CARE

Driven by concerns over both the cost of health care and the rate of cost growth, the government and private sectors have sought ways to control expenditures. Since the approach to reform by the government became politicized and failed, the private sector has embarked on a reform effort that has produced dramatic results along with a host of concerns regarding quality, freedom of choice, and operating practices.

Managed care, the practice of prospectively paying predetermined amounts of money to selected providers to maintain the health of a defined population, has been the response of the private sector to the need for cost control. It has dramatically driven down expenditures. In 1994, after decades of double digit growth, employers saw the average per-employee cost for health care coverage decline by 1.1%. Some claim that this is merely the result of shifting premium costs from employer to employee, but such shifting has been practiced for too long with little or no success to suddenly be responsible for such a dramatic turnaround. Rather, managed care has managed cost, which is precisely the outcome sought by those paying the bills for more than two decades.

The nursing profession in general, and nursing leaders in particular, find themselves at the center of the debate between doing the right thing for the patient and following the cost-constraining mandates of managed care. What should the nurse leader in the obstetrics unit do when a health maintenance organization (HMO) (an organization that assumes the financial risk for the cost of care and provides or arranges for a range of health care services to be provided to an enrolled population on a prepaid basis) expects mother and baby to be discharged 24 hours after delivery? What about the standard of care that suggests a minimum of 48 hours should pass between birth and discharge? Keeping the mother and baby in the hospital for an extra day may please the mother but upset the HMO, which in turn exerts pressure (eg, in the form of diverting admissions to a more compliant facility) on the institution. On the other hand, discharging the mother and baby too soon can leave the HMO satisfied but upset both the mother and the caregiver, who is concerned about care not given.

As the leader of the group of caregivers providing for continuity of care, the nurse leader is the only member of the clinical team able to articulate the true needs of patient care during all phases of an illness or encounter with the provider component. The nurse leader is ideally positioned to exert positive influence on the direction taken by managed care in the coming years; he or she should stand firm at times and move to compromise at others but never lose sight of the care-giving mission. To be successful, nurse leaders must understand the nonclinical, business aspects of health care; in so doing, they will better equip themselves to act as advocates for their profession and the patients for whom they care.

ROLES IN HEALTH CARE

Business transactions, from buying groceries to subscribing to a magazine, involve three roles: *orderer*, *consumer*, and *payer*, which have traditionally been exercised by a single party. In health care, these roles have historically been divided among three separate parties. The first was that of orderer, which is referred to in economic terms as a *demander*, a role traditionally exercised by a physician. The role of *consumer* was exercised by the patient. The third role was exercised by a *third-party payer*, typically an insurance company or government program such as Medicare or Medicaid. As a result of this extraordinary partitioning of the roles, price, which in most cases would act as a controlling influence, has been

unable to control demand. Consequently, the increase in the cost of health care has largely been the result of what economists refer to as *demand push* inflation.

The change brought about by managed care was to recombine two of the roles, orderer and payer, which enabled price to exercise its traditional role by stimulating or impeding the demand for health care services.

In providing health services, just as in any other business venture, it is important to remember the relationship between revenue or income and the availability of resources. The amount of revenue coming into an organization establishes the boundaries of resource availability.

ACCOUNTABILITY IN HEALTH CARE

All leaders are responsible for their actions. In health care, this responsibility takes several forms. Clinical outcomes data, Joint Commission accreditation, and patient satisfaction survey results are a few of the measurement methods. Leaders are also held financially responsible, and performance evaluation takes the form of internal financial performance reports and more formal financial statements for both internal leadership and external constituencies such as trustees and directors, regulators, and others.

Internal financial performance reports provide the data needed to manage financial and other resources as well as establish individual responsibility. These financial data are further used to produce the financial statements of the organization, which provide a summary of what transpired during a given period of time on the income statement or the financial status on a particular date on the balance sheet.

The balance sheet reports what is owned, or the *assets* of the company, and what is owed, or the *liabilities*. The difference between what is owned and what is owed is termed *equity*. Depending on the type of company, this may be referred to as owners' equity, stockholders' equity, fund balance, the capital account, or simply capital. Assets are generally categorized as current (cash, short-term securities, accounts receivable, and inventories) and fixed, such as property, plant, and equipment.

Liabilities are generally categorized as current amounts, which must be paid during the next 12 months, and long-term debts, which will not be paid during the next year.

Depending on the amount of detailed information given, a balance sheet can be displayed on a single page with assets on the left and liabilities and equity on the right or on two facing pages with assets on the left page and liabilities and equity on the right page. A third format, consisting of a vertical layout on a single page with assets at the top and liabilities and equity at the bottom, is not uncommon. Regardless of format, the amounts shown represent the *balances* of the various items on the date shown on the financial statement and thus the sheet is called a *balance sheet*.

The balance sheet displayed in Table 5–1 shows values for both the current and prior fiscal years; a fiscal year is a 12-month period designated for planning and evaluation by the organization. This provides a benchmark of sorts to help determine whether the financial picture on December 31st of the current year represents an improvement over the situation on December 31st of the previous year. It helps answer the question: has the company's leadership improved its financial condition?

Variously referred to as the *income statement, statement of revenue(s) and expense(s)*, or simply the *P&L*, an income statement summarizes the activity during an accounting period of a month, quarter, or fiscal year. The P&L presented in Table 5–2 is called a *comparative statement* because it provides a comparison with the prior fiscal year. The column headings tell that the report is for the 12 months ended, meaning the amounts shown represent activity for a full fiscal year.

The top portion of the statement deals with revenues. The amounts reported as *net patient service revenue* represent the revenue derived from health care services. The report continues with *other operating revenue*, representing income from nonpatient care operations such as interest earned on investments, gift shops, and parking lots. *Total operating revenue* is the total of both revenue streams.

The report then lists the costs associated with generating revenues. Staffing costs are always listed first. The cost of providing health insurance, pension, tuition assistance, and other nonwage compensation for employees is reported as *fringe benefits*. In some cases, these two kinds of staff-related costs are combined and reported as a single line called *salaries and benefits*.

Supplies and purchased services lines represent the expenses associated with supplies and the use of outside services, such as transcription, legal, and accounting services. *Interest expense* refers to the cost of borrowing money. Interest expense and *interest income* are never combined or netted and reported on a single line in an income statement.

The provision for *bad debts* represents the amount of revenue that will not be collected. The final expense item is *depreciation*, a noncash expense representing, in monetary terms, the portion of the life of the fixed assets consumed during the accounting period for which the P&L was prepared. The logic behind the depreciation of fixed assets is that a portion of the life of any asset is consumed in the generation of revenue. Just as the cost of supplies consumed in doing business is deducted from revenue, so the cost of that portion of the fixed assets consumed is similarly deducted. Land is never depreciated.

The *cost of operations* line is the sum of the expenses of the organization. It is deducted from the total operating revenue to arrive at the operating gain or loss, which is referred to as the *excess of revenue over expense*, if it is a gain, or the *excess of expenses over revenue*, if there is a loss.

Comparative data are of great value in reviewing financial statements. Whether the comparison is with a prior period or a budget for the reporting period, the presence of yardstick values gives the reviewer a perspective from which to measure the reported financial results. Such comparisons ensure accountability for those entrusted with the resources of an organization.

Financial statements and performance reports are prepared using the accrual basis of accounting. There are two methods or bases for recording business transactions; the *cash basis* recognizes an event only when cash changes hands, whereas the *accrual basis* recognizes events when they happen, regardless of when the cash changes hands. Most individuals handle their personal financial matters on a cash basis, recognizing an expense when the bill is paid, income when the paycheck is received, and so on. In business, however, debt is recognized when a liability is incurred, and income when it is earned. Managers must exercise caution because the natural

Table 5–1.
Hypothetical Health Care Organization Balance Sheet

		December 31, 19X2		December 31, 19X1
Current assets				
Cash		$3,100,000		$4,500,000
Marketable securities		4,000,000		4,000,000
Accounts receivable: patients net of allowance for uncollectibles		6,000,000		7,000,000
Accounts receivable: other		200,000		190,000
Inventories		500,000		600,000
Prepaid items		100,000		110,000
Total current assets		$13,900,000		$16,400,000
Fixed assets				
Land		$15,000,000		$15,000,000
Land improvements	$2,000,000		$1,900,000	
Buildings	75,000,000		75,000,000	
Fixed and movable equipment	35,000,000		33,000,000	
Total	112,000,000		109,900,000	
Less: accumulated depreciation	44,800,000	67,200,000	43,500,000	66,400,000
Total assets		$96,100,000		$97,800,000
Current liabilities				
Accounts payable	$5,600,000		$7,900,000	
Current portion of long-term debt	2,400,000		2,400,000	
Accrued liabilities	900,000		800,000	
Total current liabilities		$8,900,000		$11,100,000
Long-term debt				
Equipment leases	$1,500,000		$1,700,000	
Bonds payable	35,000,000		37,400,000	
Total long-term debt		36,500,000		39,100,000
Fund balance				
Opening fund balance	$47,600,000		$44,700,000	
Current year operating gain	3,100,000		2,900,000	
Closing fund balance		50,700,000		47,600,000
Total liabilities and fund balance		$96,100,000		$97,800,000

Table 5–2.
Hypothetical Health Care Organization Statement of Revenues and Expenses for the 12 Months Ending December 31

	19X2	19X1
Net patient service revenue	$90,400,000	$87,900,000
Other operating revenue	350,000	375,000
Total operating revenue	$90,750,000	$88,275,000
Operating expenses		
Salaries and wages	$38,200,000	$36,700,000
Fringe benefits	7,650,000	7,300,000
Supplies	20,000,000	19,500,000
Purchased services	10,000,000	10,500,000
Interest expense	1,500,000	1,400,000
Provision for bad debts	9,000,000	8,775,000
Depreciation	1,300,000	1,200,000
Total operating expenses	$87,650,000	$85,375,000
Excess of revenues over expenses	$3,100,000	$2,900,000

tendency is to manage with the same cash-basis mentality used in their personal lives.

DETERMINING COST OF CARE

As managed care assumes a more dominant role in health care, leaders must concentrate on maximizing financial resources. As revenue becomes more tightly controlled by payers and revenue growth becomes less of an option for providers, the focus must be directed at the control of expenditures. To more effectively exercise this responsibility, managers must understand the basic concepts of cost behavior, operating and capital budgeting, approaches to managing financial resources, and tools that can help with decision-making.

Classifying Costs by Behavior

One way to classify costs is by behavior. Managers must deal with three types of costs. *Fixed costs* are those that are not influenced by changes in volume or intensity of service. A department manager's salary is considered a fixed cost because the manager is paid the same amount regardless of whether volume is up or down. *Variable costs* are those that

rise and fall in response to fluctuations in business volume. Film cost in a radiology department is considered variable because the amount of film consumed will rise and fall as volume rises and falls.

Care must be taken in determining which measure of volume is appropriate for determining the relationship between variable cost and business activity. In radiology, for example, film cost may vary directly with the number of procedures. In anesthesia, the cost of anesthetic agents may be driven more by the number of minutes than by the number of surgical procedures. Thus, the cost of anesthetic agents might actually rise despite a reduction in the number of cases if the average time per case increased due to complexity (Table 5–3).

The real danger for managers lies with the third type: *semivariable costs*. These are costs that are partially fixed and partially variable. Staffing costs are the most common example of semivariable cost. On a graph, these costs resemble stair steps (Fig. 5–1). As volume rises, staffing remains fixed up to a point and then varies before becoming fixed again. The cycle repeats over and over again as volume rises and falls. If a nursing unit had a patient-to-nurse ratio of 6:1, for example, staffing costs would be fixed in the range of one to six patients. A single full-time equivalent employee (FTE) is required. A seventh patient would cause a change in

Table 5–3.
Anesthesia Supply Consumption

Month	Supply		Minutes Per Case	Cost Per Case	Total Minutes	Cost Per Minute
	COST	**CASES**				
January	$120,000	160	120	$750.00	19,200	$6.25
February	125,900	155	130	812.26	20,150	6.25
March	131,200	150	140	874.67	21,000	6.25
April	135,900	145	150	937.24	21,750	6.25
May	140,000	140	160	1,000.00	22,400	6.25
June	143,400	135	170	1,062.22	22,950	6.25
July	146,200	130	180	1,124.62	23,400	6.25
August	148,400	125	190	1,187.20	23,750	6.25
September	150,000	120	200	1,250.00	24,000	6.25
October	150,900	115	210	1,312.17	24,150	6.25
November	154,700	110	225	1,406.36	24,750	6.25
December	157,500	105	240	1,500.00	25,200	6.25

staffing—the addition of another FTE. This second FTE would remain fixed as volume grows through the twelfth patient. At that point, the addition of a thirteenth patient would set the process in motion again. In this example, the staffing cost is fixed for the six patients, becomes variable with the seventh patient, becomes fixed again for patients 7 through 12, becomes variable again with the 13th patient,

and so on. Understanding the way semivariable costs react to changes in volume is vital to decision-makers.

Classifying Costs by Type

A second way to classify costs is by type, as either direct or indirect. *Direct costs* are those that, as the

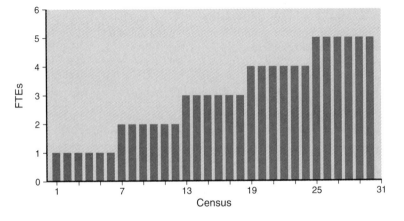

Figure 5–1. Behavior of semivariable costs. FTE, full-time equivalent employee.

name implies, are directly associated with patient care. Nursing unit salaries and supplies are examples of costs directly associated with patient care and thus are categorized as *direct costs*. *Indirect costs* are usually incurred in departments away from the point of care; examples include administrative costs in nursing, accounting, medical records, and housekeeping. Sometimes, indirect costs are referred to as *overhead costs*. Occasionally, the term *direct cost* refers to a cost directly associated with operation of a department regardless of whether the department is engaged in the care of patients. In this use, the salaries of managers, housekeepers, and clerks, along with cleaning and office supplies used in the functioning of a housekeeping department, would be classified as direct expenses.

Understanding the way costs are likely to behave under a variety of circumstances is important. What would happen if a provider's costs were 50% fixed and 50% variable, but a price regulator or payer took the view that the provider's costs were 100% variable? If volume were to decline, for every $1.00 of revenue that would be lost, only $0.50 of cost would be eliminated; only the variable costs would decrease, and by their very nature, the fixed costs would remain unchanged. In a fee-for-service reimbursement environment in which volumes are declining, this can be disastrous. An understanding of cost behavior can be used proactively and creatively to take advantage of economies of scale. The profile of fixed and variable costs must be known to determine real behavior of costs as volume changes. Also, the regulator's view must be known to determine revenue potential.

The behavior of semivariable costs is particularly important to the decision-making process. In the example of semivariable costs cited earlier, the addition of a seventh patient, if not followed by an eighth or a ninth, would be a poor choice. Revenue would increase only 16.7%, but semivariable staffing costs would increase by 100% with the addition of a second staff person. The same stair-step cycle holds true as volume declines. For reimbursement purposes, the assumption is that staff cost is totally variable when, in fact, it is not. Again, using the six-to-one ratio, a unit with 12 patients would be staffed by two nurses. If volume is reduced by one patient, the reimbursement presumption is that one twelfth of the staff is also reduced. The reality, however, is that staffing is fixed from 12 patients down to and

including the seventh patient. Staffing would not be reduced until volume dropped to six patients.

Any business that adopts a pricing strategy that gives no consideration to cost will soon find itself out of business. This is not to say that a prudent business approach cannot include prices that are less than cost. It means that cost must be understood and that management must always be aware of the difference between cost and price. To develop a price for a service, the direct costs of that service must be considered along with a portion (referred to as an *allocation*) of the various indirect costs. Several approaches can be used to determine price.

Pricing Health Care Services

Cost-Based Pricing

The first factor affecting care costs is *cost-based pricing*, the method of choice in use in health care for many years. The price for a service is a function of the costs associated with providing the service:

- The direct expense of the department or revenue center providing the service (salaries, fringe benefits, supplies, and services included)

- Indirect or overhead costs allocated to the revenue center from support departments like accounting, medical records, and housekeeping

- Depreciation expense if not included in the allocation of indirect or overhead costs

- Financial requirements for interest expense, repayment of debt, achievement of profit goals, and return on investment

- The "cost" of bad debts and other uncollectible accounts

The following information illustrates the use of relative value units (RVUs). An RVU is a measure of procedural acuity or the intensity of workload. For example, an imaging center offers three services: magnetic resonance imaging scans, each with a relative value weight of 100 relative value units; computed tomography scans, at 100 and 50 RVUs, depending on the complexity; and mammography, at 25 RVUs per procedure. Table 5–4 displays the volume of business of the imaging center in terms of both procedure counts and RVUs. The price to

Table 5–4.
Hypothetical Imaging Center Procedure Volumes

Service	Number of Procedures	RVUs Per Procedure	Total Number of RVUs
MRI scans	500	100	50,000
CT scan: routine	500	50	25,000
CT scan: complex	500	100	50,000
Mammography	400	25	10,000
Totals	1,900		135,000

RVU, relative value unit; MRI, magnetic resonance imaging; CT, computed tomography.

be charged is based on the relative value of each procedure; thus, the price for a magnetic resonance imaging scan at 100 RVUs would be four times the price for a mammogram. Table 5–5 illustrates how the amount to be charged for each RVU is determined based on the total operating costs (direct and overhead), profit target, and bad debts factor. Note that the amount for bad debts is calculated not by addition but rather by division, a technique known as *grossing up*, using the collection rate. The resulting price list is displayed in Table 5–6.

Competition-Based Pricing

A second approach, *competition-based pricing*, has entered health care as competition became a greater factor in the marketplace. As the name implies, competition-based pricing bases price on what the competition is doing rather than solely on underlying cost. In the extreme, this takes the form of sealed-bid price competition. Such is the case with HMOs and similar providers as they seek to obtain the lowest cost health services for their cli-

Table 5–5.
Hypothetical Imaging Center Price Setting Analysis

Items to be recovered via price		
Salaries and wages	$445,200	
Fringe benefits	111,300	
Supplies	150,000	
Purchased services	75,500	
Overhead expenses	300,500	
Profit target	200,000	
Total costs to be recovered	$1,282,500	Item A
Collection rate	95.00%	Item B
Total revenues to be recovered via price (item A divided by item B)	$1,350,000	
Total RVUs	135,000	Item C
Price per RVU	$10.00	

RVU, relative value unit.

Table 5–6.
Hypothetical Imaging Center Price List

Service	RVUs Per Procedure	Price Per RVU	Procedure Price
MRI scans	100	$10.00	$1,000.00
CT scan: routine	50	10.00	500.00
CT scan: complex	100	10.00	1,000.00
Mammography	25	10.00	250.00

RVU, relative value unit; MRI, magnetic resonance imaging; CT, computed tomography.

ents. Some state-run medical assistance programs use a bidding approach to obtain the lowest cost from providers.

The Medicare Prospective Payment System has brought marketplace average pricing into health care by establishing the average price itself. Rather than the providers determining the price, Medicare has established the price it will pay for each specific diagnosis and has, in effect, forced providers to achieve that marketplace average or lose money.

Private insurance companies have introduced policies for health care coverage that direct participating beneficiaries away from providers whose prices are too far above the marketplace average. This direction of beneficiaries takes the form of disincentives for the use of nonpreferred providers. For example, a visit to the "wrong" emergency department may require a copayment by the beneficiary that would have been covered by the insurance company had the patient used a "preferred" emergency department. The same kind of disincentive applies to physician services and inpatient hospitalizations. Higher copayments and deductibles are applied for the use of a nonpreferred provider. These nonpreferred providers have an incentive to reduce prices to the marketplace average or some other threshold to become preferred.

The advantage of a competitive pricing approach in health care is that management has far greater latitude in establishing prices, attracting patients, and maneuvering for survival. The disadvantage is that societal interests such as medical education, care for the poor, and the introduction of new technologies may be abandoned because of lack of funding.

Demand-Based Pricing

Demand-based pricing, which has not yet made an appearance in health care, is the third approach. The charging of higher prices is associated with high levels of demand for a product or service. Reduced demand often leads to a lowering of prices.

HEALTH CARE BUDGETING

Budgeting is a key component in the management process and understanding budgeting and the role it plays in business is essential to the proper exercise of a manager's responsibilities. Simply stated, a budget is a formal plan for the acquisition and use of resources in the future. There are four principal reasons for budgeting: increasing awareness, determining resource needs, measuring performance, and controlling operations.

The first two reasons deal with information. The proper interaction between the various levels of management and staff serves to increase awareness and knowledge. Managers who isolate themselves from the people and events for which they are budgetarily responsible have little chance of success. The second reason is to determine the types and amounts of resources needed. As a budget is prepared, a picture develops of both existing resources and additional resources needed to achieve the stated objectives. The result is a list of resource needs that can be used to focus attention during budget review and approval sessions.

The last two reasons deal with performance. A

budget provides an objective determination of success or failure by measuring the performance of both the organization and individual managers through comparison of actual results with those budgeted. Finally, the budget functions as a control technique by establishing limits and holding managers responsible for resource use consistent with those limits.

Preliminary Preparation

Before preparing the budget, several documents should be examined. The first of these is the set of *budget guidelines*. These are customarily distributed at the start of the budgeting process. These guidelines contain such elements as the budget forms, timetable, information about anticipated inflation, planned salary increases, and, perhaps most important of all, information about limits on the availability of resources. This document provides the minimum amount of information needed to prepare a workable budget.

A second document to be studied is the *organization mission statement*. Obviously, the budget must support the mission. If the mission of an organization is to serve the pediatric population in the surrounding area, for example, it might be inconsistent to divert scarce resources away from a pediatric clinic to fund a new substance abuse program for adults. The strategic plan also should be reviewed to ensure that short- and long-term initiatives are properly integrated. The use of any scarce resources for a project or program that is inconsistent with either the mission statement or strategic plan represents questionable management practice.

Finally, all of the budgets should be consolidated and reviewed a final time to ensure proper communication and integration. For example, if a hospital clinic plans to offer Saturday hours, there should be some communication with housekeeping so that its budget can reflect the need for added staffing to support the expanded operation. Problems can arise if the budgeting process is divided either by timetable (some budgets prepared, reviewed, and approved at an earlier or later date than others) or by responsibility (the chief financial officer responsible for managing the preparation of the operating budget and the chief operating officer responsible for preparing the capital budget). If budgets are not carefully coordinated, the expense and capital elements of a program may be improperly, and quite embarrassingly, misbudgeted.

Preparing the Budget

A properly prepared budget supports a manager's responsibilities to plan, organize and staff, direct or lead, and control. A well-developed budget helps leaders and managers understand expectations, organize resources and staff accordingly, and decide the leadership style best suited to a given set of circumstances. The control exercised comes from knowing what was budgeted and what was spent.

Putting the necessary time and effort into budgeting helps achieve compliance with desired constraints. It instills a sense of ownership in the workforce, building credibility among subordinates and superiors. The coordination of long- and short-term goals is facilitated. There is a better understanding of the ways in which the organization operates, and thus better management decisions are made. All of this results in better resource management.

As illustrated in Figure 5–2, the budgeting begins and ends with the goals and objectives. It may take several loops through the calculations of revenues, expenses, and capital expenditures until the budget supports all of the goals and objectives. It is virtually impossible for a manager at any level to begin with

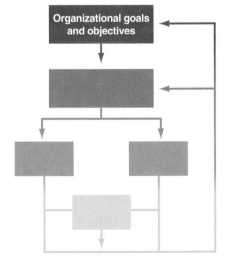

Organizational goals and objectives

Figure 5–2.

a blank page, make the series of calculations only one time, and produce a finished budget.

The process begins by conversion of the overall organizational objectives into department or unit objectives. In turn, these objectives are converted from words to numbers or the volume of business to be achieved during the budget period. Then, volume statistics form the basis of calculations for revenues, expenses, capital equipment, and construction needs.

Managers who are preparing their first budget often approach the work with the false expectation that a single pass at the calculations will suffice. When a second, third, or fourth iteration is required, they are unprepared for the additional work load or feel that the original set of calculations was inferior when such is not necessarily the case.

Analyzing Budget Effectiveness

Once the budget is completed and its fiscal year begins, attention must turn to managing the financial resources to maximize their effectiveness. As depicted in Figure 5–3, there is a cyclical nature to

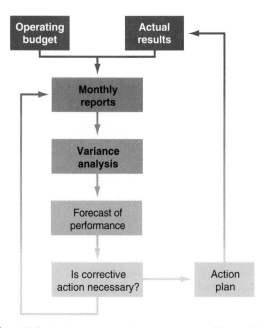

Figure 5–3. Cyclical nature of the management of financial resources.

this. Actual results are compared with budgeted expectations. The differences are analyzed. A forecast of what is likely to happen over the course of the fiscal year is made. Action plans, if necessary, are developed and put into place. A number of financial analysis techniques are available to assist managers throughout an organization to determine the cause of a fiscal performance variance or to forecast future business results.

The comparison of budget and actual results is relatively straightforward; in fact, most performance reporting systems make the comparison on both a current-month and year-to-date basis and report the variances. The key action for management is to determine the underlying cause or causes of any significant variances and, armed with this understanding, take corrective action.

For example, if medical-surgical supply spending on several nursing units is more than budgeted because of supply use, the solution may involve staff education or changes in the supply items. If the reason for the unfavorable variance is the price of the supplies, a different set of actions will be necessary. *Variance analysis* can take the guesswork out of determining whether the cause is price, use, or a combination. Variance analysis should not be confused with variance reporting. Reporting merely lists the elements that sum up to the variance, whereas variance analysis determines the underlying cause.

Most financial performance reports list dozens of line items, most of which show a variance of some sort. The best approach to reducing the amount of analytical work is to establish a performance corridor based on percentage variance from the year-to-date budget values. This approach recognizes that there will always be variances. Only those that are sufficiently significant to fall outside the predetermined corridor need to be analyzed. The advantage of a percentage corridor is that it establishes the limit in terms relative to the size of the budget.

Variance analysis should not be confused with *spending analysis*. Variance analysis is used to tell management why performance has deviated from established expectations. Spending analysis identifies how funds were used. Although large expense amounts may be a source for cost reduction efforts or cost avoidance strategies, they may not involve a variance from budget.

An adjunct to variance analysis, spending analysis

allows management to respond appropriately to the need to curtail spending. Spending analysis is nothing more than a highly detailed listing of amounts spent, categorized by type of expenditure. Beginning with the data contained in monthly performance reports, the analyst backtracks through performance reports to build the list. As a result of this effort, management is better able to understand the essential base level of spending (the amount of spending that will be incurred unless the department or operating unit is closed) and the level of discretionary spending that could be deferred or eliminated depending on the level of austerity needed. In the preparation of this analysis, any items that have been ordered but not yet received should be included. Last, seasonal spending patterns should be considered; overtime pay to cover vacancies caused by vacations in the summer months is an example of seasonal spending.

Financial Forecasting

After the comparison of actual and budgeted performance, a forecast of what is likely to happen in the short term should become the focus of management. A *financial forecast* is a prediction of the future based on historic, current, and other information.

History provides a strong foundation for a forecast; it provides an understanding of trends over time, including relationships among various aspects of the business, such as volume, supply consumption, admissions, ancillary usage, acuity, and staffing levels. The incorporation of current operating facts provides a perspective from which to view the historic data and make a judgment regarding their relevance to the future. Understanding the impact of managed care on historic inpatient use patterns, for example, is necessary to achieve realism in forecasting patient volume. Sources of information include departmental files, hospital financial reports, formal and informal records, and professional associates from outside the organization, including marketplace factors such as salary competition.

Other information rounds out the series of input for a forecast. This information, which is sometimes entirely anecdotal, includes such things as the ability of management to operate effectively in the period under examination; this may refer to the ability

of management to continue favorable performance; rectify, or at least balance, poor performance; and respond to internal and external challenges. Human intuition and plain old common sense play an important part in establishing expected outcomes.

Because forecasts represent critical, upwardly directed information, the predictions they contain must be accurate, not conservative or protective. One manager overstating the forecast for expenses can compromise others in the organization. Understatement of potentially bad news can delay remedial action until it is too late. Managers who are the recipients of forecasts should listen to what is being predicted, even if the message is an unpleasant one. It is important that pressure not be placed on subordinate managers to forecast only what they think the boss wants to hear. And the boss should not "shoot the messenger," or the messenger will stop coming. Lastly, listing the assumptions made in the development of a forecast is essential.

FINANCIAL DECISION-MAKING

A number of financial analysis techniques or decision support tools are available to assist managers throughout an organization in making decisions.

Benefit-to-Cost Ratio Analysis

One technique combines benefit-to-cost ratio analysis with net present value factoring. The *benefit-to-cost ratio*, also called the *profitability index*, is a ratio of the number of dollars of benefit to the dollars invested. In effect, it tells how many dollars are gained for each dollar invested. *Present value factoring* provides an objective restatement of future cash flows into current monetary terms. This factors into the analysis the reality that $1.00 received some time in the future is worth less than $1.00 in hand today. The ratio is determined by dividing the present value of cash inflows by the present value of the investment.

If the benefit-to-cost ratio is equal to or greater than 1.0, the investment should be made; if it is less than 1.0, the investment should not be pursued. Because it is a ratio of the number of dollars returned for each dollar invested, the benefit-to-cost ratio is particularly useful when ranking several investment opportunities.

The present value of the cash flows used in developing the ratio is arrived at by discounting them at a rate equal to the organization return on investment or return on assets. These *return on* values are also referred to as *hurdle rates* because any investment that clears this hurdle should be pursued.

A number of elements should be considered in preparing the analysis; among these are additions, reductions, or substitutions of units of service, collections, staff, supplies, maintenance contracts, and installation costs. The cash inflows, or "benefit," should be accumulated for the life of the project or length of time an investment is to be continued. For example, if a new piece of equipment will be kept in operation for 7 years, the analysis would accumulate the benefit and value it over a 7-year period. If the investment was to be abandoned in 3 years, only 3 years would be accumulated. Lacking specific knowledge, a 5-year life should be assumed for the analysis.

Break-Even Analysis

Another decision support tool is *break-even analysis*. This analytical technique determines the level of volume needed to reach the point at which net revenue exactly equals cost. At the break-even point, there is neither a loss nor a profit. As health care has moved to a competitive model for reimbursement, with prices determined as a function of marketplace forces rather than cost, break-even analysis takes on added importance.

The break-even point, which is expressed in units of volume, is a function of fixed cost, variable cost per unit of service, and net revenue per unit of service. It is calculated by dividing fixed cost by the difference between net revenue per unit and variable cost per unit.

CHANGE AND THE FUTURE

In the current environment, health care leaders must use analytical methods to support decision-making, not to the exclusion of clinical inputs but coupled with them to arrive at balanced decisions. Intuitive decision-making is no longer possible.

Given the reality of the current environment in health care and assuming that more difficulties and challenges lie ahead, how will nurse leaders be able to provide the necessary leadership for the profession, manage the scarce resources at their disposal, and advocate for patients in matters related to the provision of patient care? The answer lies in understanding the old adage that there is strength in numbers. Leaders must empower their managers who in turn must empower their staffs to be part of the process of dealing with the challenges. Rather than a single nurse leader dealing with a multimillion dollar organizational budget, an empowered team of managers and staff can exercise far greater control and stand a far greater chance of success in achieving stated objectives. To this end, a participatory management style is particularly helpful. It is far easier for a team of 30 managers from assistant directors to nursing unit managers to orchestrate and control a $30 million budget than for a single nurse leader to do so. Often, however, stressful times suggest that a highly centralized decision-making structure is the only safe approach. The reality of the current environment is such that one individual is unable to deal single-handedly with the volume and complexity of the challenges. Successful leaders will be those who are able to empower their subordinates and bolster that empowerment by carefully relinquishing control. The result of participatory management through empowerment will be a synergistic, team approach—a division of labor that improves outcomes, responds faster in time of need, and achieves success far more often than a lone individual.

Part of the empowerment process is a need for leaders to instill a sense of stewardship throughout the nursing staff. Stewardship is the recognition by managers and staff alike that resources are not theirs but rather that they are entrusted with those resources, that there is a limit on the availability of resources, and that they must squeeze the most from those limited resources to serve as many patients as possible. Stewardship is an adjunct to management; it is the responsibility all can exercise even when not functioning in a management role. It complements and supports management and is an essential element of successful empowerment.

SUMMARY

As health care moves into the next millennium, successful nurse leaders will be those who can focus on both clinical and fiscal issues and strike an appropriate balance between clinical needs and fiscal imperatives.

■ DISCUSSION QUESTIONS ■

1. What actions might nurse leaders take to evaluate the impact of staffing changes on patient care?
2. What fiscal tools might a nurse leader use to justify the certification of his or her staff in advanced life support?
3. Discuss the advantages and disadvantages of paying home health care nurses by the visit versus by annual salary.

■ LEARNING ACTIVITIES ■

1. Analyze the income and expense statement of an acute care hospital–based unit. Where does the budget vary? What factors might be responsible for these variances?
2. Follow the reimbursement process to a hospital for a Medicare patient who has been hospitalized for a total hip replacement. How much does the hospital receive for these services? What factors affect the reimbursement rate? What did it cost the hospital to provide these services?
3. Explore how home health care services are reimbursed by Medicare, Medicaid, and a managed care organization.

■ BIBLIOGRAPHY ■

Andrianos J, Dykan M (1996). Using cost accounting data to improve clinical value. *Healthcare Financial Management*.

Bailey D (1996). Budgeting skills. *Nursing Standards* 10(19):43–46.

Balicki B, Kelly WP, Miller H (1995). Establishing benchmarks for ambulatory surgery costs. *Healthcare Financial Management* 49(9):40–48.

Boyle CA (1996). Using a time-flow study to identify ambulatory surgical delays. *Journal of Post Anesthesia Nursing* 11(2):71–77.

Browne R, Biancolillo K (1996). The integral role of nursing in managed care. *Nursing Management* 27(4):22–24.

Canby JB IV (1995). Applying activity-based costing to health care settings. *Healthcare Financial Management* 49(1):50–56.

Cardona SM, Bernreuter M (1996). Graduate nurse overhires: A cost analysis. *Journal of Nursing Administration* 26(3):10–15.

Caruana R, McHugh ET (1980). Comparing ratios shows fiscal trends. *Healthcare Financial Management* 34(1):12–18.

Cleverley WO (1986). Fiscal fitness: 10 Principles for evaluating financial health. *Health Progress* 67(1):22–27.

Cleverley WO, Nilsen K (1980). Assessing financial position with 29 key ratios. *Healthcare Financial Management* 34(1):30–36.

Cohen L, Counsel CM (1996). Cost analysis of intermediate care versus intensive care for the neurosurgery patient. *Journal of Nursing Administration* 26(7):3; 26(8):18.

Conrad D, et al (1996). Managing care incentives and information: An exploratory look inside the "black box" of hospital efficiency. *Health Services Research* 31(3):235–259.

Dunn D (1996). Health care 1999: A national bellwether. *Journal of Health Care Finance* 22(3):23–27.

Forman HP, Yin D (1996). Cost analysis and the practicing radiologist/manager: An introduction to managerial accounting. *AJR American Journal of Roentgenology* 166(6):1249–1253.

Gates DM (1996). Changes in health care financing: Effects on the delivery of health care services in the 1990s. *The Journal of Cardiovascular Nursing* 11(1):1–13.

Hill NT, Johns EL (1994). Adoption of costing systems by US hospitals. *Hospitals and Health Services Administration* 39(4):521–539.

Joel LA (1996). The scapegoating of managed care. *American Journal of Nursing* 96(6):7.

Keegan AJ (1994). Hospitals become cost centers in managed care scenario. *Healthcare Financial Management* 48(8):36–39.

Khoshnood B, et al (1996). Models for determining cost of care and length of stay in neonatal intensive care units. *International Journal of Technology Assessment in Health Care* 12(1):62–71.

Lessner MW, et al (1994). Orienting nursing students to cost effective clinical practice. *Nursing and Health Care* 15(9):458–462.

Lipson DJ, De Sa JM (1996). Impact of purchasing strategies on local health care systems. *Health Affairs* 15(2):62–76.

Lubarsky DA (1995). Understanding cost analyses: Part 1. A Practitioner's guide to cost behavior. *Journal of Clinical Anesthesia* 7(6):519–521.

Meyer JW, Feingold MG (1995). Integrating financial modeling and patient care reengineering. *Healthcare Financial Management* 49(2):32–40.

Miller TR, Ryan JB (1995). Analyzing cost variance in capitated contracts. *Healthcare Financial Management* 49(2):22–23.

Moss MT (1996). Preparing nurse managers for a managed care future. *Nursing Economics* 14(2):132–133.

Mundinger MO (1996). New alliances: Nursing's bright future. *Nursing Administration Quarterly* 20(3):50–53.

Nauert RC (1996). The quest for value in health care. *Journal of Health Care Finance* 22(3):52–61.

Pierce SF, Luikart C (1996). Managed care: Will the health care needs of rural citizens be met? *Journal of Nursing Administration* 26(4):28–32.

Robbins W, Jacobs F (1985). Cost variances in health care: When should managers investigate? *Healthcare Financial Management* 39(9):36–42.

Rutledge RW, et al (1996). Cost containment strategies by private hospitals: Their effectiveness importance and use. *Journal of Health Care Finance* 22(3):1–14.

Singhvi S (1996). Using an affordability analysis to budget capital expenditures. *Healthcare Financial Management* 50(6):70–75.

Stahl DA (1996). The pulse of managed care in and beyond. *Nurse Manager* 27(4):16–17.

Stewart EE (1996). Managed care contracting issues in integrated delivery systems. *Journal of Health Care Finance* 22(3):75–83.

Tabbush V, Swanson G (1996). Changing paradigms in medical payment. *Archives of Internal Medicine* 156(4):357–360.

Talone P (1996). Ethics and managed care: Beyond helplessness. *Medical/Surgical Nursing* 5(3):212–214.

Waress BJ, Pasternak DP, Smith HL (1994). Determining costs associated with quality in health delivery. *Health Care Management Review* 19(3):52–53.

Welsh F (1995). Cost containment in emergency departments. *Healthcare Financial Management* 49(2):42–43.

White GM, Bennett T (1996). Using relative value units (RVUs) to develop your pricing schedule. *Missouri Medicine* 93(6):86–90.

6

Information Management in a Changing Nursing Environment

Christine R. Curran, MSN, RN, CNA, and Carole A. Gassert, PhD, RN

Christine R. Curran, MSN, RN, CNA, and Carole A. Gassert, PhD, RN

LEARNING OBJECTIVES

This chapter will enable the learner to:

1. Discuss the concepts of data, information, and knowledge.
2. Identify applications for individual-level and aggregate-level data.
3. Discuss the process of technology assessment in evaluating new information technology.
4. Identify the primary issues associated with emerging technology.
5. Identify appropriate technologies for the managed care environment.

INTRODUCTION

The ultimate goal of any science is knowledge. Knowledge, as an empowering concept, comes from processing data into information and information into knowledge. Nurses process and manage data, information, and knowledge to generate and support nursing decisions, develop new designs and techniques, and produce new knowledge (Graves et al, 1995). Thus, it is important to understand how nurses handle data, information, and knowledge.

Because of advanced and emerging technologies, the way in which nurses manage information and knowledge is changing. This chapter explores the concepts of data, information, and knowledge; infor-

mation and knowledge management for nurses; and the likely impact of emerging technologies in the changing health care environment.

GENERAL CONCEPTS OF INFORMATION MANAGEMENT

Collection and Documentation of Data, Information, and Knowledge

Data are discrete entities that describe objectively without interpretation. *Information* is data that are interpreted, organized, or structured. *Knowledge* is synthesized information in which interrelationships are identified and formalized (Blum, 1986, p. 35).

Data should be captured in elemental, precise forms. This type of data is called atomic-level data (Zielstorff et al, 1993). Atomic-level data are collected once and used many times (Fig. 6–1). They are stored and used for multiple purposes, some of which are not known at the time of data capture.

Data have attributes of value and type. For example, nursing data types are patient-, agency-, or domain-specific (Zielstorff et al, 1993). Information has attributes of accuracy, timeliness, and utility, such as relevance and quality. Taken together with accessibility, these attributes determine the value of information. Knowledge has the attributes of accuracy, utility, and type (Graves & Corcoran, 1989).

Data are used at both individual and aggregate levels. For example, the unit of analysis for the administrator is a patient population (*aggregate-level data*) defined by a system boundary, that is, a

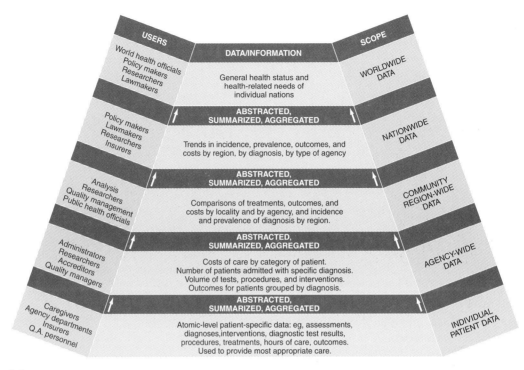

Figure 6–1. Uses of atomic-level patient data. (From Zielstorff RD, Hudgings CI, Grobe SJ [1993]. *Next-Generation Nursing Information Systems: Essential Characteristics for Professional Practice.* Washington, DC: American Nurses' Association.)

unit, division, or organization (Johnson et al, 1991), whereas clinicians tend to use more patient-specific data (*individual-level data*). Because data should be collected at the lowest possible level (atomic-level data) to serve multiple purposes, most data elements used by nurse leaders are collected on an individual basis and then aggregated.

The major source of individual clinical (patient) data in a health care agency is the medical record. Coding of the medical record provides many of the data fields for the institutional database and thus is a pivotal information source for any health care organization (Montrose and Marcoux, 1991). Because of this, nurse leaders should pay particular attention to nursing documentation and coding systems to ensure the capture of needed nursing clinical information.

The synthesis of nursing data and nursing knowledge is essentially missing from the current patient record. One cannot follow the evolution of a patient's condition across the duration of the nurse-patient relationship, condition resolution, or ex-

pected and achieved outcomes of care (short- and long-term) in any meaningful way.

There also is a need to capture the information exchanged by nurses at staff meetings, conferences, and change-of-shift report. Clinical decision-making, analysis of the decision task, and identification of supplemental information must be examined to build the knowledge base of nursing practice (Graves & Corcoran, 1988). Profession-specific knowledge is needed to form the core of the decision support systems for future nursing information systems (Turley, 1992).

Nurses have not agreed on standard terminology or a *uniform* language for documentation of nursing practice. The goal of one language for all nursing is not practical. A *unified* language, or one that is mapped to link the common meanings between terms, is more realistic. Since 1988, significant progress has been made in the development of the Unified Nursing Language System (UNLS) (McCormick, 1995).

To date, four nursing classification schemes have

been endorsed by the American Nurses' Association (ANA) Steering Committee on Databases to Support Clinical Nursing Practice for entry into the Unified Medical Language System (UMLS). These classification schemes will ultimately be separated from the UMLS to form the UNLS. They are the North American Nursing Diagnosis Association (NANDA); Omaha System: Applications for Community Health Nursing; Home Health Care Classification (HHCC); and Nursing Intervention Classification (NIC) (McCormick et al, 1994).

Nursing Informatics

The ANA designated nursing informatics as a nursing specialty in 1992. According to the ANA (1994, p. 3):

Nursing informatics is the specialty that integrates nursing science, computer science, and information science in identifying, collecting, processing, and managing data and information to support nursing practice, administration, education, research, and the expansion of nursing knowledge. The practice of nursing informatics includes the development and evaluation of applications, tools, processes, and structures which assist nurses with the management of data in taking care of patients or in supporting the practice of nursing.

Thus, nursing informatics is a practice discipline that focuses on the methods and technology of information management in nursing.

Graves and Corcoran (1989) proposed a conceptual framework for the study of nursing informatics that depicts the movement of data into information and information into knowledge. Graves (1990) subsequently enhanced this framework (Fig. 6–2) to include the purposes of management and processing of data, information, and knowledge (ie, to make or support nursing decisions, designs, and discoveries). The management of data, information, and knowledge is the functional ability to collect, aggregate, organize, move, and represent information in a way that is cost effective, efficient, and practical for the user. Management of data is the computer literacy component of the conceptual framework. The processing of data, information, and knowledge is the transformation from one form

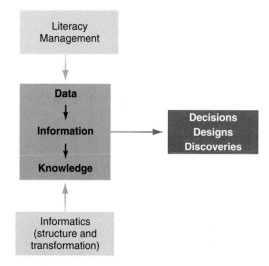

Figure 6–2. Conceptual framework for the study of nursing informatics. (From Graves JR, Amos LK, Heuther S, Lange LL, Thompson CB [1995]. Description of a graduate program in clinical nursing informatics. *Computers in Nursing* 13:61.)

or state to another, from data to information, from information to knowledge, or from knowledge to decisions, designs, or discoveries (Graves & Corcoran, 1989). Meaning is attached and value is added during processing. Processing of data is the informatics component of the conceptual framework.

Nursing informatics spans both direct and indirect health care practice arenas: clinical, education, research, and administrative settings. New roles are emerging for nurses with informatics expertise. Nurses are working as systems analysts, chief information officers, programmers, marketing representatives for computer software vendors, consultants in computer installations, and product managers, as well as continuing in the more traditional roles of nursing administrative systems coordinator or information systems specialist in health care agencies.

Nursing informatics is a branch of the health care informatics specialty. Health care information systems have shifted from a focus on financial systems to systems that include the management and coordination of health care. Integration of these systems will be paramount for maximum use of information. At the heart of this new perspective is the work under way to develop computer-based patient records. Portability of health care information across geographic areas and health care systems will be an ever-increasing pressure.

Regulatory Standards for Information Management

Health care is an information-intensive enterprise. The requirement for agencies to be producers of health care information is on the rise. According to Montrose and Marcoux (1991), this role is nearly equal in demand to the role of the agency as a provider of health care services. Federal, state, and independent regulatory bodies, such as the Joint Commission on Accreditation of Healthcare Organizations (JCAHO), as well as third-party payers, are requiring agencies to submit data elements, which, when analyzed, are believed to reflect the cost, quality, and outcomes of health care in that agency. Agencies are being compared to determine the "best" providers of care, and this information is being made available to the public.

Most nursing departments lack data structures and systems that allow for collection of data that are useful in the assessment of quality and cost of nursing care. Nurse leaders have a responsibility to ensure that cost-effective, quality patient care is being delivered by the nursing staff in their agency. Nursing databases that support decision-making for this purpose are needed.

The JCAHO added an information management section to accreditation requirements. The objectives of this addition are to assess for more timely and easy access to complete information throughout the organization, improve data accuracy, use aggregate data, have greater sharing of information, redesign information-related processes to improve efficiency, and demonstrate a balance between access and security of information (JCAHO, 1995, p. 53). Standards have a focus on key information processes and include information management planning (data integrity, security, confidentiality, uniform data definitions, staff education, and integration of systems), patient-specific data management (medical record minimum data set and patient outcome data), aggregate-level data management (data used to support managerial decision-making and research), knowledge-based information, and comparative data and information.

Table 6–1.
Elements of the Nursing Minimum Data Set

Nursing Care Elements
1. Nursing diagnosis
2. Nursing intervention
3. Nursing outcome
4. Intensity of nursing care

Patient Demographic Elements
5. Personal identification
6. Date of birth
7. Sex
8. Race and ethnicity
9. Residence

Service Elements
10. Unique facility or service agency number
11. Unique health record number of patient
12. Unique number of principal registered nurse provider
13. Episode admission or encounter date
14. Discharge or termination date
15. Disposition of patient
16. Expected payer for most of this bill

Data from Werley H, Lang N (eds). (1988). *Identification of the Nursing Minimum Data Set.* New York, NY: Springer Publishing Company.

Minimum Data Sets

Nursing Minimum Data Set

In 1977, the Nursing Information Systems Conference was held at the University of Illinois, Chicago, to foster the participation of nurses in information systems development and research. One of the subgroups at this meeting was charged with developing a basic nursing data set. The data set was developed and published (Werley & Grier, 1981) but remained dormant until a follow-up conference in May 1985 for the purpose of developing a nursing minimum data set (Werley, 1988).

The Nursing Minimum Data Set (NMDS) consists of 16 elements that are categorized into three broad groups: (1) nursing care, (2) patient demographics, and (3) service (Table 6–1). These categories were selected because they are used on a regular basis by the majority of nurses in any health care delivery setting. According to Leske and Werley (1992), the NMDS

■ Establishes comparability of nursing data across clinical populations, settings, geographic areas, and time.

■ Describes the nursing care of patients and their families in a variety of settings.

■ Demonstrates or projects trends regarding nursing care provided and allocation of nursing resources to individuals and populations according to their health problems or nursing diagnoses.

■ Stimulates nursing research using the NMDS elements alone or in integration with other systems.

■ Provides data about nursing care to influence and facilitate health policy decision-making.

Implementation of the NMDS has been hampered by the lack of a common language in nursing for nursing diagnosis, interventions, and outcomes.

Building on the NMDS, Huber and colleagues (1992) proposed a Nursing Management Minimum Data Set (NMMDS) that contains 18 proposed elements in this data set. Nine elements are collected at the unit level, and nine are collected at the institutional level. This data set is still under revision.

DeGroot and colleagues (1992) developed the Nursing Personnel Practice Data Set, which is designed to facilitate administrative decision-making related to differentiated pay and practice models. *Differentiated pay* is a system of compensation structured to pay professional salaries based on some combination of educational level, performance, position, shift, previous experience, and other select variables defined by the institution. A differentiated practice model is a system of health care delivery that delineates professional role responsibility according to credentials and skills such as educational level, type of licensure, certification, and competency. They proposed six elements: demographics, position, professional education, practice, recruitment and retention, and organizational training; some of these elements overlap with those of the NMMDS.

Other Clinical Minimum Data Sets

Several other clinical minimum data sets exist— Uniform Hospital Discharge Data Set, Uniform Ambulatory Medical Care Minimum Data Set, and Long Term Health Care Minimum Data Set (US Department of Health, Education, and Welfare, 1980a, 1980b, 1981). These sets contain 14, 18, and 24 items, respectively. Many of the items in one set are repeated in both of the other sets, validating the significance of the items. Examples of common data elements include personal identification, date of birth, sex, race, provider identification, diagnosis, disposition of the patient, and principal source of payment.

The Uniform Hospital Discharge Data Set was the first minimum data set developed; it has received the most extensive testing and revision (Pearce, 1988). Both the Medicare and Medicaid programs adopted its use in January 1975. This data set has undergone revisions since the initial implementation but continues to be a required data set for programs within the Department of Health and Human Services.

The Ambulatory Medical Care Minimum Data Set was designed to be patient specific and part of each patient's medical record. The Long Term Care Minimum Data Set has been criticized for its length, but its importance and utility have been recognized.

Taxonomies

Nursing Taxonomies

Classification systems are important because they provide an organization schema and consistent language that allow retrieval and use of data and information from automated information systems. Taxonomies are formalized structures constructed from classification systems that show interrelationships among the terms; they can be used to represent knowledge (Grobe, 1990).

Standardized vocabularies are necessary for communication among distributed information systems and to facilitate aggregate-level data analysis and outcomes research. Nurses have not agreed on standards for nursing language, particularly in the areas of nursing diagnosis, interventions, and outcomes. However, significant work in the area of nursing taxonomies is ongoing (Lang & Marek, 1990; Martin & Sheet, 1992; McCloskey & Bulechek, 1996;

Ozbolt et al, 1994; Saba, 1994; Warren & Hoskins, 1995).

Current nursing classification schemes include the NANDA, NIC, HHCC, Nursing Interventions Lexicon and Taxonomy, Omaha Community Health System, and Ozbolt's University Hospital Consortium Patient Care Taxonomy. Preliminary work is under way on a nursing outcomes classification (NOC) system by nurse researchers at the University of Iowa. Table 6–2 shows the components of each system related to diagnosis, intervention, and outcome content.

Issues that remain to be addressed regarding nursing vocabularies and classification systems include the "harmonization" of terms to form, via mapping, common terms; the need for protocols to set boundaries in the development of classification schemes (McCormick, 1995); and the need for frequent updating of these systems owing to their short half-life (Grobe, 1990). Systems to ensure data integrity, consistent processes for data collection and updating, and methods to prevent or capture missing data must also be in place before databases are used for decision-making.

Other Clinical Taxonomies

Other taxonomies in clinical use are the *International Classification of Diseases: Clinical Modification, Ninth Revision* (ICD-9-CM), Systematized Nomenclature of Medicine (SNOMED), and Physicians' Current Procedural Terminology (CPT) codes. The ICD-9-CM focuses on morbidity data for indexing medical records; there are more than 18,000 terms in this coding scheme.

The SNOMED taxonomy consists of terms used in veterinary and human medicine. Personnel in pathology departments in acute care settings are common users of this coding system. Henry and colleagues (1994) tested the feasibility of using SNOMED to represent nursing terms and identified matches for only two thirds of the terms used by nurses.

The CPT codes are a listing of procedures performed by physicians. Services are grouped into five categories: medicine, anesthesiology, surgery, radiology, and pathology and laboratory. CPT codes are used predominantly for billing purposes. Many of the procedures, however, are procedures performed by nurses but billed under physicians' names.

Conceptualizing Data for Individual Practice

Nurses excel at observation and data collection. Understanding how nurses structure clinical problems, determine relationships, and generate information is key (Curran, 1995). Experience plays a major role in one's ability to see relevance in data and information.

Butler (1994) proposed a model of human action (Fig. 6–3). At the center of his model is the two-way relationship between action and thought and the role of experiential knowledge and beliefs. For

Table 6–2.
Nursing Taxonomies by Categories of Diagnosis, Intervention, and Outcome

Taxonomy	Diagnosis	Intervention	Outcome
NANDA	×		
NIC		×	
NOC			×
Ozbolt's data set	×	×	×
Saba's HHCC	×	×	× (Discharge status in categories)
Omaha Community Health	×	×	× (Ratings)
Grobe's Nursing Intervention Lexicon		×	

Research Box 6–1
Taxonomies

Standardized vocabularies are required for communication between information systems. Nurses, however, tend to describe patient problems in terms of signs, symptoms, and medical diagnoses as well as nursing diagnoses. The Systematized Nomenclature of Medicine (SNOMED III), an existing vocabulary, includes North American Nursing Diagnosis Association (NANDA) diagnoses, nursing procedures, signs, symptoms, medical diagnoses, and pathology elements within its 11 modules. Because of this, a research study was conducted to determine whether the SNOMED III vocabulary could be used to represent terms used by nurses to record patient problems in the nursing care plan, progress note, and flowsheet (Henry et al, 1994).

Data were obtained from a total of 485 patient encounters for 201 hospitalized patients. Data were collected via interviews with the nurse caring for the patient, during intershift reporting, and through patient chart audit. A total of 4262 problems were recorded. Only data from written sources were used to test the portion of the study involving the ability of SNOMED to represent terms used by nurses to describe patient problems (1841 problems and 761 unique terms).

Overall, 69% of the terms used could be matched with those in SNOMED III; 44% were direct matches, and 25% required two or more terms to match. NANDA terms were used to describe patient problems 15% of the time in nurse interviews, 13% of the time in intershift reporting, 33% of the time in progress notes, and 35% of the time in nursing care plans.

Although it is clear that SNOMED III can be used to represent more nursing terms than NANDA alone, efforts are needed to establish a comprehensive vocabulary. This vocabulary should be interdisciplinary in nature, applicable for terms needed in the entire process of care and serve across the continuum of care. It is hoped the Unified Nursing Language System will serve this function.

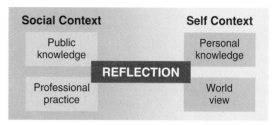

Figure 6–3. Butler's model of human action. (From Butler J [1994]. *Action to Thought: The Development of Self.* Presented at the Sixth International Conference on Thinking, Boston, MA.)

those familiar with only theoretical knowledge, what is known is limited to general principles; practice is necessary to understand the unique aspects of a situation or problem. Butler suggests that persons' actions are based on their values and beliefs and are constrained by what they experientially know. Reflection on experience, both during and after the event, allows a person to learn from that experience and is necessary to change a person's knowledge base. Reflection is an evaluative inner dialogue. External actions alone cannot bring about change in knowledge. Butler believes that more emphasis should be placed on the unexplored pathway from action to thought and less emphasis should be placed on the logical pathway of thought to action.

Tanner and colleagues (1993, p. 279) stated that "knowledge of particular patient populations is built up with many instances of knowing particular patients." Knowledge of a patient comes from an involved understanding of the patient's situation and responses to that situation. Knowledge of the patient is central to sound clinical judgment and clinical expertise.

Information has a fixed life span. As data change, information gleaned from them changes (Graves, 1993). Processing information is more complex than processing data because information has meaning attached to it. Information must be processed with this meaning intact (Graves & Corcoran, 1989). Knowledge is more stable. It is knowledge that nurses actively seek and use to deliver quality care to patients.

In this era of information overload, databases are an essential foundation for knowledge development. Nurses require data and information about specific patients under their care as well as information about their practice of nursing to reflect on practice and generate knowledge. Databases can be stored, and large quantities of data manipulated. Queries of and reports from these databases can assist nurses in developing a better understanding of the information that is available.

Most clinical information systems have not been developed from a nursing perspective. Nurses want information for the planning and delivery of care that includes alerts and reminders; the ability to review patient data by nursing diagnosis, interventions, and outcomes; and the ability for the patient and nurse to receive a schedule of activities for the day. This information is not routinely available in most systems.

Conceptualizing Data in Aggregates

Nurses generally speak about individual patient data. To what degree nurses think about or use aggregate as well as individual data to develop knowledge of nursing practice is unclear. Questions such as the number of patients seen in practice in the past year or morbidity or mortality rates of practice remain unexamined. Only when data are accumulated over time will data be available to aggregate.

Nurse leaders can help develop an aggregate level of thinking by presenting the individual nurse with reports of summary data of patients under their care for a selected period of time. Data could be listed by individual patient and include demographic information such as age, sex, and race; diagnosis; cost of care; length of stay; complications such as medicine errors and falls; and physician name. Then, reports on the basis of diagnosis, cost of care, or other summary points could be reported.

Databases for clinicians should track patients by problem, intervention, and outcome. Once sufficient patients with common medical or nursing diagnoses are entered, data could be searched for patterns such as which interventions seem to contribute to the best outcomes for patients with a particular problem.

Nurse leaders and advanced practice nurses routinely need aggregate-level data to function effectively. Population-based thinking is necessary to identify trends in patient outcomes, set or modify standards of practice, analyze safety issues, review quality and risk assessment data (eg, medication errors), and meet the health care needs of communities. Health policy decisions require data that are analyzed at the aggregate level.

Clinical and administrative databases must be integrated so nurse leaders can use both clinical and administrative data for strategic planning, decision-making, and quality monitoring. For example, data could be used to support staffing requirements for the level of patient acuity that exists, justify nursing positions based on clinical care needs, or study the effect of skill level on patient outcomes. Documented evidence of the impact of registered nurses on cost-effective patient care does not exist in sufficient quantity for the value of nursing to be irrefutable, although modest numbers of data do exist (Prescott, 1993). Linking databases will assist in the development of an information infrastructure for the organization that ultimately allows for linkages between management outcomes and clinical outcomes (Huber et al, 1992) and linkages necessary to retrieve information about the cost, quality, and outcomes of care.

EMERGING TECHNOLOGIES

Emerging technologies can be used to provide linkages, specifically information technologies used for information handling. *Information technology* is a collective term used to describe computer technologies that facilitate information handling. Information-handling activities include collecting, organizing, processing, analyzing, storing, retrieving, or managing data and information needed by nurses (ANA, 1994) in providing care to individual or groups of patients or in making decisions about care-delivery systems with aggregated patient data. Information technology may include large computer systems that are tied together or networked, portable hand-held devices that can be used by health care providers or patients to record vital data or access information, the Internet and World Wide Web, or more conventional devices such as automated telephone systems.

Technology Assessment

There has been an unprecedented increase in the development and use of technology in health care in the past two decades. Health care technology has been defined by the US Office of Technology Assessment as the techniques, drugs, equipment, and procedures used by health care providers in the delivery of care to patients. It has been further divided into physical and social components. Examples of physical components are thermometers, intra-aortic balloon pumps, medications, and computers. Methods and procedures such as protocols of care exemplify the social components of health care technology (McConnell, 1992).

New technologies have had a positive impact on patients' lives by extending life for those facing end-stage renal disease and cardiomyopathies, eradicating communicable illnesses such as polio and smallpox, and providing more independent living to those coping with severe spinal cord injuries. However, other technologies, such as intrauterine devices, have actually inflicted illness.

Current and future engineering knowledge undoubtedly will allow newer and even more sophisticated technologies to be introduced into the health care arena. Legislative initiatives have attempted to protect consumers from the adverse effects of new technologies but usually are developed after patients have been harmed. A more proactive response is for health care providers to use appropriate assessment techniques to evaluate new technologies. Pillar and colleagues (1990) proposed the use of technology assessment as a research framework that can evaluate a technology in terms of safety, efficacy, cost, benefit, and social impact. The *safety* of a technology is described as its risk-to-benefit ratio, whereas *efficacy* is the probability that individuals will receive benefit from that technology. Cost-to-benefit analysis measures in monetary terms both the benefits and consequences of the use of a technology. In situations in which dollar amounts cannot be assigned, a cost-effectiveness analysis can determine how beneficial a technology would be in terms of a health-related outcome for patients, such as perceived wellness or increased life span. The social impact involves the legal, ethical, and political issues that are introduced with a specific technology.

Happ (1996) expanded the technology assessment framework and applied it to information technology. This author represents technology assessment as the interaction of the cost, efficacy, safety, and social impact of various information technologies. The process of technology assessment is characterized as (1) identification of the technology and the environment needing to be studied, (2) testing through analysis and scientific inquiry, (3) synthesis of information to make informed recommendations about a technology, and (4) dissemination of findings. The final step in the technology assessment process is the establishment of policy regarding the use of a particular technology. As an example, Happ's model could be used to evaluate use of a portable, wireless hand-held device versus traditional computer terminals for recording a patient's vital data in a satellite clinic within a health care enterprise. The model reminds us to consider ethical issues such as privacy, confidentiality, and security of data; availability and cost of wireless transmission modalities; and potential impact of each technology on the workflow of practitioners delivering care in the clinic. Adequate technology assessment should eliminate the purchase of information technology that cannot perform as needed or add value in processing information within an organization.

Examples of Emerging Technologies in Information Management

In the past, health care organizations have focused on the acquisition of information systems. Earlier systems focused solely on the financial side of health care by providing admission, discharge, transfer, and cost capture functions. Later, systems added patient care documentation functions. The current focus is on using information collected by those systems to gain a competitive advantage. Information systems have been influenced by the need for improved decision support for clinicians, improved patient care capabilities, improved production and cost reduction, improved ambulatory or outpatient capabilities, integration of databases, and the use of local area networks (Zinn et al, 1994).

Future successes will depend on the ability of organizations to effectively use available information in a managed care environment to determine quality and outcome measures. Emerging information technology must therefore allow the (1) linkage of several different health care systems, computer-based patient records, (2) integration for enterprise-wide computing, and (3) quality improvement (Zinn et al, 1994). Emerging information technologies to be discussed in this chapter are networks, smart cards, virtual environments, the Internet, and decision support.

All of these information technologies presuppose the use of computerized patient records and point-of-care technology. Organizations that have not yet computerized information processing, including patient records, are in great danger. Changes in health care demand that prudent decisions be made and that these decisions be based on current, reliable, valid, and accurate data. If data are to meet these criteria, they must be recorded electronically at the point of origin, whether at the clinic, bedside, home, operating room, or central administrative office. In this emerging health care environment, computerized patient records and point-of-care technologies should be viewed as a routine part and cost of doing business.

Networks

As discussed repeatedly, health care organizations are moving beyond traditional hospital systems to link with health care providers throughout the community. In keeping with an expanded health care environment, the concept of enterprise systems has emerged as the next generation of information systems. Enterprise systems provide information gateways that allow dissimilar units within a health care system to connect and access information regardless of the point of patient encounter. Enterprise systems are also called community health information networks (CHINs), regional health information networks (RHINs), or health information networks (HINs), depending on the scope of the connection (Ball, 1995).

The most common term used to describe organization wide networks is CHINs. This system allows electronic exchange of both clinical and financial information by constituent members. Members may include hospitals, laboratories, care providers, employers, pharmacies, payers, nursing homes, home health agencies, imaging centers, researchers, and insurers (Bergman, 1994). Due to organizational structure, all need to share information and can do so if their computers are networked together. Underlying successful networks is the infrastructural problem of connectivity and integration or the ability to pull information together into what is called a clinical data repository (CDR). Golob (1994) describes a CDR as an "information warehouse" used to merge and store the administrative and clinical data of an organization in a common database. As a relational database, the CDR receives data from different vendor applications through a feeder that formats incoming data to match the database. Data are then independent of particular vendors, allowing different information technology tools such as report writers, graphics packages, and statistical analysis packages to access information.

Until universal standards for electronically handling data are adopted, disparate systems will need interfaces or gateways to transmit data from place to place and system to system. Standards groups are working to adopt electronic data interchange standards (EDIs). Ideally, the technology industry will support merging syntax into one overall set of standards, moving information systems to a "plug-and-play" concept similar to what exists for the telephone system. Once this is accomplished, issues of connectivity will be insignificant, and purchase decisions can be based on vendor attributes of service, cost, reliability, and creativity.

Other issues of CHINs that have surfaced are ownership and privacy, confidentiality, and security (Ball, 1995; Bergman, 1994). Discussion also has begun about whether cultural barriers can be overcome, allowing long-standing health care competitors to collaborate and share data. There is concern that different levels of CDRs will be developed to protect the competitive advantage of certain data (Appleby, 1995). In general, benefits of having data available in a CDR outweigh the skepticism that is identified; benefits include reduction in transcription errors, decrease in cost through elimination of duplication, facilitation of communicable disease reporting, determination of effectiveness of treatment (Bergman, 1994), and increased access to patient data.

Smart Cards

Smart card technology (SCT), alternately called health card technology, is gaining visibility in the United States and may assume a greater role in the changing health care environment, particularly within CHINs. Introduced in France in the 1970s, SCT involves the use of a plastic card the size of a credit card containing an imbedded microprocessor chip with sufficient memory to store and process information (Quick, 1994). In addition to the card, a SCT system requires a reading and writing device to decipher stored information and update the card, as well as a computer terminal that accesses a host computer (Alpert, 1993).

Early discussion of SCT predicted that the cards would contain a patient's medical record, allowing access to information for an increasingly mobile population (Brennan, 1987). Informaticians in France, Sweden, and Germany used SCTs as professional health cards to protect the privacy, confidentiality, and security of patient data (Allaert & Dusserre, 1994; Klein, 1994; Kühnel et al, 1994). Used in this manner, the cards add a significant and needed layer of security to information systems. The cards must contain technical features to permit authentication of the card, identification of the user as legitimate holder, access to programs as qualified, integrity of the electronic signature, association of reading or writing privileges with an electronic signature, and knowledge of holder's right to access, read, write, or update information contained in the patient files.

In the United States, the Workgroup on Electronic Data Interchange (1993) recommended that because of the cost of producing and replacing smart cards and the current lack of standards for data, simple transaction-type cards should be given to patients to identify basic information, such as name, address, contact person, and insurer). This type of card could also be used to access the patient's complete medical record stored on a CDR (Alpert, 1993). Quick (1994) used the more sophisticated smart cards in Oklahoma City for emergency health care services and record keeping. The patient's database contains information about personal choices for care, allergies, diagnoses, emergency contact, physicians, procedures, medications, and insurance. The system described is vendor specific, however, and it is not known whether information could be shared within a networked environment of disparate systems.

There are significant issues associated with SCT. As discussed with CHINs, one of the problems is integration of SCT information with other parts of the medical record. Unless information on the smart card reflects the latest encounter, decisions about care could be based on outdated or incomplete data. Critics have advocated that in essence, multi-

ple medical records would exist rather than one integrated patient record. A second issue is loss, theft, or refusal to carry cards. The population most at risk for health problems, the homeless and poor, may not be willing or able to keep up with their smart cards. An alternate means of accessing records would have to serve as back-up for SCT. A third, and probably the most controversial, issue surrounding the use of SCT and all emerging technologies is patient privacy. Most states have no laws protecting patients from unauthorized disclosure of medical information (Alderman & Kennedy, 1995; Alpert, 1993). Unless provisions are made allowing patients to limit access to sensitive medical information, SCT could facilitate access to all medical information collected and increase instances of disclosure of sensitive information. Data stored in CDRs would increasingly be available for purposes other than originally intended and without patient knowledge. Informatics organizations are working for the passage of federal legislation that would protect patient privacy.

Virtual Environments

One of the most exciting areas of development in information technology is that of producing virtual environments through virtual reality simulations and telehealth through the use of augmented reality. By definition, virtual reality attempts to eliminate obvious boundaries between the user and computer (Curran and Hales, 1995). The user is placed *within* the computer environment through a three-dimensional presentation of information that combines primarily vision, hearing, and touch (Peterson, 1992). Using special glasses and gloves, users enter the environment to manipulate the molecular structure of cancer drugs, practice surgical technique on a virtual patient, or learn to perform an invasive procedure. Virtual reality applications are found predominantly in virtual reality laboratories because of equipment costs, programming difficulties, and limited numbers of individuals able to provide technological support. Undoubtedly, health care will recognize the value of virtual reality as an information technology as it becomes more visible through the entertainment industry.

The potential uses of virtual reality simulations in nursing are endless. Physical diagnosis techniques and patient care skills could be taught using virtual reality. The addition of the sense of touch to interactive computer simulations that use audio and visual presentations would enable student and graduate nurses to practice skills to improve clinical competency. The only available nursing virtual reality program is a venipuncture program being developed by Hightechsplanations, a virtual reality development vendor. Additional virtual reality programs are planned (M. McGurn, personal communication, July 1995).

The Internet

Increased use of virtual reality in health care may also result from the phenomenal and almost manic interest in the use of cyberspace by both health care providers and the population at large. Rheingold (1993) defined cyberspace as the conceptual space in which words, relationships, and data are exchanged by people using computer-mediated communications; because cyberspace is only a conceptual space mediated by a computer interface, it is a virtual environment. Eight basic features are available through the Internet (Kuster & Kuster, 1995). Electronic mail (e-mail) transfers messages between computers that have e-mail addresses, allowing users to keep in touch with family and friends, collaborate with experts, and conduct business. Mailings lists, a second feature, include listservs and e-journals and provide forums for discussing or distributing information about specific topics. Information posted on this medium is automatically distributed to all subscribers. Usenet or newsgroups, a third Internet feature, differ from listservs by providing access only when users desire to browse messages on a host computer.

Gophers, a fourth service on the Internet, provides access to information available on computers around the world. A series of layered menus provide selections for users. File transfer protocol enables users to access and retrieve files of text, programs, and pictures. Telnet allows users to connect to another computer and operate it from his or her own keyboard. This service increases access to features not available on the user's machine. Wide area information servers (WAIS) connect with very large databases and facilitate searches using natural language queries. The final service currently available on the Internet is the World Wide Web (WWW), which uses hypertext links to access text and graphics resources throughout the world. Instead of using layered menus, WWW links to another document when key words are selected, or "clicked."

Telehealth

Expanded use of Internet services have been reported under a phenomenon known as telehealth or telemedicine. By broadest definition, telehealth is the "combined application of computer and telecommunications technologies to health care" (Brauer, 1992, p. 151) The purpose of *telehealth* is to improve the diagnosis and treatment of patients in rural and other underserved areas and to increase the attractiveness of rural areas for qualified health professionals. Brennan (1993) and Skiba and Mirque (1994) reported use of the Internet to support caregivers and patients in Ohio and Colorado. Users received information and support that reduced readmission rates for chronically ill patients. *Telemedicine* is a more restricted term that denotes "direct patient care–oriented clinical diagnostic and therapeutic activities" (Brauer, 1992, p. 152). The term *telehealth* better serves the entire health care community of providers and can include a concept Brauer calls *tele-education*, which involves services that are provider-oriented and accommodate information access and linkage with other providers. Tele-education activities include mediated continuing education, teleconferencing, and on-line consultation.

Telehealth projects have been developing for 35 years and exist in more than 40 states. The literature includes examples in which psychiatric consultation, telefluoroscopic examinations, pediatric image transmission, over-the-telephone defibrillation, and rural health diagnostic and follow-up work have been accomplished through telehealth technologies. As newer technologies are combined with existing services, the potential uses of telehealth become unlimited. One addition to Internet linkage could be augmented reality. With this technology, the user continues to interact with external reality but elicits help from a virtual reality device such as a headset or glove (Turley, 1995). Centers have reported projects to develop a glove that would allow physicians or nurse practitioners through augmented re-

Research Box 6–2

Telehealth: Computerized Telephone Interview

Computer-mediated communication is one telehealth application. Employees at Cleveland State University were randomly selected to use AVIVA, a computerized telephone interview for assessment of and advising participants about their health risks (Alemi & Higley, 1995). The program was developed by a panel of researchers active in preventive health care. Of the 96 faculty and staff chosen for the experimental group, 71% used it. Subjects called a computer and listened to prerecorded health risk questions. They answered by pressing appropriate keys on their touch-tone telephones. Certain answers activated advice being given or referral to other resources of information, such as risk-reduction programs. Because no identifying information was collected from the users, their confidentiality was maintained.

Statistical analysis showed that AVIVA was considered to be more accurate, easier to understand, more convenient, more affordable, more accessible, and easier to use than other currently available sources of health education. Despite their acceptance of the technology, employees generally were uninterested in changing health behaviors even when risks were identified. Researchers concluded that computerized telephone interviews concerning health risk are technologically viable but that the system alone was insufficient to change the health behavior of participants.

Acceptance of the technology itself has implications for nurses who are charged with reducing health risk factors among their population, but it will need to be combined with other treatment modalities to affect changes in health behavior.

of individual provider practices. With the use by practitioners of virtual offices, resistance to these newer technologies may be reduced by the time that is saved, the increased numbers of patients who are seen, and the ability to retain patients in their rural hospital settings. Legal issues such as licensing across state lines and malpractice responsibility in cases of telehealth have not yet been addressed. The federal government will not reimburse for telemedicine consultations. If such projects are to succeed, studies will need to be done to determine the cost-effectiveness of telehealth. In theory, problems of social isolation should decrease for physicians, but how patients will react to telehealth intervention is yet to be determined. Studies in which the impact of telehealth is examined must consider patient reaction to the technology.

Decision Support Systems

By definition, decision support systems combine information technology with decision-making algorithms to improve the decision-making ability of users (Brennan & Casper, 1995). Components of such a system are the dialog or user interface, database, and model base (Jacobs & Pelfrey, 1995). The interface allows a decision-maker to interact with the system and includes decision-maker and computer language and output display. In general, decision support systems prompt users for specific information required to activate its rules. The database must contain information needed to support decisions. The system combines information obtained from the user and database to activate its analytical models. By using analytical or mathematical models, the decision support system has the ability to analyze information that is received; however, the decision support system will be accurate only if the database is correct and contains up-to-date information and the models have been correctly constructed.

A new category of decision support systems is being increasingly used for making decisions in group settings. Group decision support systems facilitate the group process (Brennan & Casper, 1995). As an additional benefit, group members can be located in different settings and geographical areas and linked together through networks.

ality to palpate patients' abdomen to verify physical findings necessary to make a diagnoses.

A lack of standards, integration, and security issues holds true for telehealth projects. Additional issues of telehealth include resistance, cost effectiveness, reimbursement, malpractice liability, professional isolation, social impact, and time savings (Kane et al, 1995; Nagy, 1994). Economics may force practitioners to use information technology despite resistance to innovation, especially with the development of large enterprises and the demise

Research Box 6–3
Computer Network Support

The effect was evaluated by ComputerLink, a network system designed to support home caregivers of patients with Alzheimer's disease (AD), on confidence in decision-making, decision-making skills or ability to identify alternatives, and social isolation (Brennan et al, 1995). The system was accessed by using a computer, modem, and telephone lines. Subjects who had primary responsibility as a family caregiver for a person with AD, a local telephone exchange, and the ability to read and write English were randomly assigned to a control or ComputerLink group. The system provided information, decision support, and communication. An electronic encyclopedia contained information designed to enhance self-care and understanding of AD. The decision support was accomplished by using questions to prompt caregivers trying to make decisions. Communication included private mail, a public bulletin board, and an anonymous question-and-answer section. System users could communicate with other AD caregivers or healthcare professionals.

During the study period, caregivers generally used ComputerLink twice a week for an average of 13 minutes per session. The most significant finding is that AD caregivers who had access to ComputerLink experienced more confidence in their decisions even though their decision-making skills did not significantly improve. Despite access to ComputerLink on a 24-hour-a-day basis, AD caregivers continued to perceive themselves as experiencing social isolation. In focus groups, AD caregivers identified the ability to communicate with peers and professionals at times convenient for them, feelings of companionship, and sharing of information as benefits of the use of ComputerLink.

As the intensity of care required by patients in the home increases, it is important to explore ways technology can be used to help caregivers.

SUMMARY

Many new information technologies will have an impact on organizations and their information management. The cornerstone of each of these technologies is a system of linked information technologies. When systems within and across sites are integrated and data can easily be analyzed at both individual and aggregate levels, information and knowledge will undergo even more profound growth. To survive in the current managed care environment, nursing leaders and registered nurses must be familiar with the mechanisms to access, manage, and appropriately use a variety of information technologies.

■ DISCUSSION QUESTIONS ■

1. What nursing taxonomies are endorsed by the American Nurses' Association ?
2. What are the purposes of the minimum data set? Does the minimum data set address the needs of nurses working in managed care organizations?
3. What are some potential nursing applications for virtual reality?
4. What are the pros and cons of smart cards?

■ LEARNING ACTIVITIES ■

1. Search the Internet on the subject "Telemedicine." Note the types of "hits."
2. Visit the virtual hospital on the World Wide Web. Note the URL and create a bookmark for this site.
3. Write a clinical narrative about your practice that depicts a situation in which you learned something from the event. Reflect on how you would do things differently at this point in your practice.

■ BIBLIOGRAPHY ■

Alderman E, Kennedy C (1995). *The Right to Privacy.* New York, NY: Alfred A. Knopf.

Alemi F, Higley P (1995). Reaction to "talking" computers assessing health risks. *Medical Care* 33:227–233.

Allaert FA, Dusserre L (1994). Security of health information systems in France: What we do will no longer be different from what we tell. *International Journal of Bio-Medical Computing* 35(suppl 1):201–204.

Alpert S (1993). Smart cards, smarter policy: Medical records privacy and health care reform. *Hastings Center Report* 23:13–23.

American Nurses' Association (1994). *Scope of Practice for Nurs-*

ing Informatics. Washington, DC: American Nurses' Publishing.

Appleby C (1995). The trouble with CHINs. *Hospitals & Health Networks* 5:42–44.

Ball MJ (1995). Enterprise systems. *International Journal of Bio-Medical Computing* 39:113–118.

Bergman R (1994). Data détente. *Hospitals & Health Networks* 20:46–48.

Blum BL (ed) (1986). *Clinical Information Systems*. New York, NY: Springer-Verlag.

Brauer GW (1992). Telehealth: The delayed revolution in health care. *Medical Progress through Technology* 18:51–163.

Brennan PF (1987). Smart cards & networks: Promote access to information. *Today's OR Nurse* 9:23–27.

Brennan PF (1993). Differential use of computer network services. *In* Safran C (ed). *Seventh Annual Symposium on Computer Applications in Medical Care*. New York, NY: McGraw-Hill, pp 27–31.

Brennan PF, Casper GR (1995). *In* Ball MJ, Hannah KJ, Newbold SK, Douglas JV (eds). *Nursing Informatics: Where Caring and Technology Meet*, 2nd ed. New York, NY: Springer-Verlag, pp 287–294.

Brennan PF, Moore SM, Smyth KA (1995). The effects of a special computer network on caregivers of persons with Alzheimer's disease. *Nursing Research* 44:166–172.

Butler J (1994). *Action to thought: The development of self*. Presented at the Sixth International Conference on Thinking, Boston, MA.

Curran CR (1995). Data-driven practice: The need for clinical databases. *Clinical Nurse Specialist* 9:168.

Curran C, Hales G (1995). Virtual reality. *In* Ball MJ, Hannah KJ, Newbold SK, Douglas JV (eds). *Nursing Informatics: Where Caring and Technology Meet*, 2nd ed. New York, NY: Springer-Verlag, pp 310–319.

DeGroot HA, Forsey L, Cleland VS (1992). The Nursing Practice Personnel Data Set: Implications for professional practice systems. *Journal of Nursing Administration* 22:23–28.

Golob R (1994). Securing a bridge to the CPR: Clinical data repositories. *Health Care Informatics* February:50, 52, 54, 56, 58.

Graves J (1993). Data versus information versus knowledge. *Reflections* 19:4–5.

Graves JR (1990). *Nursing Informatics and the Future*. Keynote address for the Southern Regional Educational Board Conference, Atlanta, GA.

Graves JR, Corcoran S (1988). Identification of data element categories for clinical nursing information system via information analysis of nursing practice. *In* Greenes RA (ed). *Proceedings: Twelfth Annual Symposium on Computer Applications in Medical Care*. Los Angeles, CA: IEEE Computer Society Press, pp 358–363.

Graves JR, Corcoran S (1989). The study of nursing informatics. *Image: Journal of Nursing Scholarship* 21:227–231.

Graves JR, Amos LK, Heuther S, Lange LL, Thompson CB

(1995). Description of a graduate program in clinical nursing informatics. *Computers in Nursing* 13:60–70.

Grobe SJ (1990). Nursing intervention lexicon and taxonomy study: Language and classification methods. *Advances in Nursing Science* 13:23–33.

Happ B (1996). Applying technology assessment to information systems. *In* Mills ME, Romano CA, Heller BR (eds). *Information Management in Nursing and Health Care*. Springhouse, PA: Springhouse Corporation, pp 74–82.

Henry SB, Holzemer WL, Reilly CA, Campbell KE (1994). Terms used by nurses to describe patient problems: Can SNOMED III represent nursing concepts in the patient record? *Journal of the American Medical Informatics Association* 1:61–74.

Huber DG, Delaney C, Crossley J, Mehmert M, Ellerbe S (1992). A nursing management minimum data set: Significance and development. *Journal of Nursing Administration* 22:35–40.

Jacobs SM, Pelfrey S (1995). Decision support systems: Using computers to help manage. *Journal of Nursing Administration* 25:46–51.

Joint Commission on Accreditation of Health Care Organizations (1995). *Accreditation Manual for Hospitals. Volume I: Standards*. Oakbrook Terrace, IL: JCAHO Publications.

Johnson M, Gardner D, Kelly K, Maas M, McCloskey JC (1991). The Iowa Model: A proposed model for nursing administration. *Nursing Economics* 9:255–262.

Kane J, Morken J, Boulger J, Crouse B, Bergeron D (1995). Rural Minnesota family physicians' attitudes toward telemedicine. *Minnesota Medicine* 78:19–23.

Klein GO (1994). Smart cards: A security tool for health information systems. *International Journal of Bio-Medical Computing* 35(suppl 1):147–151.

Kühnel E, Klepser G, Engelbrecht R (1994). Smart cards and their opportunities for controlling health information systems. *International Journal of Bio-Medical Computing* 35(suppl 1):153–157.

Kuster JM, Kuster TA (1995). Finding treasures on the Internet. *ASHA* February:43–47.

Lang NM, Marek KD (1990). The classification of patient outcomes. *Journal of Professional Nursing* 6:158–163.

Leske JS, Werley HH (1992). Use of the nursing minimum data set. *Computers in Nursing* 10:259–263.

Martin KS, Sheet NJ (1992). *The Omaha System: Applications for Community Health Nursing*. Philadelphia, PA: WB Saunders.

McCloskey JC, Bulechek GM (eds) (1996). *Nursing Interventions Classification (NIC)*, 2nd ed. St. Louis, MO: Mosby.

McConnell EA (1992). Technology assessment: The road to appropriate equipment and care. *Nursing Management* 23:64A, 64B, 64F, 64H.

McCormick KA (1995). An update on nursing's unified language system. *In* Ball MJ, Hannah KJ, Newbold SK, Douglas JV (eds). *Nursing Informatics: Where Caring and Technology Meet*, 2nd ed. New York, NY: Springer-Verlag.

McCormick KA, Lang N, Zielstorff R, Milholland K, Saba V, Jacox A (1994). Toward standard classification schemes for nursing language: Recommendations of the American Nurses' Association Steering Committee on Databases to Support Clinical Nursing Practice. *JAMIA: The Practice of Informatics* 1:421–427.

Montrose G, Marcoux KA (1991). Management by information: A new imperative. *Computers in Health care* 13:49–54.

Nagy K (1994). Telemedicine: Creeping into use despite obstacles. *Journal of the National Cancer Institute* 86:1576–1578.

Ozbolt JG, Fruchtnight JN, Hayden JR (1994). Toward data standards for clinical nursing information. *Journal of the American Medical Informatics Association* 1:175–185.

Pearce ND (1988). Uniform minimum health data sets: Concept development testing recognition for federal health use and current status. *In* Werley H, Lang N (eds). *Identification of the Nursing Minimum Data Set.* New York, NY: Springer Publishing Company.

Peterson I (1992). Looking-glass worlds. *Science News* 143:8–15.

Pillar B, Jacox AK, Redman BK (1990). Technology: Its assessment and nursing. *Nursing Outlook* 38:16–19.

Prescott PA (1993). Nursing: An important component of hospital survival under a reformed health care system. *Nursing Economics* 11:192–199.

Quick G (1994). Introduction to smart card technology and initial medical application. *Journal of the Oklahoma Medical Association* 87:454–457.

Rheingold H (1993). *The Virtual Community.* New York, NY: Addison-Wesley.

Saba VK (1994). *Home health care classification (HHCC) of nursing diagnosis and interventions.* Washington, DC: Georgetown University School of Nursing.

Skiba DJ, Mirque DT (1994). The electronic community: An alternative health care approach. *In* Grobe SJ, Pluyter-Wenting ESP (eds). *Nursing Informatics: An International Overview for Nursing in a Technological Era.* New York, NY: Elsevier, pp 388–392.

Tanner CA, Benner P, Chesla C, Gordon DR (1993). The phenomenology of knowing the patient. *Image: Journal of Nursing Scholarship* 25:273–280.

Turley JP (1992). A framework for the transition from nursing records to a nursing information system. *Nursing Outlook* 40:177–181.

Turley JP (1995). Nursing's future: Ubiquitous computing virtual reality and augmented reality. *In* Ball MJ, Hannah KJ, Newbold SK, Douglas JV (eds). *Nursing Informatics: Where Caring and Technology Meet,* 2nd ed. New York, NY: Springer-Verlag, pp 320–330.

US Department of Health, Education, and Welfare (1980a). *Long Term Health Care: Minimum Data Set.* Hyattsville, MD: National Center for Health Statistics, DHEW publication No. PHS 80-1158.

US Department of Health, Education, and Welfare (1980b). *Uniform Hospital Discharge Data: Minimum Data Set.* Hyattsville, MD: National Center for Health Statistics, DHEW publication No. PHS 80-1157.

US Department of Health, Education, and Welfare (1981). *Uniform Ambulatory Medical Care: Minimum Data Set.* Hyattsville, MD: National Center for Health Statistics, DHEW publication No. PHS 81-1161.

Warren JJ, Hoskins LM (1995). NANDA's nursing diagnosis taxonomy: A nursing database. *In* American Nurses' Association. *Nursing Data Systems: The Emerging Framework.* Washington, DC: American Nurses' Publishing.

Werley HH (1988). Introduction to the nursing minimum data set and its development. *In* Werley H, Lang N (eds). *Identification of the Nursing Minimum Data Set.* New York, NY: Springer Publishing Company.

Werley H, Grier M (1981). *Nursing Information Systems.*

Werley H, Lang N (eds) (1988). *Identification of the Nursing Minimum Data Set.* New York, NY: Springer Publishing Company.

Workgroup on Electronic Data Interchange (1993). *WEDI Report 1993.*

Zielstorff RD, Hudgings CI, Grobe SJ (1993). *Next-Generation Nursing Information Systems: Essential Characteristics for Professional Practice.* Washington, DC: American Nurses' Association.

Zinn TK, Bria W, Mowry M (1994). Emerging technologies: Riding the wave avoiding the undertow. *1994 HIMSS Proceedings: Vol. 4,* pp 125–136.

Critical Concepts in Contemporary Nursing Leadership

7

Motivation and Motivational Leadership

Mary Etta C. Mills, ScD, RN, CNAA

LEARNING OBJECTIVES

This chapter will enable the learner to:

1. Distinguish between types of motivation as a determinate of specific individual actions.
2. Identify key qualities of the motivational leader.
3. Use theories of motivation to assess the work environment, evaluate the needs of individuals participating as team members, and establish effective motivational conditions for high work performance.
4. Examine means by which a leader can build a self-motivating environment.

> A man always has two reasons for doing anything—a good reason and the real reason.
>
> *J. P. Morgan*

INTRODUCTION

The ability to lead depends heavily on understanding what will move people to perform. A true leader is someone who is self-motivated to achieve and able to energize others to achieve.

Clinical leadership offers many challenges; one is to recognize the effect of personal and professional needs on the motivation of staff to tackle tough jobs and reach outcomes important to the organization. Such recognition fosters empowerment through approval, satisfaction, accomplishment, and self-esteem, which fuel individual motivation. For example, nurses who make themselves available for unscheduled shift coverage or volunteer to provide home care for their acute care patients may be doing so for many reasons. Responsibility to patients, reciprocal coverage for other staff, the ability to earn extra money, or fear of a poor evaluation may be factors in the decision. In these examples, each motive, although different, may lead to the same behavior.

THE ART OF LEADERSHIP

The art of leadership includes the ability to understand what drives individuals to take specific actions and to create opportunities for them to meet personal and organizational needs at the same time.

Motivational leadership can occur at any level of the organization. A beginning clinical nurse may exhibit as much or more leadership than formal leaders in his or her ability to move others to take action. Unlike the formal authority that comes with line positions, power to influence rests within individuals, exclusive of their positions.

MOTIVATION: WHAT IT IS AND WHAT IT IS NOT

Motivation implies action and energy. The root of the word *motivation* is *motive*, which in turn comes from the Latin word that means *to move*. Regardless of the reason—fear, money, accomplishment—if individuals are trying to perform, they are motivated. In the absence of action, individuals are not considered to be motivated even if they express desire, interest, attitude, or morale. The fact is that wanting to do something does not always result in moving to do so.

Motivation may be protection- or achievement-oriented. Employees who perform just well enough to keep out of trouble, to protect job security and salary, or to protect gains made by short-lived performance efforts are protectively motivated. These individuals generally are evaluated as meeting only minimal levels of safe performance. Achievement-motivated individuals, on the other hand, make an effort to produce at a high level over extended periods of time.

Because motivation comes from within, it is important to realize that although leaders can create conditions that favor high employee performance, they cannot ensure that others will respond in the desired manner. In other words, the adage, "You can lead a horse to water, but you can't make him drink," is still true. Nevertheless, leaders are identified by their ability to make things happen.

KEY QUALITIES OF A MOTIVATIONAL LEADER

Motivational leaders consistently demonstrate a number of qualities that develop gradually over time in response to successes and failures in achieving desired responses from others. Such qualities can also be evaluated and developed through training (Bennis & Nanus, 1985; Dunne & Erlichs, 1988; Henderson, 1995).

Key qualities of the motivational leader (Fig. 7–1) include knowledge and skill, effective communication of ideas, confidence, commitment, energy, insight into the needs of others, and an ability to take the action necessary to achieve goals important to others.

Knowledge and Skill

Knowledge and skill of the clinical nurse leader come from preparation in the responsibilities of

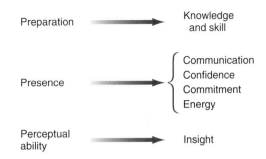

Figure 7–1. Characteristics of motivational leaders.

health care delivery and organizational duty; this might include specialized knowledge in areas such as patient health care requirements (process and outcome), planning, financial responsibilities, and human resource management. More than baseline knowledge, the motivational leader also has the ability to evaluate the likely success of actions in accomplishing goals and is able to support or suggest changes in directions that will lead to the desired outcomes.

Effective Communication of Ideas

Effective communication of ideas permits the motivational leader to capture the imagination and energy of others. This involves the ability to convey ideas clearly and in such a way that they can be heard positively. In this sense, the use of public language becomes critically important. How something is said becomes as important as what is said. For example, if the leader knows that budget reductions must be made and wants staff involvement in creating and implementing a solution, the means by which the message is delivered can make the difference between success and failure. A notice circulated to staff soliciting ideas will cause rumors and conjecture in addition to making staff feel isolated from the real process of resolution. A meeting in which the leader states, "We're going to have to cut back," may imply that staff efforts to date are not being valued and that the workload will be greater. A better choice would be to convene the group "to discuss ways to make it easier to meet patient needs while using less money." This method implies that patient needs remain the central concern and that there is an expectation that staff involvement can lead to an inventive means of both relieving workload and saving money.

Confidence

Confidence comes from an internal sense of security that one is competent to make a statement or take action and that there is a reasonable chance of success in accomplishing something of value. When the leader is both knowledgeable and confident, a lot of "natural drive" exists to take action. The motivational leader is secure enough to have a lower need to control and, as a result, is able to encourage autonomy, participation, and the empowerment of staff in decision-making. The combination of knowledge and confidence also enables the leader to deal with the ambiguity inherent to all complex organizations.

Leaders who fail to have this combination of skills are often autocratic and may be micromanagers. Operating from a sense of insecurity or a need for recognition, they may respond to others in a way that is devaluing.

Leaders who are comfortable with their abilities to set valid directions while having the power or influence to get a job done rarely need to use it like a club; rather, they use formal and informal authority to support their plans and actions and engender in others a sense of importance in moving ideas forward.

Commitment

Commitment is the internalization of an idea and a resulting drive to accomplish specific goals. A leader can be committed to developing something as intangible as an "atmosphere of professionalism" or as tangible as a professional compensation plan. The mere setting of a goal does not indicate motivational leadership—it is the ability of the leader to translate the importance of the goal to others and to elicit actions from them supportive of reaching the goal.

Energy

A high energy level is also necessary to empower and fire the imagination of others and constantly invent and move ahead in anticipation of future events as well as of current needs. Different styles of energy can be motivational in various situations and with different personalities of staff. What makes someone appear to be a "high energy leader" in a particular situation may make him or her seem "pushy and aggressive" in another situation. The energy to adjust style and approach while persisting in the attainment of the goal is a critical success factor.

Insight into the Needs of Others

Insight is the acute awareness of the reason behind events and an ability to anticipate results of actions. When a leader is able to put goals into a context that has real and personal value to each individual, conditions for motivation will exist. For example, if a staff member has a personal need to view herself as being in charge, establishing the individual as chair of an important committee to develop something of value to the patient care unit could engender positive action.

Although there are many styles of motivational leadership, abilities to listen, reserve judgment, give direct and positive feedback, recognize individual value through respect for others, and use humor can be additional key qualities.

As health care systems focus on integration of services across a continuum, so are leadership responsibilities shifting from technical duties to a focus on human relations management and operations. In many of the organizational models under development, the role of the leader is to facilitate, coordinate, and integrate services and staff and represent the organization. Models such as professional practice and shared governance especially depend on the clinical leader to produce an environment that fosters autonomy in decision-making and provides the skills, resources, and information necessary for other individuals to make this transition.

Patient-focused care and collaborative care models are designed to restructure the care-delivery process. These models depend on interdisciplinary organization and delivery of care, which maximize each staff member's contribution to patient care. Practice roles are expected to enable providers with different specialties to fully participate in care. For example, a dietary aide might be responsible for assisting in patient ambulation as well as dietary

Research Box 7–1

Empowerment as a Motivator

McNeese-Smith (1995)	Enabling others to act; increased employee job satisfaction and organizational commitment.
McDermott, Laschinger, & Shamian (1996)	Positive correlation between staff nurses' perceptions of empowerment and their perceptions of manager's power.
Wilson & Laschinger (1994)	Perceived empowerment leads to organizational commitment.

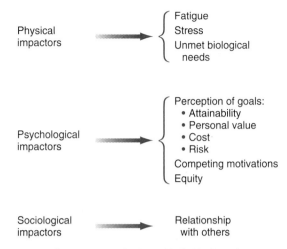

Figure 7–2. Evaluation of individual needs.

support. The leader of an interdisciplinary staff with these altered practice roles will find it necessary to transform and build new working structures and interstaff relationships.

Leadership qualities influence how new care structures are designed, put into place, and made responsive to the complex needs of workers. The leader must provide the essence of positive change that attracts and retains staff and ensures dependable role performance and innovative and spontaneous behavior.

THEORIES OF MOTIVATION

In broad terms, the determination of how to establish motivational conditions depends on an accurate assessment of the situation to be affected and evaluation of the needs of persons who must participate in the process. Work motivation studies have relied heavily on understanding how people use their intellectual or perceptual abilities to analyze and interpret their and others' thoughts and actions. These theories emphasize the importance of understanding the ways in which individuals process information to make choices and decisions. In addition to psychological needs, physical and sociocultural needs underlie behavior (Fig. 7–2).

Physical Needs: Fatigue, Stress, and Biological Factors

Physical needs contribute to work motivation by supporting or hindering an individual's ability to

accomplish the job. For example, fatigue may result from extended shifts or the stress of working under the pressure of time constraints or inadequate preparation. When Selye (1956) first discussed the general adaptation syndrome (the body's response to stress), he specifically noted the direct relationship between psychological pressure and physical symptoms. Under these circumstances, staff may instinctively draw back from the activity that is causing the stress or may become ineffective in their activities.

The need to meet basic physical needs was addressed by Maslow (1987) in his need-hierarchy theory. In the use of this theory, the leader evaluates whether working conditions permit staff to satisfy basic needs such as hunger, thirst, or sleep. For example, extensive overtime expectations or staffing shortages that make breaks for personal care impossible require immediate evaluation and action. If these problems are left unattended, the quality of performance and morale will decline and resignations will increase. Even if a direct solution, such as increased staffing is not possible, staff can be involved in determining ways to restructure the workload to accommodate these basic requirements. In itself, the realization that the leader is aware of the problem and able to empower others toward an actual intervention can be motivational.

Psychological Needs

In a work setting, people can be expected to perform better to the extent that goals are difficult, specific, and attractive. Several theories have been advanced that may be helpful in motivating others through the identification of—and response to—their needs.

Force-Field Theory

Consider the ability of people to have a broad perspective. The classic *force-field theory* of Lewin (1938) indicates that the extent to which people can view the total issue with which they are dealing improves their opportunity to gain insight into the solution of the problem. If the leader can set goals that another individual considers personally attainable, motivational energy can be stimulated. High performance levels would be dependent on the leader's providing feedback. Concrete rewards such as performance-based merit increases, self-scheduling, and shared governance, could stimulate commitment to goals. However, to the extent that staff members are unable to attain goals because of constraints such as their own personal or professional limitations or organizational policies or procedures, they may become less motivated.

Expectancy-Value Theory

Building on this logic, the *expectancy-value theory* (Vroom, 1964) and achievement-based materials (McClelland, 1951, 1978; Rotter, 1954, 1966) indicate that in situations in which more than one behavior is possible, the individual will choose the behavior with the largest combination of expected success and value (Petri, 1986, p. 219).

A leader can use value-expectancy by evaluating what is important to a specific individual and designing a means by which that individual can achieve her or his own goal while also fulfilling the leader's goal. For example, offering a means for employees to gain-share (personally gain financial benefit from reducing organizational expenditures) may meet an employee's needs for increased earnings and autonomy while meeting the leader's needs for down-sizing the organizational budget and freeing resources for other uses (Hammer, 1988). Similarly, re-engineering care systems to make them more efficient and effective may operate to expand an individual's scope of authority and meet needs

for professional growth and autonomy (Hammer & Champy, 1993; Kohn, 1994).

In using this approach, it is important to consider several specific factors: the person's perception of (1) his or her own capability of acquiring a desired goal (involving knowledge, skill, and competence), (2) the value of the goal, (3) the probability of the value being fully realized, (4) the cost (ie, personal, financial), and (5) the risk (ie, esteem, status, safety) (Dwyer, 1988).

In some instances, a clinical leader who expects her or his actions to be well received by staff is surprised to find just the opposite. For example, the expectation by some managers that all nursing staff will be enthusiastic supporters of professional practice models that give staff members a fixed salary rather than an hourly wage and empowers them to negotiate their schedules with other staff may not be well received. Although the appeal of personal control over work scheduling can be expected to motivate nurses to make a commitment to a particular unit and raise personal satisfaction, the concept of a fixed salary in which staff receive no differential or overtime pay may prove to be a disincentive to those focused on obtaining greater income by working more or different hours. Therefore, motivational factors may prove to be highly variable among individuals.

Another important factor is to consider the match between individual and organizational needs and values. For example, knowing that people hold different perspectives on abortion must enter into staff interviews for positions in obstetics/gynecology. An absolute lack of motivation will exist for staff who are opposed to abortion yet are hired with the unspecified expectation that they participate in an abortion procedure. In the event that an applicant desires the position but objects to the role, *cognitive dissonance*, or competing motivations, is set up. To reduce dissonance, the individual must change his or her opinion or behavior.

Equity Theory

Individual motivation is also affected by whether people feel they are being treated fairly. This situation has been addressed within the *equity theory* (Adams, 1965; Greenberg, 1983) and involves the evaluation of what one puts into a job versus what one gets out of it in comparison with some other relevant person (Klinger & Nalbandian, 1985). Inputs might include education and skills in the work itself, whereas outcomes include wages, promotions, and future opportunities. This becomes especially important as managers or self-managed groups consider system operations (eg, scheduling, patient, and committee assignments) and rewards (eg, pay levels, differentials, bonuses, and leave time) as they will be applied to individuals. A major source of employee complaints and grievances originates with a perception by an individual that he or she is not being treated as well as others under the same circumstances.

One means of providing motivational structures while attending to equity is to construct self-determined systems. Flexible benefit packages in which each employee is able to select the type and distribution of benefits, such as health insurance, leave time, and tax-deferred spending accounts, is an example of motivational incentives that appeal to individual values. These plans have been promoted in the literature (Lawler, 1987) and found to be successful (Cohn, 1988).

Motivation-Hygiene Theory

Some individuals are self-motivated to grow and constantly expand their horizons. Self-actualized people (Maslow, 1987; Rogers, 1959) are more likely to be independent of their environment. They characteristically demonstrate full use of talents and potentials, perception of reality, acceptance and a sense of kinship with others, spontaneous behavior focused on problems and ends, comfort with solitude, freshness of appreciation, deep interpersonal relationships with rather few individuals, philosophical humor, and creativity.

The self-actualized individual is internally driven and depends much less on being motivated by another person. Because satisfaction is internal, this individual will more likely respond to a collegial approach and to an organizational climate in which there is greater job responsibility and independence.

This approach is supported by the *motivation-hygiene theory* of Herzberg et al (1967), which stresses the importance of job enrichment to improve the meaningfulness of assignments, perceived significance, and worker autonomy. By restructuring the work environment to meet at least some of the aspirations of staff, leaders may upgrade staff skills, match them to tasks, and provide adequate resources and information. Actions are, in fact, required beyond job enrichment to include reorganization of work through matching of job requirements with professional abilities and creating practice models in which staff truly collaborate in the design of patient care and organizational systems.

Sociological Influences

At times, the environment of the job in itself is a motivating force beyond anything the nurse leader can offer. The need to be liked by others and a sense of belonging to a select group may fulfill needs for affiliation or self-esteem. In this event, the need of staff to meet the expectations of the peer group may take precedence over the job. Maslow (1987) referred to this as the third (belonging) and fourth (self-esteem) stages of the need hierarchy.

The basic notion here is that people have a felt need for personal power, sense of achievement, competence, and independence. Beyond this, there also is a need for social status, recognition, attention, and appreciation that is part of group membership.

The clinical leader's evaluation of what will motivate staff must include identifying how much peer influence enters into staff behavior. Peer pressure can both support and undermine goals that have been set. In a goal-supportive environment, staff as a team can be exceptionally effective and positive in their work by developing innovative and quality approaches to managing care. When the leader and staff share equally in this process, the patient care unit, whether community- or acute care–based, can be expected to experience positive results such as low staff turnover, high patient and physician satisfaction, and quality patient outcomes.

Unfortunately, staff teams may also be socially supportive of each other but not focused on meeting goals of the health care organization. In this event, certain groups of staff may form a clique that operates to provide mutual personal support in the work environment but only to the extent that it protects job security.

To assess and develop a plan of action, the leader must decide whether opportunities can be structured to facilitate individual motivation to achieve or whether the only way to support necessary changes is to temporarily separate the group. This action involves a degree of risk because if it is not well planned, the group may unite in opposition to the leader. One solution would be to evaluate individual skills and needs in consideration of unit goals. A restructuring of staff teams or work design, or both, could then be developed specifically to give individuals an opportunity to simultaneously meet their own needs and the goals of the unit. For example, the establishment of mentor/staff teams in which experienced nurses with advanced skills work with staff to lay the groundwork for new and more productive relationships may adequately address this need.

Because work experience has a major impact on personal growth, leaders need to create an organizational climate that helps staff become self-actualized. Increased job responsibility and independence are examples of ways to do this. Organizational re-engineering may change the working environment in ways that support this growth (Hammer & Champy, 1993). This involves examining how work is actually done and streamlining it to increase efficiency and effectiveness. It changes not only the process of work but also how personnel are selected, assigned, and empowered to self-manage.

Human Resources Model

In a changing health care environment with an increased diversity of patient expectations and needs, care settings, and providers, organizational redesign has become a major area of focus (Blouin & Tonges, 1996; Schneider et al, 1996; Strasen, 1994). Increasingly, there is an emphasis on "productive" work designs based on the *human resources model*. Early work in this area can be traced to McGregor (1960), who proposed that the approach that managers took to motivating employees was based on their assumptions about employee behavior. He suggested that the emphasis in the traditional model was on external rewards and that close supervision implied that employees would not work unless controlled through the use of rewards or punishment. He labeled managers of this type to be operating on the basis of *Theory X*.

In contrast, *Theory Y* became the essence of the human resources model in which workers were seen as being able to derive satisfaction from the work itself and make commitments to organizational goals. The rewards of this type of organization—self-direction and self-control—were more personal; in addition to the usual salary and leave benefits were the abilities to meet self-esteem and self-actualization needs through imagination and creativity in the solution of problems. These traits, rather than being attributed to only a few people, were considered to be broadly distributed throughout the population.

Theory Z was proposed by Ouchi (1981) as a combination of McGregor's theories X and Y. Ouchi suggested that people have both characteristics pertaining to both theories X and Y rather than characteristics of only one theory and that the involvement of employees is essential for any organization to excel. In Theory Z, the manager is responsible for creating an environment in which there is a philosophy of mutual commitment and continual development of the individual. As discussed by Smith (1984, p. 33), Japanese management concepts incorporate "(1) permanent employment, (2) infrequent evaluation and promotion, (3) nonspecialized career paths, (4) implicit control, (5) collective decision making, (6) work group responsibilities, and (7) holistic concern for employees." This model involves a significant investment in the development of human resources.

A human resources organizational design would give workers control over the total job. Quality control would therefore take place at the level of the person providing the service. Compensation would be based on knowledge, abilities, and team work rather than the accomplishment of specific tasks. In this environment, each manager acts more as a coordinator of resources than as a planner and controller. As a result of being broadly included in the information loop, systems of organization would be jointly designed by persons at all levels of the organization.

Shared governance is one example of how a health care organization can extend full decision participation to its members. Broadly shared governance gives nurses collective responsibility and accountability for their practice by shifting decision-

Research Box 7–2
Organization as an Influence

Smeltzer, Formella & Beebe (1993)	Work restructuring resulted in a 20% reduction in the nursing operations budget.
Strasen (1994)	Reengineering via function following form leads to improvements in quality, service, and financial outcomes.
Havens & Mills (1992)	Staff nurses' involvement does not ensure their influence on practice.

making from the nurse executive acting alone to the practicing nurses in the department acting in consensus (Porter-O'Grady, 1992). The principles behind shared governance models include self-direction, autonomy of practice, flexibility, and career growth.

These principles become especially important in an era of rapid organizational change and transformation. In an effort to streamline the process of work, many organizations are redesigning themselves through a process of re-engineering. The goal of this process is to significantly reduce time and/or cost, increase revenue, improve quality and service, and reduce risk (Kohn, 1994). For example, re-engineering may take several specialist jobs and create one case manager position that gives an individual responsibility for an entire process (Hammer & Champy, 1993). This allows individuals with the knowledge required to make decisions about work the power to change it.

APPLICATION OF THEORY AND ESTABLISHMENT OF MOTIVATIONAL CONDITIONS

There are realities involved in designing an organization able to accommodate complex patient needs and multiple levels of worker preparation, skills, life stage, and professional requirements. In addition to leadership, which was discussed earlier in this chapter, there are five broad categories of conditions

necessary to establish favorable motivational patterns (Table 7–1).

Norm Design

Anyone entering an organization expects that there will be some organizational definition of the "rules of the game." No matter how broadly defined, the standard operating procedure of the system—whether a system of care delivery or a system of organizational decision-making—must be clearly articulated (verbal and written) to the members of the organization. Even if the rule is that there are no rules, this must be clearly presented.

External Rules

External rules such as state nurse practice acts, professional association standards, Joint Commission on Accreditation of Healthcare Organizations (JCAHO) accreditation guidelines, National Committee on Quality Assurance (NCQA) standards, legal requirements of care, and federal and state employment laws can be expected to guide the practice of nursing in the legal sense. Clinically, nurses are held to accepted practice standards in which they are judged according to what other professionals would do under like circumstances. In this regard, the clinical leader must ensure that the external rules against which the organization as a whole will be judged are known by its members. This is the basis for many organizational, departmental, and unit-based policies and procedures.

Internal Rules

Internal rules, such as policies, procedures, and protocols, will normally be developed as either a mechanism to ensure compliance with, or provide further definition of, external rules or a means of controlling and standardizing behavior. To the extent that internal rules are truly generated internally, they are also subject to change. In other words, no rule should be considered permanent and unchangeable. Clinical leaders need to be flexible enough to use the human relations model and encourage higher-order staff motivation when appropriate. To the extent that this occurs, internally

Table 7–1.
Establishing Motivational Conditions

Standard Benefits	Incentives	Professional Environment	Interpersonal and Social Factors	Leadership
Salary	Compensation	Organizational structure	Organizational climate	Preparation
Leave time	Gain-sharing			Confidence
Insurance	Self-management	Autonomy Job definitions	Cohesive work groups	Energy
Guaranteed benefits	Performance-based compensation Nonfinancial	Division of labor Multidisciplinary alliance		Commitment Insight Communication
Cafeteria-style benefit plans	At-risk pay Revenue sharing Professional practice Bonuses based on budget savings Clinical ladder Leave benefit incentives Professional incentives	Reduced levels of structure Clinical ladders Development of assistive roles for patient care Self-managing teams Managed care and case management	Professional practice peer review Vision Quality circles Problem-solving teams Delphi technique	Specialized knowledge Staff decision-making Listening Positive Respect Humor
Attract, retain, and reward staff	Reduce organizational costs	Enhance patterns of interaction and communication	Operations improvement Staff empowerment	Direction setting Staff autonomy and empowerment
Competitive status of the organization	Enhance quality and productivity	Personal freedom	Creative energy	Anticipation of results
Security, self-esteem	Reward performance Employee influence on work	Professional autonomy Productivity Care continuity	Professional growth Trust and respect Team building	Human relations focus

designed rules can be developed that maximize resource use and quality care while promoting an environment in which employees are progressive and committed.

Although orientation of new staff is important to the communication of these policies and procedures, a clear and consistent approach must also be taken by the clinical leader. Consistency is not intended to reflect an unwillingness to make situational decisions but instead to ensure clear sensible rationale for the choices made.

Rules, or norms, are intended to serve as a basis for predictable performance of critical work processes that protect the legal status of the organization and its members and provide quality patient outcomes. For example, there is an expectation that staff working with patients will be knowledgeable and competent to provide cardiopulmonary resuscitation as necessary. By virtue of the responsibilities assumed by the health care system and its members, patients have a right to expect timely and expert response in this area. Another example is that there must be adequate staffing coverage for patient care. Whether the norm is that the leader develops a schedule around specific policies or that the staff organizes their own pattern of coverage, the norm will be that sufficient coverage is provided.

Although norms rules in and of themselves provide some motivation, the rationale and methods of their implementation are more important. As seen on the basis of several motivational theories, motivation can be stimulated by working with staff to establish a system in which they have latitude in decision-making and objective setting. This may occur through techniques such as participative management (Maier, 1963), quality circles (Mills, 1990), professional practice (Zelauskas & Hower, 1992), and shared governance (Minnen et al, 1993; Porter-O'Grady, 1992), all of which are examples of the decentralization process.

Standard Benefits

The organization as an entity offers benefits as a tangible means of attracting, retaining, and rewarding staff. The motivational consequences of benefit plans rests with their ability to make an organization competitive with other organizations to attract and retain staff. Sufficient rewards may also allow the organization to attract more highly prepared staff. However defined, organizational reward systems must be logically structured and made uniformly available.

Incentive Rewards

The drive to reduce organizational costs while enhancing quality and productivity has led to the development of innovative incentives to stimulate employee motivation to achieve high personal and organizational goals.

Compensation techniques are being initiated that in essence are based on value and need theories. For example, in place of automatic salary increases, exempt (professional) employees might be offered a combination of lower base pay and "at-risk pay," which varies with success in saving money or generating revenue. If the unit performed well financially, the employee could earn a far greater amount than he or she gave up in base pay. This would be similar to investing in stocks that could return a much higher rate of payment than the initial investment made. Similarly, *gain-sharing* is based on employee participation in the design and implementation of processes that reduce costs while enhancing quality and efficiency (Mills, 1990). Employees can benefit from organizational savings that they have created. As a result, performance can be expected to improve, and commitment to the goal is increased.

Professional practice often combines the elements of gain-sharing and shared governance by providing incentives for nurses to assume full responsibility for providing nursing services to their areas of responsibility in exchange for salaries, bonuses, and self-management (Crowley, 1988). In place of using contract agency nurses or paying overtime and shift differentials, staff members receive a base salary and organize their own routines and shift scheduling to provide full-service coverage to patients in their area of responsibility. In return, they receive bonuses based on salary and wage savings, supply savings, and increased revenues from patient volumes in excess of projections.

Performance-based compensation may tie financial incentives to individual performance. By giving staff a route of professional and financial recognition based on an achieved level of competency, a personally rewarding career route can be made available.

Nonfinancial motivational factors can also be performance-based; these may include leave benefit incentives as extra time off for educational advancement or professional development. Staff who have special interests in specific clinical fields might be given incentives to develop patient and staff educational programs in these areas or to participate in committee work that develops standards of care management or organization-wide policy.

Each of the techniques discussed provides a work design that is essentially self-reinforcing and empowering. Not only is performance rewarded, but also the employee has a direct influence on designing the goal, the means by which it will be reached, and the nature, type, and quantity of the reward.

The leader in this type of environment will function to empower staff and evaluate and monitor progress toward organizational goals. To do this, the leader must understand the short- and long-range goals of the organization, which include business and strategic plans, compensation strategy, and personnel needs and mix. The program must be developed to fit the individual nature of the organization.

Professional Environment

Studies of job satisfaction and expressed needs among hospital nurses (McNeese-Smith, 1995; Weisman, 1980) have explored the relationships among satisfaction, turnover, and performance. As a motivational element, job satisfaction has been defined as the degree of positive effect toward the overall job or its components. It does not, in itself, ensure achievement motivation because satisfied employees may be contented with the status quo. In instances in which performance and satisfaction are concurrently high, autonomy has been found to be one of the most significant factors (Benefield, 1988; Goodell & Coeling, 1994). Other factors have included internal locus of control and employees' perception of the manager's leadership behaviors, such as challenging process, inspiring shared vision, and role-modeling (McNeese-Smith, 1995).

Autonomy, which is the control over work through independent decisions, can be influenced by the clinical leader through promotion or control of choice. Environmental events, such as organizational norms, standard benefits, and incentive re-

Research Box 7–3
Role of Job Satisfaction

Goodell & Van Ess Coeling (1994)	Autonomy positively influences job satisfaction.
Lucas, Atwood, & Hagaman (1993)	Professional satisfaction and satisfaction with the organization are predictive of turnover.
Zavodsky & Simms (1996)	Enthusiasm and interest in work are significantly related to having a variety of experiences and to enhancement of patient wellness, pace, recognition, personal growth, and development and technology.

wards that promote either self-determined or controlled behaviors, have been discussed. In the context of professional organizational structure, the leader influences the nature of the environment in which work occurs.

Basic to the environment is the job itself and the means by which the worker can influence what is to be done and how it is to be accomplished. As a result, job definitions should be built by working groups that are composed of a blend of staff who know the institution and its resources and philosophy, are intricately aware of patient needs and care processes, and can contribute constructively to group decision-making. Whether through the design of clinical ladders that recognize advanced competence or the creation of new patient care support roles, jobs must include variety and sufficient complexity to use and challenge skills and abilities. The purpose of this effort is to motivate staff.

To further improve the motivational climate, attention must also be given to the division of labor. In addition to individual roles and job descriptions, alliances between individuals that create multidisciplinary and multirole work teams must be encouraged. By giving information and responsibility for self-managing teams, flexibility and autonomy can be maximized.

Managed Care and Nursing Case Management

Managed care and nursing case management are examples of processes organized around these principles. As defined by Zander (1990), *nursing case management* provides continuity by linking tasks, shifts, and departments. It suggests a continuity of provider by linking people across clinical settings. In this latter case, as described by Zander, nurses in staff roles are given authority as clinical leaders to manage patients in specific diagnostic categories throughout an entire episode of care. These nurses work in a formal collaborative practice with attending physicians. The model is designed to go beyond unit management or nurse management to form a continuum of care for the patient; it can therefore create *units without walls* and, as Zander indicates, "the equivalent of hospitals without walls."

The strategy of case management is to formally join specific nurses across units into group practices and link these practices with specific physicians. The result will (1) improve continuity of care delivery; (2) create financial and other resource savings; (3) increase nurse satisfaction, morale, and retention; (4) provide a flexible, adaptable system; and (5) decrease traditional barriers between nurses in various clinical areas (Zander, 1988). It is an example of one approach to create a motivating professional environment.

Interpersonal and Social Factors

One of the most important responsibilities of the clinical leader is that of participating in the selection of personnel and establishing a climate that enhances motivation. In professional practice settings, new applicants are interviewed through a peer review process that empowers staff to recommend employment decisions and provide a test of "chemistry" at the same time. The usefulness of this approach is to match interpersonal needs and create group strength. The final decision is generally that of the manager, who selects from staff recommendations. Groups, however, ultimately influence norms by defining expectations and creating peer pressure to conform. The leader who is sensitive to this fact can set the tone for a climate in which

collaboration to meet unit goals becomes an important value for each staff member.

The clinical leader has a major role in facilitating group efforts by creating the vision that attracts people who can help realize and achieve it. Naisbitt and Aburdene (1985) named this critical process *alignment*. When alignment happens, the group of people "transcend their personal limitations and realize a collective synergy that surpasses expectations based on past performance."

Controlling the Spin and Building the Team

In government circles, *controlling the spin* means making sure that communications and actions are clearly interpreted in the way in which they were intended. The way in which a leader sets new directions (Table 7–2) is as much a part of establishing a motivational climate as the structure itself.

A rule of thumb often repeated in education is to "tell them what you're going to say, tell them the information, and tell them what you told them." Clear communication at every stage of growth and change is a key feature in having others understand, participate, and buy into decisions. There are several techniques that can be helpful in this process.

Quality circles and *focus groups* are frequently used to bring together staff to discuss ways to improve job performance through problem-solving and direction setting. Although quality circles have been criticized for the time, training, and education costs involved, they have also been shown to yield significant operations improvements (Mills, 1990).

Similar to quality circles are problem-solving teams. According to Dailey (1990), these teams are

Table 7–2.
Building the Team

Group process techniques	Quality circles
	Problem-solving teams
	Delphi technique
	Focus groups
Leadership mechanisms	Delegation
	Recognition
	Collegial relationship

"a blend of quality circles, team building, delegation of authority for problem solving," and cost identification. The difference is that the focus is on middle managers rather than on all levels of employees and the implied use of a shorter-term approach to specific problems.

The *Delphi technique,* or *nominal group process,* is useful to quality circles, operations improvement, and problem-solving teams. This method, which originates from the approach of the Rand Corporation to generating creative "think tank" ideas, provides a way of accessing ideas from each member of a group without influence from other group members (Whitman, 1990). For example, with this technique, each group member writes down several ideas that he or she thinks would be useful in identifying or solving a specific problem. Through controlled feedback, the group leader solicits and records one idea from each person, continuing around the group until all ideas have been listed. Further controlled interaction is used to merge and clarify ideas and organize them by priority through objective individual ratings that are summarized as basic statistics.

In each of the methods discussed, autonomy is facilitated through flexibility and the choice that comes with self-regulation. The use of these interpersonal and social factors can be key to making the organization more autonomy-based (Deci & Ryan, 1987).

The very nature of quality circles, Delphi technique and problem-solving teams dictates that a climate that supports individual involvement in creating the work environment be nurtured. This must become part of the nature of the organization.

Even in a situation in which a high degree of autonomy exists for individuals, there usually is a motivational leader who is able to rally others to action and control how events are interpreted. The result can be unanimity of direction rather than fragmentation.

The most difficult part of developing staff and building the team is knowing how and when to delegate responsibility for action. Delegation means assigning to someone else the duty and authority to accomplish something. It also entails trust that the duty will be performed and a willingness to give necessary freedom. This can be especially difficult for someone who is relatively inexperienced. An inexperienced nurse, for example, may find it diffi-

cult to delegate to others what is still new and uncomfortable. Skill is frequently built by personally doing the job. Learning a skill while still reasonably delegating it to others is an art. Assistance with this process can come from a mentor who is able to provide guidance and support.

The way in which delegation is structured in work design must enable full participation on the part of all workers and maintain sufficient job complexity and variety to keep members committed and motivated to reach desired goals. Rather than a complicated hierarchy, a more streamlined approach of communication across departments will need to be developed around which delegation can occur. This process will be assisted by computer information systems. The effect will be to reduce middle management as an administrative structure and increase the emphasis on clinical leadership and self-management. This will further reinforce the human resource model approach, which uses networks, entrepreneurs, and small teams. (A complete discussion of delegation is given in Chapter 10.)

Frequently, it is also helpful to privately evaluate which individuals seem to be particularly efficient and effective in their roles as measured on the basis of patient and staff satisfaction, patient outcomes, organization, balanced perspective, and relative calm in performance of duties. These individuals, regardless of their position, may be leaders. Enlistment of their support by recognizing their abilities, including them in decision-making, and delegating agreed-on additional responsibilities may be a start. This approach is frequently motivational in gaining support from others. Ultimately, a collegial relationship may develop out of mutual respect, support, and professional collaboration. At this level, each person further facilitates the motivation of the other. Mutual dialogue, planning, and coordination of work are important components of this process.

DEVELOPING SELF-MOTIVATING ENVIRONMENTS

To be effective, an organization must be able to attract and hold people in a system who are dependable in their work performance and have innovative and spontaneous behavior (Katz, 1971). Having a critical number of the right people who are highly motivated to accomplish the work of an organization is key. Staff must be willing to take action, even unusual action, when necessary to improve the quality of patient outcomes. This spontaneous behavior can create the very innovation that makes the service being provided distinct and favorably received. For example, the nurse leader who spontaneously releases staff during periods of low census may at the same time improve morale and conserve resources for a time of greater need. Another example involves the leader with the foresight to develop service integration between care settings across which staff might be more consistently and effectively used. A case in point is the obstetrical service that adds and links community-based home visits and lactation support and counseling.

Beyond planning and delegating, leaders must empower others through the assignment of authority to decide to act rather than only follow directions. Staff members will feel empowered when the leader not only delegates the task but also accepts their advice and guidance. Many leaders begin to feel threatened or uncomfortable at this point; it is one thing to motivate and another to accept the results. For example, if staff are empowered to redesign the organizational structure of a patient care service, the leader must be willing to give significance to the changes that are recommended. In one institution, for example, a dilemma was created by staff who insisted that allowing them to totally manage the ventilatory requirements of patients who underwent open-heart surgery as necessitated by the patient's condition was more desirable than waiting for respiratory therapy to intervene on a standard schedule or on-call basis. Although the nursing staff wanted to take full patient responsibility, operations management would not relinquish the function, and conflict resulted. Realizing that the system valued cost-effective quality care, the staff proceeded to calculate the value of their service in terms of expense, revenue, and patient outcome. This approach satisfied management's concerns, and the service was changed. By giving these staff members a reasonable chance of success in having ideas implemented, the leader empowered them to achieve. Following success in creating their own role in respiratory care of patients, the staff developed an idea for an intra-aortic balloon pump transport team, for which they gathered interdisci-

plinary and administrative support. The idea was successfully marketed.

The ability of organizational members to create an environment in which they are continually motivated to achieve signals a dynamic system. The way this occurs is through vision and organizational transformation.

VISION OF THE FUTURE

Envisioning the future is an art at best. Still, through an awareness of the economic environment, demographic trends, innovations in technology, and competitive forces, it is possible to piece together some key future factors that will have an impact on the organization. Staff involvement in creating a future vision is essential. More important than reliance on current data is the consideration of future needs and the development of a sense of what the organization should be in the future.

The development of this future vision marks an opportunity for staff to express ideas and form commitments. Like a self-fulfilling prophecy, this vision can lead to an evaluation of the organization and opportunities for redesign and change.

Transformation is a rethinking of how things can be done. Rather than tinkering with the system to gain incremental improvements, it involves basic reworking to change the system. This means opening options for totally new approaches. It requires motivational leaders with a strong sense of self and an ability to welcome change and uncertainty. Interactive planning and idealized redesign are examples

---

Research Box 7–4
Research Informs Practice

Ingersoll et al (1995)	Implementation of professional practice has administrative implications for information, readiness, and roles.
Rizzo et al (1994)	Cultural patterns and work characteristics can be used to redesign care delivery.
Hood & Smith (1994)	Transformational leadership enhances quality of work life.

of a motivational approach to meeting that challenge. Interactive planning is a proactive and participative means of making a plan rather than just coming up with a plan. It targets a specific purpose of mission and, through reference projections (forecasting what will happen if nothing is changed) and environmental analysis (determining the extent to which services are needed and will be supported), leads to a plan design. This approach is intended to be a coordinated system-wide effort on the part of organizational members that is not limited to top administrators. Idealized redesign, in its simplest form, is a response to the question, "If the organization were totally destroyed, how would you reinvent it to ensure success in the current environment?"

Work must be designed to maintain the greatest motivational element for patient care providers—a work design focused on self-actualization achieved through meeting patient needs. Most people employed in health care have an acute sense of the organizational purpose, that of providing care. The sense of having made a personal difference for someone in need remains the most powerful motivator in health care (Zavodsky & Simms, 1996). Future work design directions for clinical leaders must not lose this focus. It must be noted, however, that although this factor may keep people in the field of health care delivery, it will not necessarily keep them in a particular organization.

Organizational Design

Several approaches to organizational design are emerging from the fields of behavioral science and administration; they involve creative ways of reconfiguring the organization to ensure viability through the use of effective planning that incorporates all committed and productive employees, and they are built directly around the discussed motivational elements.

Lattices and Matrices

Through a symbolic cross-hatching of horizontal and vertical lines, a lattice organization (Naisbitt & Aburdene, 1985) allows people to deal with others across the organization. It operates to reduce the traditional hierarchy and give motivational autonomy and recognition to employees. Leadership in this system emerges naturally as people make commitments and take responsibility for their actions.

Amoeba Diagrams

Morgan (1993) describes the drawing of organizational lines according to actual working relationships and business dependencies. In a health care environment, this would be akin to drawing a free-form shape around the clinical leader, clinical nurses, dietary aide, pharmacist, laboratory technician, housekeeper, and physician for a given patient population. This active series of working relationships is considered an organizational unit charged with specific goals of care integration. The formal recognition of this suborganization changes working relationships and can strengthen motivation within interdisciplinary collaboration.

Entrepreneurship and Intrapreneurship

Many of the motivationally based work redesign applications depend on creating an environment that supports and encourages *intrapreneurial* ventures. In this arrangement, employees are given autonomy to develop and implement new ideas and to benefit financially, personally, and professionally from their efforts. *Entrepreneurship* goes one step further in that the employee or group of employees become independent of the organization to undertake and manage their own ventures. Entrepreneurs create these new businesses within the organization.

An example of intrapreneurship is a staff-created and -managed clinic for abused children that was developed by nurses who formulated a multidisciplinary team business plan and patient identification and treatment procedures. An example of entrepreneurship is one in which nurses left hospital employment to establish a home health agency for community-based care. The intrapreneurial counterpart to this would be the development of a subsidiary nursing corporation within a hospital that nurses would manage under contract to the hospital.

NURSING RESEARCH ISSUES IN MOTIVATION

The health care paradigm is rapidly shifting from acute care and episode-based payment to primary care and a capitated (flat fee per client) payment environment. It is also shifting from a model of disease unpredictability to a model of disease predictability in which genetic evaluation and intervention and immunotherapy will play an increasing role. The results of these new technologies are anticipated to further reduce acute care hospitalization and increase primary, ambulatory, and home health services.

As the nature of health care services shifts, the need for nursing will continue to grow and evolve. The changing nature of where and how care will be delivered will also raise important issues for future motivational research. Key research issues will in part focus on the most effective means of organizing new service environments and evaluating the impact of these structures on health care providers and their clients. Transformed systems will also require the motivation of individuals to change the service delivery site in which they practice and expand their scope of practice and the relationships they will have with new practice partners (as case managers). Further understanding of how best to maximize performance and personal satisfaction and achievement will make these new organizations stronger and more effective in the management of patient care.

SUMMARY

Motivation is the basis of human behavior. At a time when health care institutions are experiencing a rapid rate and pace of change, the need to maintain a creative, committed, and productive workplace is of paramount importance. The role of the clinical leader is growing as health care delivery diversifies into multiple patient treatment sites and traditional models of organization change to flattened organizational designs based on human resource management. The hallmark of leadership is an ability to motivate others to develop and achieve established goals and a sense of personal accomplishment and satisfaction.

Motivation by definition is the force within the individual that influences strength or direction of behavior. Work motivation specifically concentrates on processes that influence job-related behavior; this is important in the context of organizations

because to be effective, organizations must be able to attract and retain people in the system who have dependable performance and innovative and spontaneous behavior.

Theories of motivation have been under development for more than 90 years. Resulting research has shown that there is no single motivational scheme that can encompass all behavior; rather, individual motivation is shaped by a complex array of physiological, psychological, and sociological factors.

Motivational leaders must be instrumental in establishing conditions that support staff motivation, build effective teams, develop self-motivating environments, and stimulate constantly renewing systems. Leaders may be at any level of the organization and may have significant influence rather than formal authority. In finding ways to make organizational, personal, and professional goals consistent, it is possible to merge interests and stimulate motivation.

■ DISCUSSION QUESTIONS ■

1. What is the difference between achievement and protection motivation?
2. How can personnel assessments be used to structure motivational conditions?
3. What are the motivational strengths of management styles related to Theories X, Y, and Z?
4. How could motivational leadership skills be identified and developed?

■ LEARNING ACTIVITIES ■

1. Identify an occasion on which you were particularly proud of an achievement. List the three key conditions that motivated you to reach this goal.
2. Select one *individual*, and consider what drives him or her to produce high-quality work. Design a work request in a way that would motivate that person to achieve.
3. For *a team of staff* charged with a specific objective, assess how the group can be given personal, professional, and tangible and/or intangible incentives to achieve.

■ BIBLIOGRAPHY ■

Adams JS (1965). Inequity in social exchange. *In* Berkowitz L (ed). *Advances in Experimental Social Psychology,* Vol. 2. New York, NY: Academic Press.

Arkes HR, Garske JP (1982): *Psychological Theories of Motivation.* Monterey, CA: Brooks/Cole Publishing Company.

Benefield LE (1988). Motivating professional staff. *Nursing Administration Quarterly* 12:57–62.

Bennis W, Nanus B (1985). *Leaders: The Strategies for Taking Charge.* New York, NY: Harper & Row.

Blouin A, Tonges M (1996). The content-context imperative: Integration of emerging designs for the practice and management of nursing. *JONA* 26:38–46.

Bracken RL, Christman L (1978). An incentive program designed to develop and reward clinical competence. *JONA* 8:8–18.

Cohn BA (1988). Glimpse of the 'flex' future. *Newsweek* August 1:38-39.

Crowley CM (1988). Self-governance picks up new believers. *Centerpoint* Spring:2–3.

Dailey RC (1990). Strengthening hospital nursing. *JONA* 20:24–29.

Deci E, Ryan RM (1987). The support of autonomy and the control of behavior. *Journal of Personality and Social Psycholgoy* 53:1024–1037.

Dunne R, Erlichs (1988). MBA management development program for middle level nurse managers. *JONA* 18:11–15.

Dwyer CE (1988). Changing people's behavior. *In Strategic Management.* Philadelphia, PA: Management and Behavioral Science Center.

Festinger L (1957). *A Theory of Cognitive Dissonance.* Evanston, IL: Row, Peterson.

Goodell T, Van Ess Coeling H (1994). Outcomes of nurses' job satisfaction. *JONA* 24:36–41.

Greenberg J (1983). Motivation: The force behind behavior. *In* Baron RA (ed). *Behavior in Organizations.* Newton, MA: Allyn and Bacon.

Hammer M, Champy L (1993). *Reengineering the Corporation.* New York, NY: Harper Collins.

Hammer TH (1988). New developments in profit sharing gain sharing and employee ownership. *In* Campbell JP, Campbell RJ (eds). *Productivity in Organizations.* San Francisco, CA: Jossey-Bass, pp 328–366.

Havens D, Mills M (1992). Staff nurse empowerment: Current status and future projections. *Nursing Administration Quarterly* 16:58–64.

Henderson M (1995). Nurse executives: Leadership motivation and leadership effectiveness. *JONA* 25:45–51.

Herzberg F, Mausner B, Snyderman BB (1967). *The Motivation to Work.* New York, NY: Wiley.

Hood J, Smith H (1994). Quality of work life in home care: The condition of leaders' personal concern for staff. *JONA* 24:40–47.

Ingersoll G, Brooks A, Fisher M, et al (1995). Professional practice model research collaboration: Issues in longitudinal multiple designs. *JONA* 25:39–46.

Katz D (1971). The motivational basis of organizational behavior. *In* Hollander E (ed). *Current Perspectives in Social Psychology.* New York, NY: Oxford University Press, pp 570–587.

Klinger DE, Nalbandian J (1985). *Public Personnel Management Context and Strategies,* 2nd ed. Englewood Cliffs, NJ: Prentice-Hall, p 211.

Kohn D (1994). The role of business process reengineering in health care. *Topics in Health Information Management* 14:1–6.

Lawler EE (1987). Pay for performance: A motivational analysis. *In* Nallantian H (ed). *Incentives Cooperation and Risk Sharing.* Totowa, NJ: Rowman and Littlefield.

Lewin L (1938). *The Conceptual Representation and the Measurement of Psychological Forces.* Durham, NC: Duke University Press.

Lucas M, Atwood J, Hagaman R (1993). Replication, validation of anticipated turnover model for urban registered nurses. *Nursing Research* 42:29–35.

Maier MRF (1963). *Problem Solving Discussion and Conferences: Leadership Methods and Skills.* New York, NY: McGraw-Hill.

Manthey M (1973). Primary nursing is alive and well in the hospital. *American Journal of Nursing* 1:83–87.

Maslow AH (1987). *Motivation and personality.* New York, NY: Harper and Row Publishers.

McClelland DC (1951). *Personality.* New York, NY: William Sloane.

McClelland DC (1978). Managing motivation to expand human freedom. *American Psychology* 33:201–210.

McDermott R, Laschinger H, Shamian J (1996). Work empowerment and organizational commitment. *Nursing Management* 27:44–47.

McGregor DM (1960). *The Human Side of Enterprise.* New York, NY: Harper and Row Publishers.

McNeese-Smith D (1995). Job satisfaction productivity and organizational commitment. *JONA* 25:17–26.

Mills ME (1983). Core-12: Impact of flexible scheduling on staff fatigue and quality of care. *Nursing Research* 32:356–361.

Mills ME (1990). Operations improvement. *JONA* 20:40–46.

Minnen T, Berger E, Ames A, et al (1993). Sustaining work redesign innovations through shared governance. *JONA* 23:35–40.

Morgan G (1993). *Imaginization.* Newbury Park, CA: Sage Publications.

Naisbitt J, Aburdene P (1985). *Re-inventing the corporation.* New York, NY: Warner Books.

Oldham GR (1982). Work redesign. *National Forum* 62:8–10.

Ouchi WG (1981). *Theory Z: How American Business Can Meet the Japanese Challenge.* Reading, MA: Addison-Wesley.

Petri HL (1986). *Motivation: Theory and Research.* Belmont, CA: Wadsworth Publishing Company.

Porter-O'Grady T (1987). Shared governance can help the bottom line. *Aspen's Advisor* 1:6–7.

Porter-O'Grady T (1992). *Implementing Shared Governance: Creating a Professional Organization*. St. Louis, MO: Mosby.

Rizzo J, Gilman M, Mersmann C (1994). Facilitating care delivery redesign using measures of unit culture and work characteristics. *JONA* 24:32–37.

Rogers CR (1959). A theory of therapy personality and interpersonal relationships as developed in the client-centered framework. In Koch S (ed). *Psychology: A Study of Science. Volume 3: Formulations of the Person and the Social Context*. New York, NY: McGraw-Hill.

Rotter JB (1954). *Social Learning and Clinical Psychology*. Englewood Cliffs, NJ: Prentice-Hall.

Rotter JB (1966). Generalized expectancies for internal versus external control of reinforcement. *Psychology Monographs* 80:1–8.

Schneider B, Brief A, Guzzo R (1996). Creating a climate and culture for sustainable organizational change. *Organization Dynamics* 24:7–19.

Seyle H (1956). *The Stress of Life*. New York, NY: McGraw-Hill.

Smeltzer C, Formella N, Beebe H (1993). Work restructuring: The process of decision making. *Nursing Economics* 11:215–222.

Smith HL (1984). Japanese management: Implications for nursing administration. *JONA* 14:33–39.

Strasen L (1994). Reengineering hospitals using the "function follows form" model. *JONA* 24:59–63.

Vroom V (1964). *Work and Motivation*. New York, NY: Wiley.

Weisman C, Alexander CS, Chase GA (1980). Job satisfaction among hospital nurses: A longitudinal study. *Health Services Research* Winter:341–365.

Wilson B, Laschinger H (1994). Staff nurse perception of job empowerment and organizational commitment: A test of Kanter's theory of structural power in organizations. *JONA* 24(suppl):39–47.

Whitman NI (1990). The committee meeting alternative: Using the Delphi technique. *JONA* 20:30–36.

Zander K (1988). Nursing group practice. *Definition* 3:1–3.

Zander K (1990). Differentiating managed care and case management. *Definition* 5:1.

Zavodsky A, Simms L (1996). Work excitement among nurse executives and managers. *Nursing Economics* 14:151–155, 161.

Zelauskas B, Hower D (1992). The effects of implementing a professional practice model. *JONA* 22:18.

8

Clinical Leadership in Nursing: The RN as Integrator

Sarah S. Detmer, RN, MS

LEARNING OBJECTIVES

This chapter will enable the learner to:
1. Differentiate between the concept of leadership and the concept of management.
2. Discuss the current health care environment and its impact on nursing management.
3. Discuss how culture affects nursing practice.
4. Discuss leadership strategies to build an empowering environment for nurses.

INTRODUCTION

A leader is a picture painter. The leader of an organization sets direction from a platform of commonly held values within the culture of the organization. The effective leader builds commitment, loyalty, and ownership through sharing the organization's vision and mission and encourages creativity in designing ways to fulfill them. Leaders are focused on doing the right thing, whereas managers are focused on doing things right.

All nurses are leaders. All nurses, whether administrative or clinical practitioners, lead patients toward improved health outcomes while motivating and supporting staff. Regardless of the role the nurse is playing, each nurse builds commitment and ownership in patient care and in the organization as a whole.

In these times of very fast change and uncertainty in health care, leadership in any setting has its challenges and its opportunities. If the leader of a health care organization, a nursing service, or a patient care unit within the nursing service can facilitate a common desired picture of the perfect unit with its membership, loyalty and alignment will follow and creativity and learning will flourish. New ways of providing care to patients in a cost-effective manner will develop to meet the health care challenges of our time.

This chapter focuses on the differences and commonalities between leaders and managers, reviews leadership styles, and discusses the importance of organizational culture in the building of empowering environments that foster satisfaction and motivation in the changed health care environment. A unique focus is on developing nursing leadership that celebrates clinical excellence.

DEFINITIONS OF LEADERS AND MANAGERS

If leaders are picture painters, managers are problem solvers whose energies are directed toward goals, resources, structures, and the management of people. A manager uses leadership qualities to achieve results so that people can continue to contribute to the vision and the direction of the organization. Managers can and do provide leadership, depending on their approach. From the manager's perspective, the task at hand is to get things done and to do so with the loyalty and goodwill of the employees. Managers and leaders are similar in how they think and act and in what motivates them. Managers are organized, whereas leaders may create chaos and uncertainty with change and creativity. Managers facilitate and negotiate while leaders are constantly opening up new ideas to additional opportunity. In the ideal world, managers and leaders embrace the same values, qualities, and characteristics.

Leaders are the keepers and promoters of the values of the organization. "Doing the right thing" requires consistent attention to values. A leader's behavior reflects those values at every turn and in every decision, in every promotion and in every interaction with people, in the way he or she sets scheduling priorities, assigns and supports work, and acknowledges people. The entire membership of an organization, whether it is of a whole country, a patient care unit, or a team on that unit, watches the leader for signs of what is important and what is valued. Differences and similarities between leaders and managers are presented in Table 8–1. This list is not exhaustive, and the similarities between leaders and managers can and do overlap.

Consider, for example, the staff nurse taking care of a newly diagnosed diabetic patient. While the nurse is managing care for the patient, she is also assessing the patient's clinical values and coaching and facilitating the patient's compliance with the diabetic role. The nurse listens carefully for concerns and difficulties the patient may encounter and subsequently searches for creative ways in which to manage the patient in a fiscally effective manner.

Table 8–1.
Comparison of the Qualities of Leaders and Managers

Leaders	Managers
Vision	Implement
Values	Operationalize
Role model	Go by the recipe
Teaching	Follow the rules
Coaching	Direct people
Facilitating	Plan by the rules
Listening	Get the job done
Stimulating creativity	

Such creativity is important in today's health care environment, because the demands of managed care focus on quality, cost, and outcomes of care.

THE IMPACT ON NURSE LEADERSHIP OF CHANGES IN NATIONAL AND LOCAL HEALTH CARE DELIVERY

The nurse leader of today has advanced to a full member of the health care team. With the enormous rate of change within the national and local health care delivery environments, the nurse leader must be looking to the future along with colleagues around the conference table to position the institution for an appropriate role in health care delivery. There are times when the nurse leader must prioritize values to maintain standards while reducing the cost of patient care. At these junctures, generating creative ideas and new approaches to care from within the organization is critical. Leaders must be willing to break the mental models of how care is delivered and explore other ideas of accomplishing the organization's mission. The nurse is the leader of that effort and needs the support of the entire staff, both managers and staff nurses, to continue to provide care while searching for new, less expensive models.

If, in fact, the organization must face reductions in staff and ultimately implement layoffs, the leadership is much less able to consult staff members. Staff jobs are at stake, and confidentiality becomes the driving value in the interest of protecting those who will lose positions. Crisis environments are much less likely to permit nurse leaders and managers to engage in deliberate planning or to allow for creativity and testing of new models.

Just as nursing staff members watch the behaviors of a nurse leader to signal values, so the leadership staff watches the behaviors of the executive team members to signal their values. Financial choices, organizational structure choices, leadership selection, and decision-making behavior all tell the organization's staff what is important to the leadership, which in turn further complicates the job of the nursing leadership. Clarification of values, team realignment, and focus on patient care become critical in times of change and uncertainty. Nurse leaders must refocus the staff on the things they see as most important in their jobs. The staff nurse, as a clinical leader, must also be aware of these values and organizational directives as he or she manages patients.

FORMAL AND INFORMAL LEADERSHIP

Everyone has had the experience of watching a group of people come together in support of an objective or a cause. Within the group there are formal and informal leaders. There may be a formally elected or appointed leader such as the chairman of an organization elected by the membership, a vice president of nursing who is appointed by the chief executive officer, or a nurse specialist leading a team in the operating room. There are others in the group who take on various roles, including that of an informal leader. The informal leader has the same creativity and ability to articulate ideas that the formal leader has in an organization. Informal leadership surfaces even in groups of children around a common interest. A Little League baseball team is a case in point. Teamwork to win is a high motivator. Individual players will surface in informal leadership roles on the team. The spirit of the team overcomes any individual ambitions.

Sometimes an individual exercising informal leadership in a nursing work group can advance the cause of the concerns of the workers of a particular shift, or the concerns of a union, or the concerns of a staff regarding patient care standards. Informal leadership in a group provides a natural resource for staff creativity and new mental models of care delivery. An astute unit manager recognizes the creative potential in the informal leaders and can tap that energy. For example, a licensed practical nurse (LPN) who has had 20 years of experience in three different settings brought to the attention of the unit manager that supplies and equipment needed for patient care were not readily available. All of the staff were seeing delays in care delivery as everyone was having to collect supplies constantly. Stocking supplies in patient rooms daily became a nurse's aide role that had not been considered before. The organization and timeliness of care improved remarkably, as did patient and staff satisfaction. Advancing new ideas and concerns is best accomplished in an open environment rather than one that is adversarial. There are informal leaders in every group. The effective nurse manager understands who they are and nurtures and develops their leadership to maximize their contribution to the mission of the organization.

Consider the competent staff nurse who steps forward to assist others in the organization of the care of their patients. She understands the workload measurement system and gets angry when representatives of the staffing office will not listen to her recommendations for staffing. Because she is articulate, the rest of the staff members share her discontent. The unit manager recognizes her ability and invites her to represent the unit on a staffing standards committee for the surgical services. The nurse not only feels recognized but she also has been given the opportunity to have a positive impact on the staffing of the entire service and to increase her contribution to the effectiveness of the organization.

LEADERSHIP STYLES IN CLINICAL PRACTICE

Leadership in clinical practice is of primary importance in patient care delivery and outcomes. Leadership style is defined as a distinctive or characteristic manner of performance (Gillies, 1989). Leadership style is important in building a culture that values clinical excellence. Some styles are motivating and empowering, whereas others create uncertainty, fear, and confusion.

Specific Leadership Styles

Four styles of leadership are described in the literature: autocratic, democratic, participative, and laissez faire. The *autocratic* style of leadership is task-oriented and directive. The leader uses his or her power and position in an authoritarian manner to set and implement organizational goals. Decisions are made without input from staff. In the *democratic* style of leadership, the leader uses personal and positional power to create ideas and input from staff and subordinates. Democratic leaders value the input of staff and motivate them to set their own goals and plan their own work in an effort to control their own practice. Democratic styles best empower staff toward excellence because this style of leadership allows nurses an opportunity to grow professionally. *Participative* leadership suggests a compromise between the authoritarian and the democratic styles. In participative leadership, the manager presents his or her own analysis of problems and proposals for actions to members of the team, inviting critique and comments. The participative leader then analyzes the comments and makes the final decision. The *laissez faire* ("let alone") leader abdicates leadership responsibilities, allowing staff to work without assistance, direction, or supervision. Staff members plan, implement, and evaluate their work in any way they see fit (Gillies, 1989).

LEADERSHIP OF THE MANAGER

Leading staff nurses is a critical challenge for the nurse leader. Whether the registered nurse is a team leader on a particular shift, or the nursing executive for the entire organization, the tasks are the same. If the nurse leader is providing the vision, the alignment around the vision, and the avenue to "do the right thing," the manager will "do things right." The nurse leader must resist the temptation to spell out the details of how to reach a patient care goal. Instead there must be expectations that allow the staff to use their own expertise and clinical knowledge to design the best ways to get there. Staff development, the ownership of unit goals, the appreciation of clinical knowledge, and the selection of strong staff are key ingredients in creating an environment in which staff can flourish.

Perhaps the most important structure is staff development. To do things right, staff members must be clinically expert and sound critical thinkers. They cannot alter procedures if they do not have a solid background in pathophysiology or the function of specialized equipment. Unit leaders must also be clinical experts to provide support and to teach and coach nurses. The unit manager is the leader of the unit and, as a leader, maximizes the creativity of the staff. To understand the unit leadership role and to implement it, management development is crucial. The nurse leader must not only use formal classroom training but also must be the unit leader's teacher or coach and role model on a daily basis as the unit leadership skills and staff's clinical skills are continually improved.

The nurse leader, whether formal or informal, a team leader or a nurse executive, tolerates mistakes and uses errors in judgment as opportunities for dialog and coaching. The nurse sees the development through both formal classroom education and teaching and coaching as a long-term effort of continual improvement. Because the nurse executive has the broad view within the organization, there is an opportunity to help others understand the whole from a systems viewpoint. If staff nurses have been made aware of the larger health care picture, then they can provide leadership in developing cost-cutting measures as well as improvement in clinical practice.

Ownership

In providing the unit manager with teaching and coaching skills, the nurse leader builds unit pride and ownership for the manager. In turn, pride and ownership can be translated into unit-based and self-directed work teams. There is increasing evidence of improved patient care in organizations in which both managers and staff have ownership for the success or failure of the unit. That ownership creates an environment in which creativity is fostered and individual patient and family care needs are met more satisfactorily. If the work group is aligned around a common set of values and expectations with regard to patient care, then staff will be committed to meeting those expectations and ultimately to the success of the health care institution.

For example, the intensive care unit (ICU) nurses in the community hospital in one town had been in the habit of enforcing visiting hours that were very restrictive to families. The nurses were concerned that families get in the way of efficient care and they relied on rules to keep families at bay. The leadership embraced a new philosophy regarding patient and family satisfaction and looked for opportunities to improve. A few informal nurse leaders in the ICU proposed a policy that leaves the visiting hours open and in control of the individual nurse. Hence, the nurse could make the decision about whether or not the presence of a spouse, a parent, or a child would improve the patient's outlook. The nursing staff, while initially reluctant, began to see the clinical advantages of the new policy to the patients and were willing to own the responsibility for making visiting-hour decisions. Patient and family satisfaction improved; the families felt more involved and better informed; and the confidence of staff to make patient-centered decisions improved as well. When the staff share the value and put patients in the center of their decisions, the change comes easily and patients get better care.

BUILDING A CULTURE TO SUPPORT EXEMPLARY PRACTICE

The unit leader virtually determines the quality of care delivered to a group of patients. The nurse executive also determines the culture in which that quality will be delivered. The organization of the work and the direction of the clinical practice as a whole rest with the clinical leader and with the clinical knowledge that is intrinsic on the unit.

Identifying Values

The nurse manager articulates the expectations of staff through identification of values of care delivery and by bringing staff together around those values. For example, if technical expertise is the primary focus, everything revolves around that expertise, including education programs, performance evaluations, documentation formats, and quality assurance measures. If, on the other hand, the technical expertise is a given and patient education and self-care are important, then the education, performance evaluation, documentation of expectations, and quality measures reflect the self-care philosophy. In a home health agency, the nurse manager can lead staff members to an expansion of their clinical roles by providing additional clinical education in physical assessment, pathophysiology, pharmacology, and medical management. Through this education, a more thorough patient assessment and subsequent medical and nursing intervention will occur in a more timely way, preventing further deterioration and hospitalization of fragile patients. Patients get better care and the total cost of a spell of illness may be decreased.

If continuity of care and concern is a value held by the clinical nurse leader, the implementation of a case-management model that extends beyond the inpatient unit and the hospital walls may result. For example, a nurse manager on an oncology unit listens carefully to two staff nurses as they voice their concerns about a family's ability to handle a patient's care at home. Additional intravenous therapy is expected to be part of the plan of care at discharge. Because the staff is patient-focused and very concerned for the patient's welfare, a decision is made to keep the patient for an extra 2 days for family teaching, which adds to the cost of the patient's care. In subsequent discussions, the advantages of a case-manager role are explored by the staff nurses and the manager. The role is envisioned as including a home follow-up component to ensure continuity and quality of care as well as continuity of concern. The role is successfully implemented on the oncology unit with improvements in patient, physician, and nurse satisfaction. In addition, a shortened length of stay for new patients is realized. Without both formal and informal clinical leadership that articulates the values of exceptional patient care, the care becomes mundane, routine, and task-oriented. Quality suffers and patient and family satisfaction declines.

Selecting Staff

One of the ways of strengthening the leadership of a patient care unit is to be very careful about the selection of staff, including managers. In times when nursing layoffs, down-sizing, and the use of assistive staff add to the pressures of hiring, careful selection is much more difficult. The urgency of getting patients taken care of tends to override the careful evaluation of candidates. The sorting of qualified candidates starts with the review of resumes. Talking with former employers can enlarge the picture as well. However, the definitive activity is the interview. Aside from practical experience, the next most important issue to approach is the articulation of values, which is supported by action. A discussion of heroes is one way to understand the values of a candidate. Conversations describing "what if" scenarios also can be helpful. The "fit" in values between the candidate and the existing culture and leadership is critical to the success of a new leader as well as to the success of a staff nurse.

The identification of one's own values and how they are reflected in the workplace is a very important part of any job, whether in leadership or in clinical practice. When interviewing for a position, one must evaluate the leadership skills and the values of the supervisor for a "fit."

If the head nurse is more interested in the schedule or the completion of tasks than in the larger patient picture, the "fit" may not be the right one for a patient-oriented staff nurse. If the bulletin board is full of directives, the environment may not be one in which the nurse will feel valued and creative. What the unit manager says about the goals of the unit over the next month or the next year, how involved the staff feels in the decisions of the unit, whether there is a designated clinical expert to whom staff looks for support and improvement, who the role models are, and whether there is a preceptor program designed to provide a thorough orientation are all examples of questions and observations the candidate nurse should pursue. Effective leadership involves the clear articulation and interpretation of the values and direction of the organization as well as the flexibility to encourage creativity and participation in accomplishing goals in getting there. Selecting strong leadership is a challenge for the individual searching for the right job, as it is for the institution searching for the right leader.

DEVELOPING THE ENVIRONMENT FOR CLINICAL EXCELLENCE

Exemplary clinical excellence cannot be attained without the commitment of the clinical staff. Staff members must be passionate about patient care to critically evaluate and constantly improve their practice, both their technical expertise and their patient and family interactions. Because the commitment to excellence must come from the staff, the clinical leader must not only build a staff with such commitment through performance evaluation and staff selection, but also encourage creativity and research in the clinical arena. Once the committed staff is present, the ultimate system supporting clinical excellence and continuous improvement is peer review and self-governance.

Nurturing staff commitment to patient care and clinical excellence starts with concurrence about what is really important. Senge (1990) outlines a process for personal mastery and vision, both as an individual and as a group, that is useful in achieving agreement about what is important. Alignment of values in this process leads to a commitment to a shared direction. From this commitment, the group can agree on goals and short-term objectives to achieve their vision. Because the vision is important to everyone, energy becomes focused and creative problem-solving can occur. The alignment around values is crucial to the focus and the energy of the group. The alignment also moves a group away from a negative and energy-wasting "we-they" polarization and into a more positive communication and joint planning mode. The work group moves from a victim's position of being directed to being a creative and empowered staff energized by the passion of shared commitment.

As an example, two different experiences in the same intensive care unit are presented. In one experience, the unit is led by a new, inexperienced manager who struggles without much support in her new role. Although she is clinically very experienced and competent, the staff she attempts to lead has different standards by which they work. Her approach to leadership is autocratic and non-negotiable, and the strong staff fights the clinically correct changes in standards and procedures at every move. The environment becomes punitive and negative. Staff turnover increases, and professional satisfaction and commitment fall to an all time low. Because staffing is accomplished with temporary, expensive agency and contingency staff who lack commitment to the work group, quality of care falls and costs soar.

Under a different leadership, the environment changes. Alignment is accomplished through creating opportunities for the staff to articulate what is important to them. They begin working together to accomplish their goals, starting with peer review in testing clinical competence, which is usually a threatening process. Because of their new focus on and commitment to patients and clinical excellence rather than their focus on working against the manager, staff nurses develop a new level of energy and professional satisfaction. Many return to school for further education, and some unit-based research activities begins. Staff turnover decreases, and physician-nurse collaboration improves. Critical thinking becomes the norm, and individualized, improved patient care results.

To lead a professional group toward a vision of clinical excellence, an environment must be created in which critical thinking skills are highly valued. Every patient is not the same, and adequate data for the evaluation of patient status and subsequent intervention is as critical in home care as it is in the intensive care unit. Collaboration with medical staff and other allied health professionals requires comprehensive levels of patient care evaluation to select appropriate interventions and treatment. Confidence in evaluating patient status is developed with experience, and the expectation that the patient's status will be evaluated critically should be shared by all staff. Critical thinking skills can be developed through education, role-modeling, peer review, and continual quality improvement. Each of those approaches requires an open environment in which each staff nurse feels confident and creative enough to evaluate critically and improve continually.

Unfortunately, while excellent progress may be made in the internal environment of an individual unit or agency, the system within which the group must operate may not be so progressive. In almost every situation, there are external or systemic impacts on what happens in a group and vice versa. As a result, team members must not only become critical thinkers in evaluating patient care, but must also become systems thinkers in evaluating both the internal and external systems within which they work.

Senge (1990) outlines a format for thinking systemically. Unintended consequences arise from decisions that are not thought through, and delayed responses within the system can block opportunity for correction. For example, if in the interest of cost-containment, the number of housekeepers is decreased and the work is rearranged, the increased delay time in cleaning and preparing a room for an admission may result in patient and family dissatisfaction. The increased stress may negatively affect the patient's recovery.

Although the decision about housekeepers seems removed from quality of clinical care, it has an effect from a systems viewpoint. Nurse leaders must frequently look for work-shift decisions when fellow administrators are attempting to become more efficient by eliminating positions. Those who know the most about the systems impact of decisions are the front-line people, whether they are nurses, housekeepers, or physicians. Just as important is the systems impact of transfer policies designed in the emergency department. If the timing of transfers is planned to keep space available for new patients, and the inpatient units are not prepared, the back-up frustrates everyone, including the patients involved.

The primary role of the unit leader in these environments is that of facilitator and teacher or coach. It is impossible for a creative staff in an open environment not to make mistakes. If there is a commitment to continuous improvement, then there must be a commitment to learning, which can only happen if the staff takes calculated risks and learns from the results. The role of leadership in this environment is to consistently review the values and ask questions of the staff so that maximal critical thinking and systemic thinking has taken place and that values are not inadvertently being violated.

The teaching or coaching role is one of inquiry and education as opposed to directive. For example, if a staff wants more control over the work schedule, the unit manager might ask for volunteers to develop standards for staffing that meet their agreed-to patient care standards. The group would outline what coverage needs to take place and what kind of clinical talent must be present to meet patient care objectives. The group might even create the rules for the scheduling process, such as who gets to fill in the schedule first or who is going to be on call if there are more patients than predicted. The unit manager could post some examples of schedules so that staff could self-schedule to meet standards while maintaining control over the process. The unit manager is a teacher rather than a director, a coach rather than an autocrat, helping staff to focus on the values that they hold important to their profession.

Structures for an Empowering Environment

In any work group that feels empowered, there are restrictions on the scope of decisions that the staff may make. Many of those restrictions are imposed from outside the institution. The Joint Commission on Accreditation of Health Care Organizations sets standards that they expect each hospital to meet and looks for evidence that the hospitals are meeting those standards. Many of the standards are processes and give maximum opportunity for unit-based decision-making. For example, the nurse surveyor looks for evidence of patient education as well as an adequate problem list. The surveyor needs to see that subsequent actions in response to the problems are identified, evaluated, and documented. The surveyor looks for an interdisciplinary approach to patient care and especially to quality assurance. Within the Joint Commission scope, the unit manager needs to help the staff understand the reasons for standards and assist in meeting them in the most creative ways. In the obstetrical services, the state department of health maintains the regulatory power over standards for these units and surveys at least annually. The staff should know what the standards are and be able to document how the unit meets these standards.

Decision-Making in Leadership

There are other times when the decisions about the operation of a unit seem to come from sources other than the staff itself. Vroom and Vetton (1973) developed a decision tree that assists in understanding of the decision levels (Table 8–2). The decision tree helps staff understand the forces that impact their environment. Most nursing leaders today make

Table 8–2.
Vroom and Vetton Decision Tree

Decisions may be reached in one of the following ways:

- The leader makes a decision without consulting anyone and assumes full accountability
- The leader makes a decision after informally consulting one or two people in the organization
- The leader makes a decision after convening a task force to analyze the problem
- The leader makes a decision with direct reports
- The leader asks direct reports to decide on a solution and agrees to support the decision

every effort to move as far down the tree as possible to create an empowering environment.

Fear of Power

One of the most inhibiting factors in hospitals and health care settings currently is fear of power. Many staff are afraid to express their views because of fear of reprisal or fear of loss of status in the work group. This fear is present all through the organization. Staff is afraid of managers and managers may be afraid of staff. Administrators may be afraid of the state or the Joint Commission. Physicians may be afraid of their colleagues who have power on the credentials committee. An organization that is riddled with fear cannot be creative. An organization that is riddled with fear cannot be empowered. An organization that is riddled with fear cannot be a learning organization interested in continuous quality improvement.

Fear in an organization has a very deleterious effect on the power of the organization as a whole. Ryan and Oestrich (1991) talk at length about the high cost of fear to the organization. The primary enemy of fear is trust. Every manager and leader should strive to build trust and enhance communication. Secrets, closed-door sessions, surprise decisions, and lack of participation feed fear and undermine trust. Cycles of mistrust feed on each other until commitment is gone and staffs are permanently in a we-they, victim's mentality. Mistrust is further inflamed by inappropriate decisions that ignore the best opinions of front-line caregivers, managers, and patients.

Effective leadership involves the wise use of power. Bennis and Nanus (1985) describe power as the basic energy to initiate and sustain action, translating intention into reality. Power is not synonymous with control but rather with mobilizing effort to a common and valued end. Effective leaders align employees around a vision of opportunity and change in the organization and focus their energy and resources. "Vision is the commodity of leaders and power is their currency" (Bennis & Nanus, 1985, p. 18). Such power should not be feared but nurtured in the organization.

Misuse of personal power can create fear in the organization and make alignment and commitment of employees impossible. Covey (1992) observed that coercive power is generated out of the fear of both the supervisor and the staff. The supervisor is afraid she or he will not get compliance or respect without the threat of force, and the staff nurse is afraid of reprisal. An example is the staff nurse on the night shift who, because of experience, is always in charge. In making assignments, she consistently provides herself with the lightest load and regularly takes a 2-hour nap at 2 AM. The newer staff members are afraid to reveal her practices for fear their workloads will further increase, and the charge nurse's passive-aggressive behavior will jeopardize patients. This scenario can go on for months. Staff may even leave without revealing the difficulty. The challenge for the manager, if she does not fire the charge nurse for sleeping, is to redirect the fear-inducing power of the charge nurse into positive, principle-centered power that focuses on an organizational set of values, nurturing commitment rather than fear.

The impact of coercive fear in all situations saps the energy of staff away from creativity and commitment to patient care. Such fear, whether generated by a staff nurse or a supervisor, increases silence, turnover, and the loss of potentially committed people.

The same fear of reprisal inhibits the accurate reporting of patient care incidents and errors. If, in the inappropriate use of power, a supervisor "disciplines" rather than "teaches" under such circumstances, the opportunities for improving clinical practice will be lost. Staff energy will be focused of covering up rather than on correcting the systems problems that contribute to an error or incident. Rewarding and encouraging creativity, which improves systems and clinical judgment, focus staff energy in positive directions.

CELEBRATING CLINICAL EXCELLENCE

Recognition comes in various forms and from various sources. In health care, recognition comes from patients, fellow colleagues, and leaders. One of the most obvious forms is money. Clinical ladders provide not only financial compensation for excellence but also public recognition to patients, staff, managers, and physicians. Although money is a motivator and a recognition, the ongoing confidence resulting from promotion on a clinical ladder can further enhance performance. For the ladder to work well, it is important that the clinical behaviors be embraced by the entire staff. Most ladders gain credibility by being staff-developed. The leader's responsibility in such a case is to create the vision and let the staff committee develop the tool. The ladder has the added advantage of articulating the most important clinical values of the organization. It also sends a very strong message that excellent clinical practice is so important that it is worth more money. Ladders are a celebration of clinical excellence.

Recognition celebrations are another way to promote clinical excellence. Many health care institutions have an annual celebration in which individual staff members are identified by their peers for their patient care and teamwork. "Nurse of the Year" celebrations enhanced with a motivating outside speaker focus attention on role models and help to underscore values.

LEADING CLINICAL STAFF

Thinking and Planning Role

Each individual nurse manager brings unique strengths and weaknesses to the role. It behooves the nurse leader to spend time with each staff nurse to accomplish two objectives:

- Outline and agree on expectations in the relationship.
- Create a strategic plan for the unit that grows out of the commonly embraced values of the patient care unit.

Although this "thinking" time is difficult to find, it is very important for the development of the staff as well as the success of the nurse manager. Identifying expectations in the relationship will help the staff understand what the unit leader needs in the way of information for the larger unit picture. It is also a way to help the leader identify what the staff needs in the way of guidance and reassurance.

The planning sessions help both the unit leader and the staff define the role of the unit within the larger organizational structure, including both clinical care and development of culture. For example, if a nurse manager is trying to lead a staff toward a self-governance model and the administration is against developing a salaried model, the direction the nurse manager takes may be quite different. She or he may focus on clinical empowerment rather than compensation or management. If the staff opposes the idea of being salaried when both administration and the unit leader want to move in that direction, the leadership may need to back off and take more time to build trust. Forcing the issue will undermine relationships, whereas involving the staff in the design of the model will build trust and confidence.

The unit leader is in fact the chief operating officer of the patient care unit. It is the leader's responsibility on a day-to-day basis to see to it that the nursing staff have what they need to deliver care and that the nurse-power is present with appropriate clinical expertise to provide safe and effective care to patients and families. The nurse manager operates within the framework of the mission of the institution and of the nursing service. The leader and the staff together identify their mission in the bigger picture and create the ownership necessary for good teamwork.

Teaching and Coaching Role

In adopting a teaching and coaching role in relationship to the staff, the unit leader is in a perfect position to serve as a role model. Peters and Austin (1985) outline five coaching roles: educating, sponsoring, coaching, counseling, and confronting.

The *educating* role requires great flexibility because each staff member needs something different. Those needs come out in day-to-day activities, and some can be identified in discussions about role expectations. Listening is a major talent in the teaching and coaching role. A very effective technique involves asking the appropriate questions to bring the person to his or her own conclusions about a problem. When this technique is successful, the staff nurse is then encouraged to use the same approach with her patient care team, resulting in more staff ownership, better patient care decisions, and less dependence.

Sponsoring leads the staff into new territory. The development of a unit-based quality assurance program is an excellent example of sponsoring. The unit leader selects a staff nurse with leadership skills

and an interest in quality improvement. The staff nurse works closely with the quality assurance department to develop unit-based criteria, with the help of a small unit committee. The RN keeps the unit leader informed and looks to the manager for prompting and for ideas. In reality, the unit leader lets the staff nurse manage the project and stands by to coach and encourage. Careful attention should be paid to allowing the staff to take full credit for projects that the unit leader sponsors. Understanding when to "let go" and permit the staff to own the project is key to successful sponsoring.

Coaching and *counseling* are approaches designed to develop and fine-tune clinical as well as leadership skills. For example, the staff nurse team leader has a multidisciplinary team to manage a caseload of 50 patients, 10 of whom are less than 1 week out of hospital care. There are three people available on the team on a certain day, the team leader, a nurse's aide, and a physical therapist. The 10 newly discharged patients require an assessment to confirm continuing progress. After reviewing the clinical status of the patients with all team members, the physical therapist agrees to see four of the rehab patients, while the nurse assistant visits three patients needing personal care, one of whom is a rehab patient. The team leader will visit two newly admitted patients and one long-term hospice family in need of pain management review and support. The remaining two newly discharged patients are postpartum families who needed a lot of teaching on their initial visits. The mothers and babies were doing well, but the team leader's priorities usually include newborns. Frustrated by the heavy visit load, the team leader consults the area manager for support. The manager reviews the distribution of work with the staff nurse and walks through possible options as the nurse perceives them. With the coaching of the manager, the nurse feels safe in making phone assessments for the two postpartum families with a follow-up visit and teaching plan the next day.

Leading a patient care team in any environment requires a firm knowledge of the team's clinical ability, a clear understanding of the plan of care, and an ability to rearrange priorities based on patient need and safety. The coach leads the staff to their own answers, reinforcing critical thinking skills and sound clinical judgment.

Confrontation is the most adversarial of the techniques discussed. Usually confrontation occurs when one member of the staff has not met the agreed expectations. An example is the situation involving a staff nurse team leader responsible for a team of four who are caring for a patient load of 16 patients on a pulmonary medical-surgical unit. The team includes a respiratory therapist, a nurse's aide, and an LPN who gives medications. The patient load is heavy and the team needs to be highly organized to complete the work of the morning and review the plan of care for all 16 patients. The respiratory therapist leaves the unit to retrieve missing equipment without reporting off to the team leader and is gone for 30 minutes. The team has made a commitment to the principle that each member will report off to a team leader before leaving the unit. The team leader must confront the therapist and remind members of the commitment to patient care and good communication. While there were no untoward consequences from the team member's oversight in this example, the values of the team are reinforced and the need for the rule acknowledged in a productive and positive way. If there is not agreement because of a difference in values or priorities, then the "fit" of team members comes into question and the commitment of the individual members is a problem.

Confrontation provides the opportunity for the unit leader to bring out the individual nurse's role expectations and to evaluate progress against goals. A review of performance gives the unit leader the framework within which to provide straightforward feedback to the staff nurse and assess chances for success in the role. Methods for new levels of support for the nurse can be identified. Assessment of the nurse's "fit" on the patient care team can be evaluated. A confrontation interchange provides the unit leader an opportunity to explore the culture of the unit with the staff and to help the individual understand the formal and informal expectations of the team. The structured format of an evaluation creates a point of entry for the unit leader to help the nurse adjust to the culture and become a more integral part of the unit team.

LEADING ALLIED HEALTH COLLEAGUES

One of the most important relationships in the delivery of patient care is the nurse's relationship with the allied health and support departments. If directors of those departments are patient-focused, their staff will likely be patient-focused as well. If the departments see their customer as the patient, then the timely delivery of service, the collaboration with nursing staff, and the trust that builds around shared values is evident. If, on the other hand, there is a sense of competition and each department is worried about whether they are doing more work than the others, the focus on patients is gone and dissension builds. Collaboration with allied departments at the level of unit leadership is critical to the role-modeling process at the staff level. Once again, staff watch the behavior of the leaders and interpret what is important from their behaviors.

If departments are working well together, there is a mutual respect and an enhancement of clinical depth. If the pharmacist and the nurse are focused on clinical practice and patient care, the pharmacist brings additional clinical depth to the nurse in education about drugs while the nurse shares patient information with the pharmacist that enhances clinical judgment and job satisfaction. Individual relationships with staff in the allied health department give the nurse a chance to build alliances that provide mutual support and collaboration. The result is improved patient care.

For example, a physician has ordered intravenous antibiotics for a patient with pneumonia. The order gets to the pharmacy by computer, but 4 hours later the drug has not arrived. The exasperated nurse calls the pharmacist to inquire about the delay, only to reach a defensive and frustrated pharmacy clerk who explains that they are very busy. To the detriment of the patient's status, the antibiotics arrive 2 hours later. If the nurse had shared the urgency of the patient need with the pharmacist, the priorities within the department may have been altered. The drug would have arrived in a timely fashion. The patient would have been the customer instead of the exasperated nurse. Smooth teamwork results in improved communication and patient-centered alliances.

As we shoot the sacred cows we protect regarding patient care delivery models, we can come together around a patient-focused care model. Alliances with other departments can be enhanced as trust builds and values are shared. Because a true multidisciplinary approach requires the best thinking of all allied health departments, the planning of new models should involve the best of the clinical thinkers from each department. Imagine the challenge of identifying everything that needs to be done for a patient and having the best, most cost-effective person there to do it. Such planning requires that everyone leave egos and fears at the door and work from a blank sheet of paper. It requires that the entire team come together around what each member is are passionate about with respect to patient care and create new ways to deliver that care. It demands strong alliances and teamwork at the bedside for best patient care.

It is in the climate of the well-functioning team that the nurse has a major voice. The team must function not as individuals but as a unit, with some of the following characteristics:

- Team members collaborate rather than compete.
- Each team member brings individual styles, ideas, and biases to the group.
- Each team member represents and advocates for the patient from a unique clinical perspective
- Team members can agree to disagree.
- Team members understand one another's style, ways of perceiving, and differences in language.
- Each team member is accountable to himself or herself, to the other members of the team, and to the patient and family.
- Leadership moves around the team from member to member, depending on the issue at hand.

Within these parameters, each team member carries a leadership role that is important to the organization of the patient's care.

SUMMARY

Clinical leadership in today's health care institutions must be multitalented and diverse. Nursing leaders must be clinically competent to be credible while assuming the roles of politician, planner, coach, educator, financier, and diplomate. They must be team builders, patient advocates, and statisticians. Leadership and staff must be passionate about what they believe in with regard to patient care and health care delivery. Although the central focus may be on patients and staff, clinical leaders must understand and be able to articulate the cost-versus-quality is-

sues and how they fit into the future financial structure of our health care system. The nurse is the integrator of care whether leading a patient care team or a multidisciplinary management group.

■ DISCUSSION QUESTIONS ■

1. Discuss the impact of environment on nursing leadership.
2. Compare and contrast the traditional and current roles of leaders and managers.
3. What is the importance of informal leadership in the clinical environment?
4. Compare and contrast the styles of nursing leaders that you know.
5. How does the culture of an organization influence clinical practice?
6. Discuss ways in which nursing leaders can build an empowering environment.
7. How should decision-making occur in nursing unit operations?
8. What impact can the fear of power have on clinical leadership?
9. Discuss the roles of nursing leaders as integrators of care.
10. What are some creative ways to celebrate clinical excellence?

■ LEARNING ACTIVITIES ■

1. You are an internal nursing consultant who helps new managers adjust to their role. Deidre B. has called you for help because she is unable to effect change on her nursing unit. You know a large part of Deidre's problem is her immediate director who is controlling and refuses to allow her staff any autonomy. Other managers have confided this to you. How can you help Deidre?
2. Your nursing unit has recently done an exemplary job in redesigning their model of practice. You want to reward them by celebrating their clinical excellence. You take this plan to your immediate supervisor who refuses to acknowledge their work, stating that she cannot "promote one nursing unit over another and show favoritism." How would you handle this situation?

■ BIBLIOGRAPHY ■

American Hospital Association (1993). *Nursing Leadership: Preparing for the Twenty-first Century*. Chicago: American Organization of Nurse Executives.

Ashton J, Wilkerson P (1996). Establishing a team based coaching process. *Nursing 95* 27(3):48n–48q.

Bellman GM (1993). *Getting Things Done When You Are Not in Charge*. New York: Simon & Schuster.

Bennis W, Nanus B (1985). *Leadership Strategies for Taking Charge*. New York: Simon & Schuster.

Charns MP, Smith-Twekesbury LJ (1993). *Collaborative Management in Health Care: Implementing the Integrative Organization*. San Francisco: Jossey-Bass Publishers.

Covey SR (1992). *The 7 Habits of Highly Effective People*. New York: Simon & Schuster.

Covey SR, Mervill AR, Merrill RR (1994). *First Things First*. New York: Simon & Schuster.

Drucker PF (1992). *Managing for the Future*. New York: Truman Talley Books/Dutton.

Fritz R (1991). *Creating*. New York: Fawcett Columbine.

Gillies DA (1989). *Nursing Management: A Systems Approach*. Philadelphia: WB Saunders.

Koeckeritz J, Stockbridge R, Zann C (1995). A leadership development series. *Nursing Management* 26(10):48ii–48ll.

Mcdermott K, Laschinger K, Shamian J (1996). Work empowerment and organizational commitment. *Nursing Management* 27(5):44–47.

Peters T, Austin N (1985). *A Passion for Excellence*. New York: Random House.

Ryan K, Oestrich D (1991). *Driving Fear Out of the Workplace*. San Francisco: Jossey-Bass Publishers.

Sanders B, Davidson A, Price S (1996). The unit nurse executive. *Nursing Management* 27(1):42–45.

Senge PM (1990). *The Fifth Discipline*. New York: Doubleday.

Senge PM (1994). *The Fifth Discipline Fieldbook*. New York: Doubleday

Stark J (1995). Critical thinking: The road less traveled. *Nursing 95* 24(11):53–56.

Trofino J (1996). Vision: A professional model for nursing practice. *Nursing Management* 27:43–47.

Vroom V, Vetton (1973). *Leadership and Decision-Making*. Pittsburgh: University of Pittsburgh Press.

9 Time Management

Betsy Frank, RN, PhD

"If I could save time in a bottle, the first thing that I'd like to do . . ."

Jim Croce, *Time in a Bottle*

L E A R N I N G   O B J E C T I V E S

This chapter will enable the learner to:
1. Identify factors that affect an individual's use of time.
2. Discuss factors that facilitate and inhibit the effective use of time.
3. Analyze factors that have an impact on time management strategies in the clinical area.

INTRODUCTION

As Jim Croce's song reminds us, time, for most, is a precious commodity (Fig. 9–1). All nurses have competing demands on their time. At any one instant nurses are employees, students, spouses, parents, children, or any combination of these. A particular nurse may have been assigned a paper for a class, but she is scheduled to work the next 4 days in a row. And, on one of those days she wants to go watch her child's school play after the workday is done.

In the work environment, patients, other nurses and health care providers, supervisors, and those who are supervised make what seem like impossible demands on any one nurse. In a typical shift on a busy medical-surgical unit, a staff nurse might have to admit five patients and discharge eight as well as supervise other health care personnel. If the work environment is a home health agency, the nurse may have to give care to six clients and do intake assessments on two others, all in 8 to 12 hours. Those in managerial roles might have to attend several meetings, prepare reports, and counsel personnel.

It is no wonder time management is a popular topic at seminars and in the literature. Stephen Covey's (1989) *The Seven Habits of Highly Effective People* and Kenneth Blanchard and Spencer Johnson's (1983) *The One Minute Manager* have been best sellers for nurses and other busy people.

Most nurses are looking for that one bottle to

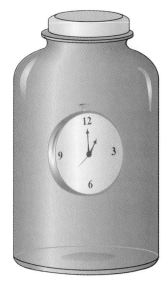

Figure 9–1. Time in a bottle.

115

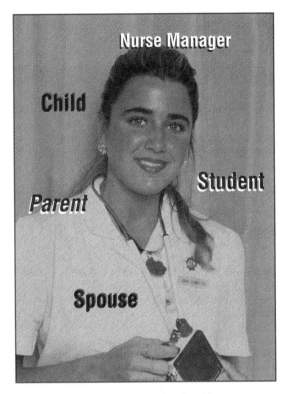

Figure 9–2. The multiple roles played by nurses.

package all their precious time. After all, if they can manage their time better, they can become more effective in their jobs and in their personal lives (Fig. 9–2).

INFLUENCES ON THE USE OF TIME MANAGEMENT STRATEGIES

Before nurses can make adjustments in how time is used, it is necessary to understand their personal inclinations for managing that time. Then, they can choose time management strategies that are most likely to fit with their own preferences.

Edward Hall, a noted anthropologist, and his coauthor (1990) point out that how time is managed may be a factor of cultural upbringing. They define two primary time management styles. Persons who have a monochronic orientation are often of Northern European extraction and are very time-oriented.

They like to do one thing at a time. Deadlines are important, as is adherence to well thought-out plans. Interruptions are most irritating to those with monochronic time preferences. Personal space is also most important.

Polychronic time-oriented people often have Mediterranean, Latin American, African-American, or Arabic cultural backgrounds. They can do many things at once, are easily distracted, and in fact tolerate interruptions. Deadlines are goals, not absolutes. People with polychronic orientations can change plans more easily than those with monochronic time management styles (Bluedorn et al, 1992).

Davidhizer, Giger, and Turner (1994) note that tendencies toward a monochronic or a polychronic time management style are ingrained through childhood experiences. In families and in schools, certain styles of time management are rewarded. Davidhizer et al (1994) also state that in response to stress, one may alter time management strategies to adapt to circumstances such as going back to school. Marriage partners may change the way time is handled to match spousal preferences.

Problems in the workplace can arise when co-workers do not understand how others view time. When those who can handle many tasks at once work with some who cannot, anger and conflict may arise. The nurse who can handle an admission while checking physician orders may express dismay at the person who can only do one task at a time. Nurses who are monochronic by nature get irritated with a cluttered work environment. They may also be the ones who are always picking up after others. Of course, no one has a "pure" time management orientation. However, understanding personal inclinations, as well as others' preferences, may go a long way in dissipating conflict due to differences in time management styles.

The way time is handled may also be gender-related. Hessing (1994) interviewed clerical workers and found that these women closely linked their own timetables with those of the other members of their households. While the work schedule was at the center of the day's events, other activities such as housework, child care, and the like were tightly woven into a deliberate pattern. Often women constructed more time by doing several tasks at once. For example, they did laundry while helping with their children's homework. These women also planned ahead for emergencies.

One might surmise that since most nurses are women they may have unique abilities that allow them to function effectively in a high-stress work environment. In any work setting, staff nurses and managers plan and implement a variety of routine activities that can be interrupted at any time with urgent matters that require immediate attention.

Another way of looking at time management is to consider it in a larger sense. Covey (1989) challenges his readers to think of time management not just as managing time, but as managing one's personal life. According to him, day-to-day organization is important, but so is long-term planning. Covey recommends that one remain in tune with long-term goals as daily activities are carried out.

Think about the job held or potential future employment. Does the current or future job fit with long-term career goals? Does this job allow integration of all the roles played? If not, perhaps a job change is on the horizon or a potential job may not be the one to achieve.

Consider Cathy, who has been a nurse for 20 years. Her children are in elementary and middle school. She is not ready to pursue advanced education, but is very committed to her nursing career. She has been working day shifts as a clinical manager, but finds that she cannot attend her children's sports events or volunteer in their classrooms. A managerial position opens up on nights. She applies and is accepted. Now she finds she can sleep during the day, participate in her children's after-school activities and, on her days off, school day events, **and** have a rewarding career.

DIAGNOSING OUR PERSONAL TIME MANAGEMENT STYLE

Most time management diagnostic tools are rooted in the American business culture, which has a primarily monochronic outlook. If one takes into consideration different styles, scoring of these tools must be interpreted with caution. Nevertheless, these tools are useful in that they do point out personal time management preferences.

Take a moment and complete the diagnostic tool in Table 9–1. When scoring the instrument, score a

Table 9–1.
Diagnostic Test: You and Time

	Often	Some-times	Rarely
1. Do you handle each piece of paperwork only once?	☐	☐	☐
2. Do you begin and finish projects on time?	☐	☐	☐
3. Do people know the best time to reach you?	☐	☐	☐
4. Do you do something every day that moves you closer to your long-range goals?	☐	☐	☐
5. When you are interrupted, can you return to your work without losing momentum?	☐	☐	☐
6. Do you deal effectively with long-winded callers?	☐	☐	☐
7. Do you focus on preventing problems before they arise rather than solving them after they happen?	☐	☐	☐
8. Do you meet deadlines with time to spare?	☐	☐	☐
9. Are you on time to work, to meetings, and to events?	☐	☐	☐
10. Do you delegate well?	☐	☐	☐
11. Do you write daily To-Do Lists?	☐	☐	☐
12. Do you finish all the items on your To-Do List?	☐	☐	☐
13. Do you update in writing your professional and personal goals?	☐	☐	☐
14. Is your desk clean and organized?	☐	☐	☐
15. Can you easily find items in your files?	☐	☐	☐
Subtotal			
	× 4	× 2	× 0
Total			

4 for every item placed in the "often" category, 2 for those items scored as "sometimes," and zero for those marked "rarely." A score of 49 or above indicates being highly organized and in control most of the time. A score in this range probably also indicates a monochronic time orientation. A score below 24 might indicate frequent frustration and disorganization. However, a score in this range may also indicate tendencies toward a polychronic time orientation, which may appear to others as evidence of disorganization but which, in fact, may really indicate competent handling of one's time.

TIME MANAGEMENT IN THE WORK ENVIRONMENT

Whether nurses work in an acute care setting, home health agency, or long-term care, an 8- to 12-hour shift never seems to be enough time to complete all that is assigned. In addition to giving direct care in an acute setting, home health care agency, or clinic, an individual nurse may have a committee or inservice meeting to attend. Charting and paperwork will consume much of the day. It is a daunting task, especially since most nurses chose their career to deliver direct patient care.

With budget constraints in the current health care environment, however, many organizations have redesigned how care is delivered. Now more than ever, nurses must have the skills not only to organize personal time in the workplace, but also to coordinate the activities of other workers. In fact, the roles of staff nurse and manager are blended in many cases. Chapter 10 will help with the specifics of coordinating the work of others.

FACTORS THAT INHIBIT EFFECTIVE TIME MANAGEMENT

In lives that often seem frantic, several things may inhibit effective time management. Marrelli (1993) identifies three behavior patterns that keep managers and others from using time wisely. They are procrastination, perfectionism, and lack of prioritizing.

Procrastination has often been viewed as a block to effective use of time. How often are cumbersome

Research Box 9–1
What Do Nurses Do in the Work Day?

Data obtained through a work sampling technique were collected from six specialty units in a large hospital. Each unit was observed for a 7-day period, with data recorded in 15-minute time blocks during an 8-hour shift. The work sampling checklist was developed by the staff at the study hospital and from a review of the literature. Observations were placed in the following categories: (1) with patient, (2) patient chart, (3) preparation of therapies, (4) shift change activities, (5) professional interaction, (6) miscellaneous clinical, (7) checking physician orders, (8) unit-oriented inservice, (9) paperwork, (10) phone communications, (11) supplies, (12) miscellaneous nonclinical, and (13) unknown. Interrater reliability for the observations ranged from 91 to 100%. Results showed that in an 8-hour shift, 31% of the time was spent with patients. Forty-five percent of the time was spent in indirect clinical patient care, including charting and preparing therapies. Nonclinical activities such as obtaining supplies and doing paperwork accounted for 10% of the time. Finally, 13% of the time was spent in miscellaneous activities such as breaks, and 1% of the time could not be categorized. The authors recommended that support personnel be increased so that nurses could delegate nonclinical activities. They also suggested that paperwork be computerized to increase the number of clinical activities performed by professional nurses. Whether implementation of these tactics as part of re-engineering efforts will increase nurse satisfaction, maintain or increase quality, and decrease costs remains to be seen.

Data from Hendrickson G, Doddato TM, Kovner C (1990). How do nurses use their time? *Journal of Nursing Administration* 20(3):31–37.

tasks such as writing a report put off in favor of doing the easy jobs such as filing or sorting through e-mail? For some, having a deadline only frustrates and prevents task completion. However, for others, deadlines help to create plans or prioritize the "to do" list. Some nurses work better under pressure, while others need lots of lead time to get a job done. Knowing how managers and their staff work with respect to deadlines can lead to better teamwork. The goal is quality work outcomes no matter when the task is done.

Perfectionism is a common personality attribute in nurses. Perhaps nursing education supports this trait because students learn early on that mistakes in the clinical arena can in some instances be harmful to patients. However, wanting to be perfect and having the desire to do a job right are two different things. Perfectionism can lead to procrastination for fear of making a mistake or it can cause nurses to do a job over and over again to get it just right. In either case, a better product might not result. In essence, quality must be balanced with the economic and personal costs that are incurred when tasks are delayed by perfectionism (Forsyth, 1994).

Having reasonable standards for practice helps to alleviate the need to be perfect (Forsyth, 1994). Consider a nurse manager who must write a performance appraisal. The human resources department has provided guidelines for completing the appraisal. If the guidelines are followed, the employee should have a reasonable evaluation of job performance. The manager could spend an hour or so writing the appraisal, which is based on data gathered throughout the evaluation period. Or, the manager could spend 4 or 5 hours trying to get each word perfect. So, the question could be asked, does perfection in wording lead to a more accurate performance appraisal? The answer is, probably not.

Not being able to *prioritize* may also impair one's ability to be an effective time manager. If nurses are coordinating care given by themselves and others, they need to be able to determine what has to be done immediately and what can wait for a later time in the workday or workweek. Again, consider Cathy, the night nurse who is the charge person for a busy medical nursing unit. When she comes to work at 7:00 PM, she attends the change of shift report. Immediately following the report she needs to work with her staff to assign patient care appropriately. If she has her own patient assignment, she has to plan how she will give care while coordinating the care others deliver. Since she is a charge nurse, she should make rounds on all patients, including her own, right after report so that she can learn about anything that might require her attention. What would happen if she just began to give care to her own patients first? She might lose her ability to anticipate events that would demand action on her part. Such a situation might include assisting with a discharge at 9:00 PM that evening at the same time medications for her patients are due to be given. Her rounds would give her the opportunity to see what needs to be done for the patient going home. Then, she would not be surprised when the patient is going out the door and some portion of the discharge activities was not completed.

Covey (1989) also suggests that prioritization should take into consideration one's life goals. He places activities into four categories: (1) important and urgent, (2) not important but urgent, (3) not important and not urgent, and (4) important but not urgent. He advises that top priority should be given to activities such as relationship building and acting on new opportunities. These activities are in the "important but not urgent category." His contention is that importance is related to outcomes and relationship building will have more impact on work and personal life outcomes than attending to some mail and answering some phone calls. Covey does not suggest, however, that one ignore urgent activities, just that urgency should not dominate how time is spent. If one is always concerned with urgency, stress and burnout may result and long-term goals may get relegated to that never-accomplished list.

TIPS FOR EFFECTIVE TIME MANAGEMENT

With some understanding of how personal styles and time-wasting behaviors influence time management, nurses can choose the most appropriate strategies to enhance their time management effectiveness in their personal and work settings. The strategies discussed here are compiled from the many tips suggested in the myriad articles and books written about this quintessential topic of concern for nurse managers.

Keep a Time Log or Calendar

A daily hour-by-hour log can help to give structure to the multitude of things that must be accomplished (Ryan et al, 1994). For instance, such a log could help nurses to organize administration of medications and treatments, teaching sessions, home visits for their patients, and committee meetings.

A monthly calendar provides structure for the

day-to-day things in work and personal lives (Marrelli, 1993). A pocket calendar may be useful if it needs to be readily at hand for appointments away from one's office or patient care unit. A wall calendar is important if several people need to coordinate schedules. Reviewing the monthly and daily calendars can give a sense of how overall time is spent and may give clues for how time could be used more efficiently.

Daily "to do" lists help to prioritize what needs to get done and help to focus on the outcomes to be accomplished. The list also helps one to reorganize when urgent matters intrude on plans.

Focus on Getting Started While Keeping the Goal in Mind

Nurse leaders and their staff need to balance these into two seemingly disparate approaches. Puetz and Thomas (1995) propose that getting started allows motivation to propel activity toward task completion. However, Thompson and Huston (1994) suggest that looking at the final goal allows for thinking backwards and breaking down a task into manageable parts. Their advice is to think of the last task before job completion. If that is known, then one can identify all the other tasks that must precede.

Anticipate

By taking a few moments of each day and the beginning of each week and trying to think of those things not planned for or not known that may arise, one can plan for the unexpected. Thus, like the women in Hessing's (1994) study, nurses could be more flexible in dealing with urgent matters. For leaders, being in close contact with staff allows them to be aware of anything that might lead to work absences. Back-up staffing plans can then be made.

Organize That Paperwork

Know what to keep and what to throw away (Van Auken, 1995). Do files need to contain every agency newsletter? Probably not. But notification of policy changes should always be kept in a readily accessible place.

Traditional time management wisdom warns that each piece of paperwork should be handled only once (Ryan et al, 1994). In reshuffling papers many times, important items may get lost. If possible, reply immediately to requests, post important items, or file important items so that they can be easily retrieved. Anything that is not important should be thrown away.

Use Resources Wisely

Technology has greatly enhanced the ability of all health care professionals to communicate effectively and efficiently. By using voice mail and electronic mail, one can communicate with colleagues within and outside the employing organization without regard to the actual presence of the other person at the time a message is sent. Likewise, messages can be retrieved and answered during time that is personally convenient.

Technology, however, has not replaced the written word. Hard copies of references such as procedure manuals, kept readily at hand, can help leaders, managers, and staff to quickly locate needed information (Kroll, 1993). As such manuals become computerized, more hardware will be needed to access the information. Likewise, routine information could be placed in a memo book or on the computer. Thus, time could be better spent with communication that really needs face-to-face contact (Van Auken, 1995).

Having adequate supplies and putting in place a system for monitoring the need for replacement of materials is another essential element of efficient time management. How irritating is it if staff have to wait for supplies that should be readily available? Or, what if the manager is in the midst of compiling a report and the printer cartridge runs dry?

Colleagues are resources as well. Promoting teamwork can go a long way toward achieving organizational goals effectively and efficiently (Van Auken, 1995).

Be Positive and Attentive to Personal Needs

Attitude can affect a manager's ability to use time judiciously (De Baca, 1987). Feeling overburdened leads to feeling tired and hinders one's ability to be productive. By trying to refocus negative attitudes, one can see problems as challenges rather than road blocks to success.

Nurse leaders and others should also make time each day for attending to their own health (Lynch, 1991). Reading something for fun, taking a walk, or going to an aerobics class helps to manage stress. And, during the workday, making time for breaks is essential to one's long-term well-being. One effective strategy for assuring personal time is to write down the activity on a personal calendar (Thompson & Huston, 1994).

Learn to Say "No"

Only so much time is available to spend (Pagana, 1994). Nurse leaders and others may feel guilty if they refuse to take on extra duties. However, one needs to decide whether what is requested can be accomplished effectively in the time given. If one needs to acquire new skills and knowledge, can that be done, or is the acquisition even desired, given long-term goals?

Keeping a list of every committee one is on and every project to be completed can help nurse leaders to see when one more task is just too much. Van Auken (1995) goes so far as to say, when one commitment is added, another should be deleted. This caveat could apply to longer-term obligations as well as daily meetings. Do you need to be present at all scheduled meetings? Could information be gained through meeting minutes instead, if personal input to decisions made at some meetings is not needed ?

Conduct an Effective Meeting

Meetings in and of themselves can be time wasters. To promote efficient meetings, prepare an agenda that outlines the reason for the meeting, and stick to the agenda. Start the meeting on time and end it on time. Although some free-flowing conversation is necessary for team building, the meeting chairperson should redirect conversations that get too far afield of the topic at hand (Forsyth, 1994).

The place where meetings are held can also promote effective time management. A conference room may be a better meeting place than an office where the telephone may interrupt conversation (Forsyth, 1994).

End the Workday on Time

Lynch (1991) counsels nurses to end the workday as close to on time as possible. By prioritizing tasks to be done on a daily basis, one can gain some sense of what has to be done today and what can wait until another day. Since the workload is always expanding, one cannot realistically expect to complete all that is required each day. Staying longer and always taking work home may indicate that a lot of time has been wasted during the day.

STRIKING THE BALANCE

Each of these tips can help managers use time effectively and efficiently. However, the tips used are only good if they are integrated into one's personal style and the culture of the workplace. Davidson (1995b) even warns that the traditional tips may not actually be as useful as advertised. He invites individuals to create breathing spaces that are suited to the fast-changing health care environment. Breathing spaces, according to Davidson, help leaders to be flexible and handle the beforehand instead of aftermaths.

The key to understanding breathing spaces is to balance efficiency with what is effective (Fig. 9–3). In other words, a particular strategy may help save actual time, but may hinder overall effectiveness. For example, traditional wisdom suggests that paperwork should be handled as little as possible. Davidson (1995a) says, however, that some papers should be handled more than 20 times while other papers should not touch the desk. Traditional thought suggests that working smarter not longer is beneficial. Davidson submits that for some creative projects, working longer is the smart thing to do. Finally, he agrees with Covey (1989) that slowing down may actually be more efficient than working at an accelerated pace. Spending more time at one point may save time at a later date. Taking a few extra moments to organize one's day and analyze how chosen time management strategies fit with personal cultural and gender styles, as well as workplace characteristics, and to think about how each

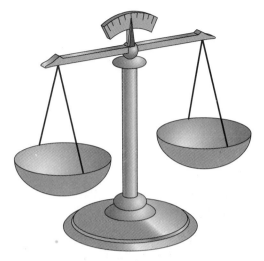

Figure 9–3. Striking the balance.

week or month fits into one's life plan will yield greater rewards than living moment to moment or day to day.

SUMMARY

Time is a precious commodity. How we spend it can have lasting impact on our overall lives. Yet, in the midst of busy days, we often cannot see how we can accomplish all we want and need to do. Taking a few moments to plan daily activities and periodically taking stock of our life goals and using time-management strategies that fit our personal style can help all of us to be more effective and efficient time managers.

■ DISCUSSION QUESTIONS ■

1. Your coworker Mary appears scattered, always doing multiple tasks at one time, such that you cannot tell what is being done. You, on the other hand, tackle one task and finish it before going on to another. Discuss the factors that shape the use of time by yourself and others.
2. You work in a busy educational services office at a visiting nurses' association. You are having trouble tracking the workflow in your office. Discuss ways in which you and your coworkers could

better coordinate schedules and keep track of the multiple activities that arise from your office and others.
3. You are considering going back to school. Using Covey's framework and ideas, identify what should influence your decision to go back to school and propose ways to overcome any obstacles.

■ LEARNING ACTIVITIES ■

Case 1

Donald is a unit coordinator for a 20-bed subacute unit at a community hospital. He has been on vacation for 1 week and returns to work on a Friday. On his first day back at work his staff, in addition to himself, are one RN, two LPNs, a nursing assistant, and a unit clerk. It is 7 AM and Donald must deal with the following items:

1. A stack of mail with return addresses as listed
   a. Hospital foundation
   b. Vice president of patient care services
   c. Educational services
2. A phone message saying that the weekend RN just called to say she will be out this weekend for a family funeral.
3. Team assignments need to be made.
4. A float nurse is assigned for 8 hours of a 12-hour shift and the staff has requested that she stay the entire 12-hour period.
5. The LPN has been assigned second lunch and she refuses, saying, "I always go to second lunch and I am tired of it!"
6. A crash cart needs checking.
7. The glucometer needs calibrating.

Prioritize the activities with regard to what needs immediate attention and what can wait. What time management strategies can Donald use to prioritize these activities? What might influence his decisions?

Case 2

Beth is a 33-year-old RN and single mother, enrolled in a bachelor's program. Today is her class night. However, she has been asked to attend a meeting at her place of employment, and her 8-year-old son is playing in a soccer game. He has complained that she has not attended many games this season. Of the three events, which one should Beth attend?

1. What strategies should she use to determine what event to attend?
2. Are there any strategies she could use to help reduce her conflict when making decisions regarding future events that may compete for her time?

■ BIBLIOGRAPHY ■

Alexander R (1992). *Common Sense Time Management.* New York, NY: AMACOM.

Blanchard K, Johnson S (1983). *The One Minute Manager.* New York, NY: Berkley Books.

Bluedorn AC, Kaufman CF, Lane PM (1992). How many things do you like to do at once? An introduction to monochronic and polychronic time. *Academy of Management Executive* 6(4):17–26.

Covey SR (1989). *The Seven Habits of Highly Effective People.* New York, NY: Simon & Schuster.

Croce J (1971). Time in a bottle. Available from: Denjac Music Co., MCA Music, New York.

Davidhizer R, Giger JN, Turner G (1994). Understanding monochronic and polychronic individuals in the workplace. *Clinical Nurse Specialist* 8:329, 334–336.

Davidson J (1995a). Roasting the sacred cows of time management. *The Prairie Rose* 63(3):10a.

Davidson J (1995b). Managing the beforehand: The benefits abound. A key breathing space principle. *The Prairie Rose* 63(3):11a.

DeBaca V (1987). So many patients, so little time. *RN* 50(4):32–33.

Forsyth P (1994). *First Things First: How to Manage Your Time for Maximum Performance.* London: Pittman.

Hall ET, Hall MR (1990). *Understanding Cultural Differences.* Yarmouth, ME: Intercultural Press.

Hendrickson G, Doddato TM, Kovner CT (1990). How do nurses use their time? *Journal of Nursing Administration* 20(3):31–37.

Hessing M (1994). More than clockwork: Women's time management in their combined workloads. *Sociological Perspectives* 37:611–633.

Kroll BN (1993). A good manager has to delegate. *RN* 56(2):23–26.

Lynch M (1991). P-a-c-e yourself: Tips on time management. *Nursing 91* 21(3):105–107.

Marrelli TM (1993). *Nurse Manager's Survival Guide: Practical Answers to Everyday Problems.* St. Louis, MO: Mosby.

Pagana KD (1994). Teaching students time management strategies. *Journal of Nursing Education* 33:381–383.

Puetz BE, Thomas DO (1995). Procrastination: A symptom of mental blocking. *RN* 58(8):22.

Ryan A, Weston S, Mangan P (1994). Professional development: Time management. *Nursing Times* 90(29):9–12.

Thompson BA, Huston JL (1994). How to break down tasks so they don't break you: Coping with overwhelming demands on your time. *Health Care Supervisor* 12(3):39–43.

Van Auken P (1995). A new strategy for time management. *Supervision* 56(1):3–6.

10 Supervision and Delegation

Enrica K. Singleton, DrPH, MBA, RN

LEARNING OBJECTIVES

This chapter will enable the learner to:

1. Understand the supervisory process and apply the concepts of supervision and delegation to clinical practice.
2. Describe the role and work tasks of a supervisor.
3. Describe the importance of appropriate delegation in today's health care environment.
4. Apply Fine's model of task analysis to redesign roles and tasks when planning and delivering patient care.

INTRODUCTION

The restructuring of the nursing organization within health care organizations, especially the change in the skill mix, has created the imperative for registered nurses to understand the supervisory process and master the skills of supervision and delegation. In addition to being responsible and accountable for their own practices, nurses must acknowledge the accountability they hold for the performance of other members of the health care team, particularly assistive and unlicensed personnel.

There is both legal and professional accountability in the supervisory process. Legal accountability is manifest when a supervisor is held responsible for the acts or omissions of subordinates in the event of a legal action against the organization. For example, if an unlicensed staff member left the side rail down on a bed and the patient suffered an injury, the supervisor could be named in a malpractice action. Professional accountability differs from legal accountability. For example, in the above situation, because the tasks had been delegated appropriately to a competent, trained staff member, the supervisor met the professional expectations of her role; that is, the supervisor was professionally competent. From the standpoint of professional accountability, as opposed to legal accountability, it is unlikely that this event would result in any professional or licensure censorship by a state board of nursing. Both types of accountability are present in acute, long-term, and community settings and are critical for successful patient care outcomes in the reformed health care system.

The supervisory process encompasses the concepts of *supervision* and *delegation*. Supervision and delegation are best described as control techniques that oversee work processes. These concepts have been part of nursing management for years. According to the still relevant definition offered by Beach (1985; p. 341), supervision is "the function of leading, coordinating, and directing the work of others to accomplish designated objectives." Supervisors seek to have groups accomplish the required work of the organization in a timely fashion as they seek to promote satisfaction and high morale among employees. Swansburg (1990) expands the definition of supervision, suggesting that supervisors must be concerned with what workers must know to perform their jobs competently. Assisting staff to acquire these skills is part of the supervisory process. Swansburg distinguishes between traditional supervision and modern supervision but acknowledges that both approaches involve planning work, making decisions, issuing detailed instructions to subordinates, and inspecting results.

Delegation, a part of the supervisory process, seeks to assign appropriately the work tasks to the best qualified individual. Modern supervision adds to these responsibilities an attention to a philosophy based on human dignity, individual differences, and growth potential.

In the traditional sense, supervisors and delegators are middle managers with responsibility for linking top- and first-line management layers. The supervisory process applies the concepts of supervision and delegation to all staff members who monitor and assign patient care. Supervisors report to managers above them and are reported to by staff. As managers of patient care, supervisors have knowledge that extends beyond traditional nursing care to organizational systems. In this chapter, the supervisory role is discussed from a clinical management perspective, and the supervisory process is seen as a vital function that occurs within the framework of patient care and human resource planning. Supervision and delegation are influenced by an organization's approach to job design, personnel policy and procedures, position descriptions, personnel recruitment, selection, transfer, promotions, layoffs, training, and personnel evaluation. In the final analysis, the delivery of quality nursing care is the ultimate purpose of supervision and delegation.

The purposes of this chapter are to examine the concepts of supervision and delegation and to suggest mechanisms to best allocate the work of nursing. An emphasis is placed on the assignment and supervision of work tasks in a changing health care environment.

THE SUPERVISORY ROLE

The concept of supervision, when discussed from the perspective of role, is, according to Bolman and Deal (1991; p. 144), "a position in a group or organization that is defined by expectations and the way the person who occupies a particular role is *expected* to behave in ways that fit the role." The supervisory role is what Stevens (1985) describes as an achieved role; the position is viewed as an accomplishment. Stevens (1985) further suggests three components of the role: the sociological, that is, what others expect from a person in this position; the rationalized, that is, the job function and re-

sponsibility as detailed in the job description; and the personal, that is, defined as how one chooses to enact a role based on one's uniqueness. The way supervisors portray their roles to others conveys their philosophy of supervision.

Hayes (1987) suggests that staff members view supervisors as powerful, with considerable authority in resource allocations and management decision-making. Historically, supervisory competence was the prime source of supervisory power, but now this competence is threatened continually because of the rapid pace of technological change. Modern-day supervisors spend a great deal of time attending to the business side, as opposed to the clinical side, of their areas of responsibility. Accordingly, their position grants them power to distribute materials and funds, redistribute workloads, redesign work processes, conduct performance appraisal procedures, and recommend pay raises.

Supervisors hold managers accountable for their performance in accomplishing the work required in their areas of responsibility. To effect this performance, supervisors must have the education, the skills, and the desire to achieve the objectives associated with the supervisory role.

Supervisory roles are examined from a historical, mentoring, networking, and power perspective.

Time-Honored Supervisory Roles

Supervisors must choose the approach to supervision that best meets their own management styles. The historical role of supervisors, as described by Mitzberg (1975), provides guidance to those who are seeking to establish or define their role. A supervisor's particular uniqueness and strengths determine the roles he or she models most frequently. These roles are defined in Table 10–1.

Although not exhaustive, this list provides one framework of roles for supervisors. Staff expectations of a supervisor's future behaviors usually are based, at least in part, on messages the supervisor sends through role-modeling behaviors. It is important to note that staff will mimic a supervisor's behaviors. For example, if supervisors handle disturbances through mediation and problem-solving, their staff can be expected to model similar behaviors when they handle disturbances. According to Bidwell and Brasler (1989), the modeling is passive.

Table 10–1.

Time-Honored Supervisory Roles

Figurehead: symbolic head with ceremonial functions

Leader: director of subordinates to goal achievement

Liaison: builder of communications networks

Monitor: scanner of the environment to keep abreast of changes pertinent to the job

Disseminator: distributor of information to appropriate personnel

Spokesperson: representative speaker for the area of responsibility

Entrepreneur: initiator of new projects

Disturbance handler: mediator and problem-solver

Resource allocator: distributor of resources

Negotiator: mediator between individuals and groups in the setting

The imitator identifies with the role model and internalizes and adopts the model's standards. If supervisors wish to push for the development of certain behaviors, they may choose the more active role of mentor.

Supervisors as Mentors

Mentoring leaders are role models who actively teach, coach, develop, and critique staff by guiding and facilitating career growth. Mentoring in nursing occurs when new graduates model their practices after an experienced nurse whose talents, skills, and quality of caring for patients are appealing. In essence, the new graduate admires and wishes to emulate the behaviors of the senior staff member.

The mentoring process may be formal or informal, but the supervisor who chooses the mentor role has special characteristics, which may include expert clinical skills, knowledge, experience, a desire to nurture, and an emotional commitment to his or her profession (Research Box 10–1).

Fields (1991) indicates that although mentoring is a popular phenomenon in nursing, it is not new.

Research Box 10–1

Mentor Characteristics

Darling's research using the "Measuring Mentor Potential Questionnaire" showed that the best mentors were at or near the top in one of the inspirer roles (model, envisioner, and energizer) and in the investor and supporter roles.

Darling LAW (1985). Becoming a mentoring manager. *The Journal of Nursing Administration* 15(6):43–44.

She identifies historical nurse leaders who had mentors; for example, the relationship between Nightingale and Sir Sidney Herbert, Secretary at War for the British government, was that of mentor and student.

The mentor-student relationship is always in transition, redefining itself and constantly undergoing adjustment. Frequent changes in the health care delivery system can lead to an atmosphere of uneasiness and role strain between the mentor and student. This strain is considerable when a mentor-student relationship begins without adequate attention to the "psychological fit" of the involved parties. Supervisors must assess potential relationships between mentors and students to prevent stressful relationships.

Supervisors as Holders of Power

Power may be conceptualized as the ability to change behavior regardless of whether individuals want their behavior changed. Successful nurse supervisors have learned to use some or all of their sources of positional power. The sources of supervisory power, as identified by Stevens (1985), are outlined in Table 10–2.

In this period of decentralization, in which important decisions are made at lower levels of the organization, positional power can provide a beginning point from which a supervisor's staff responds to management decisions.

Legitimate power is delegated by the administration of an organization and is directed towards persons who work within the organization. Expert power is implied in supervision and offers supervisors credibility. Decision-making and knowledge

Table 10–2.

Elements of Supervisory Power

- Knowledge and expert power of nursing, management, technology, and trends in nursing practice
- Network relations and links to informal channels within or outside of the institution
- Resource control with knowledge of access to resources and power to distribute or withhold same
- Decision-making or problem-solving ability with positional authority to dictate adherence to decisions
- Vision and leadership in one's craft, with the ability to identify, communicate, and pursue goals

power may be used when making decisions about patient care. Network power is used to stabilize and position nursing in times of organizational change and adaptation. Resource control is demonstrated when supervisors limit the number of unlicensed assistive personnel that can be assigned to a patient care area. A supervisor's use of positional authority is demonstrated as priorities are established for distributing financial and material resources. Ideally, in decentralized structures, supervisors and staff should work together when making some decisions.

An appropriate use of supervisory power is critical for staff satisfaction, patient outcomes, and continued organizational success. Supervisory power must be used to monitor health care trends and predict changes that will occur in areas of designated responsibility. The supervisory process directs that power be used correctly and wisely to influence and persuade staff to design strategies to promote quality, cost-effective patient care in a changing health care market.

The use of supervisory power depends largely on what has been the traditional role of supervisors in a health care organization. Power depends on the organization's culture of symbols, rituals, language, assumptions, and the overt behaviors that reflect organizational values. For example, consider a supervisor who is in an organization in which upper management values centralization and makes day-to-day operational decisions. In this setting, the nurse supervisor will have difficulty promoting empowerment to make situational decisions at the unit level, even though many decisions should be made by those who are closer to the source of activities.

If attempts are made to empower staff in such settings, the supervisor must be prepared to bolster staff morale if edicts from those in higher administration overturn staff decisions.

Supervisory Relationships

Relationships in the supervisory process are pivotal to the outcomes of patient care. Good supervision builds strong relationships, increases motivation, and enhances staff commitment to quality. Inadequate supervisory relationships can cause resentment, a lack of motivation, and chaos. Consider a scenario in which the nurse case manager lacks the power to negotiate with insurers about the length of time a patient will need in acute care. If a direct supervisor refuses to acknowledge the expert power of the case manager and the nurse's knowledge of the patient's need for additional resources, then the nurse case manager's power is being usurped by the supervisor. Supervisors are expected to analyze the roles they assign to staff and respect the power in the staff nurse role. Role behaviors in health care organizations must be within the constraints of licensure laws and statutes governing employment. For instance, without a standing order, a supervisor cannot order a staff nurse to discharge a patient without the knowledge and consent of the patient's physician, as this act is outside of the domain of nursing practice.

If supervisors are comfortable in the leadership role and are trusting of their staff, they are comfortable with strong managers, associates, and subordinates. A mutual respect for and knowledge of others' strengths and weaknesses can enhance the supervisor-staff relationship.

Supervisors and Networking

Networking and network building are important functions for supervisors. Building positive interagency relationships with groups, organizations, and institutions is important in the changing health care environment. Supervisors in health care organizations build and establish relationships that are formal or informal based on a negotiated discreet exchange ("I give you something, you give me something."), coercive and based on fear ("You give me this or else I'll . . . ."), or cooperative and purposive, based on a coalition for a common cause or goal.

Effective supervisors recognize the use of utilitarian, coercive, purposive, personal, and formal/legal strategies as they approach their duties in the health care organization. The importance of networking with colleagues in pharmacy, radiology, laboratory, and administration cannot be underemphasized as health care continues to change under managed care directives.

Identifying and cultivating strengths among staff and peers can help a supervisor accomplish an agenda. Successful performance brings the nurse supervisor's professional reputation to the attention of physicians, pharmacists, quality management coordinators, social workers, and other professionals. This is particularly important in managed care, as all disciplines and departments must work together to facilitate an early discharge of patients. On the strength of image and reputation, supervisors will experience greater ease in becoming very purposeful in working with small teams of people to accomplish organizational tasks. Consider the supervisor who leads a mock institutional survey in preparation for a visit from the Joint Commission for the Accreditation of Healthcare Organizations (JCAHO). This kind of activity can give the supervisor visibility, recognition, and an enhanced image for nursing throughout the organization.

SUPERVISORY WORK TASKS AND JOB FUNCTIONS

Supervisors historically have been charged with four work functions in an effort to accomplish the work of the organization. These functions are planning, organizing, controlling, and evaluating. Other supervisory functions are related to the adherence of standards.

Planning and Organizing

Planning

Planning is one of the basic functions of management. It is a process that is influenced by the purpose and mission of the organization, the philosophy of nursing care, unit goals, objectives, policies, and procedures. In addition, it is affected by the allocation of human, financial, and material resources, the nature of the patients/clients/customers, and the expectation of the payer groups. All managerial functions, such as organizing, staffing, directing, and controlling, require planning. A formal plan requires that managers commit to paper the ideas that guide their actions. For example, in managed care, cost containment is a critical issue. A supervisor might want to write, in conjunction with other departmental staff, a plan for reducing the length of time patients with certain diagnoses remain in the hospital or develop a critical path to recognize potential variances in patient care. (A complete discussion of critical paths is given in Chap. 3.) Planning occurs at all levels of patient care and supervision.

Organizing

The supervisory process implies coordination of resources to achieve efficient and effective goal attainment. This *organizational* function encompasses all activities necessary for delineating organizational goals, assembling human and material resources, structuring work and authority relationships, establishing communication channels, and adapting organizational responses to internal and external demands.

In the newly designed health care delivery system, supervisors must master the organizing function to restructure and reformulate the interfaces between changing human and material resources in a reasonably short time. The dictates of managed care with the accompanying fiscal constraints make this an important organizational function.

Controlling and Evaluating

Supervision carries with it the responsibility to exert *controls* in the environment to measure the outcomes of work processes. Control functions include attention to work flow systems, information systems, patient care delivery models, staff vacation and holiday time, staff remuneration, and promotion. Many control functions are delineated in organizational policy and procedures.

Evaluation assists with determining the nature of

these controls and is usually a set of procedures or guidelines used to assess the work outputs to gain information about work goals, activities, outcomes, impact, and costs. For example, an evaluation of staffing patterns on a particular unit can assist supervisors to determine the appropriateness of the current pattern of practice or to establish criteria for an acceptable staffing pattern and personnel mix. The supervisory process uses systematic procedures to evaluate periodic performance as well as examine the utilization of resources and services within the organization. A more detailed discussion of performance management can be found in Chapter 17.

Control and Evaluation of Organizational Standards

Standards are descriptive expectations that measure performance in specific areas. Standards convey organizational values. Values and standards guide dimensions of the structure of the organization, health care practices, the nursing personnel system, and human resource development.

Stevens (1985) discusses standards for quality control of patient care from the perspective of structure, process, and outcome. Structure-based standards address the way subject matter is systematized; for example, "there is a fail-safe system for removing outdated supplies from nursing units." Process standards measure the actions of the subject matter; for example, "the nursing division reassigns staff on each shift according to the classification system." Outcome standards measure the results as opposed to the process; for example, "absenteeism is reduced 50%."

Standards may be internal or external to an organization. For instance, an organizational standard may be an agreed-on decision to practice a case management delivery system, while national standards may be standards for clinical practice. Standards are used to plan and evaluate work processes while serving as a control mechanism for assuring appropriate outcomes. Standards may be measured against defined criteria and norms.

Standards are not evaluation instruments, but they do provide a yardstick for examining the quality of services provided. Hence, supervisors and leaders who are responsible for health care delivery systems must know the standards that are important to nursing and related health care disciplines.

EXTERNAL STANDARDS. Standards are derived from a variety of sources—federal, state, and local units of government, licensing agencies, accrediting organizations, professional organizations, trade associations, institutions (personnel policies), departments, patient care units, and individuals. Statements of standards must be readily available to personnel on patient care units. Standards provide a basis for measurement that is objective, achievable, practical, and flexible. Standards can be broken down into criteria that become the basis for measuring performance.

Standards requiring supervisory attention include education and practice standards determined by state boards of nursing. Supervision involves monitoring compliance to these standards and identifying staff whose practices vary from these standards. Supervisors and professional nurses should be aware of state law and associated penalties for nurses who violate standards of practice.

Many health care institutions voluntarily seek accreditation by JCAHO. This accreditation is a mark of distinction that implies that an organization meets the same external standards as similar groups across the nation. JCAHO standards focus on performance and outcomes. For example, one of its standards states, "The goal of the leadership function is for organizational leaders to provide the framework for planning, directing, coordinating, providing and improving health care services that are outcomes" (JCAHO, 1994; p. 29). Joint Commission representatives visit an organization and perform an audit to assess compliance to its standards. The Joint Commission has specific standards affecting nursing service that require nursing supervisors to work directly with staff to meet these criteria. Adherence to JCAHO standards is mandatory for organizations to maintain this premier accreditation.

Another set of important standards that requires supervisory oversight in evaluating nursing services is the American Nurses' Association's *Standards for Organized Nursing Services and Responsibilities of Nurse Administrators Across All Settings* (1991). A mock review of the nursing organization using these standards allows supervisors to identify areas of strength and weakness. If areas of noncompliance with standards are noted, the nursing organization can make plans for implementing corrective action. Supervisors and staff at all levels must assume responsibility for meeting accreditation and professional standards.

INTERNAL STANDARDS. *Internal standards* for nursing service are developed by nursing leaders, managers, and staff in the organization. Standards are found in an organization's personnel or departmental policies, nursing procedures, and organizational structure. Criteria for determining when an internal standard has been met are developed by the organization.

Koontz and Weihrich (1988) identified eight types of standards established by most organizations. They are given in Table 10–3.

Organizational standards are critical to the organization as the health industry continues to reform. Strategic planning and goal standards provide current check points and future directions for the organization. Standards relating to revenue, finance, and cost expenditures are becoming increasingly important to nursing services because of the need to decrease the cost of patient care. The standards for

Table 10–3.
Common Organizational Standards

Physical standards: patient acuity ratings to establish nursing care hours

Cost standards: cost per patient day

Capital standards: review of monetary investments or new programs

Revenue standards: revenue per patient day for patient care

Program standards: guide for development and implementation of programs to meet client needs

Intangible standards: staff development and personnel orientation costs

Goal standards: outline of qualitative goals in short- or long-term planning

Strategic plan standards: outline of checkpoints in developing and implementing the organization's strategic plan

evaluating nursing personnel are also important and implied in patient outcomes. A complete discussion of performance standards is given in Chapter 17.

THE SUPERVISORY PROCESS AND DELEGATION

A critical component of the supervisory process is delegation. In the traditional bureaucratic organization, there is one person at the top of the pyramidal structure. Since it is obvious that this person cannot do all of the work of the organization, the work must be delegated. Delegation starts at the top management level: the supervisor delegates work to immediate staff who in turn redelegate all or part of this work to their staff. The components of delegation may include participation on organizational task forces and committees, and the assignment of duties and responsibilities of patient care with the authority needed to complete the tasks. Delegation is important, as it frees the manager or supervisor to do other managerial tasks. Delegation can empower staff, generate greater commitment, and foster professional growth and pride. Delegation provides a mechanism to train employees to take on larger projects and greater responsibility (Research Box 10–2).

Effective delegation requires that supervisors know the abilities, strengths, and weaknesses of their staff. Supervisors must also trust the judgment

Research Box 10–2
Competency Needed in Delegation

Chase conducted a study of nurse manager competencies. She sent questionnaires to 300 members of the American Organization of Nurse Executives from small, medium, and large hospitals and received a response rate of 70.3%. The executives rated 53 competency statements on two scales, knowledge and understanding, and ability to implement and/or use. Delegation was in the 10 highest ranked competencies on both scales that contributed to the effectiveness of first-line managers.

Chase L (1994). Nurse manager competencies. *Journal of Nursing Administration* 24(45):56–64.

of staff members who make decisions. The following example reflects the attention to the belief, vision, trust level, and caring components of delegation.

CASE EXAMPLE ◆

The vice president for nursing services has called a meeting of nurses who are in management positions. She calls the meeting to order and, after greetings, says, "We have an excellent staff development department. I have called this meeting because I want you to meet our new director of staff development, Dr. May Stewart. Many of you met her during the interview process. Dr. Stewart brings a distinguished career in staff development to our organization. She will be responsible for department operations and accreditation. Please give Dr. Stewart your support. She will provide the details of this endeavor."

From this presentation, the assumption is that the vice president and the director have a shared vision and the vice president believes that the director can accomplish the task at hand. The goal is perfectly clear. One can also assume that the vice president cares about helping the nursing staff meet their educational needs. In actuality, the vice president has placed positional strength behind this director and has delegated authority for day-to-day operations. The psychodynamics clearly established the relationship among the leader, the followers, and Dr. Stewart, the delegatee.

Ultimately, supervisors are responsible for the conditions and outcomes of the operations that are within their spans of control. As supervisors practice delegation, the supervisory process allows them to become highly skilled in organizational operations and the coordination of the activities of subordinates.

Supervisors educated during the primary nurse era, when total accountability for patient delivery was a focus, may have more difficulty mastering effective delegation techniques. On the other hand, nurses whose education or practices exposed them to team nursing are more comfortable with the delegation and supervisory process. Therefore, when supervisors advocate developing a nursing sys-

tem that incorporates supervision and delegation of responsibility to various levels of care-giving personnel, they must be prepared to communicate with staff whose orientations have given them different levels of experience and knowledge. A complete discussion of delivery models and the supervision of patient care is given in Chapter 3.

Delegating and Decision-Making

Supervision and delegation activities require constant decision-making. Competent decision-making is intrinsic in the managerial functions of planning, organizing, controlling, and evaluating work processes. Supervisors who are able to make effective decisions and delegate decision-making authority to qualified staff are far more productive in meeting organizational goals and objectives.

The decision-making process may be as simple as deciding who will attend a continuing education conference or as extensive as redesigning a model of patient care delivery. Regardless, the decision must be made based on an extensive examination of the problem or need and on comprehensive data-gathering and analysis of the immediate and far-reaching effects of the decision. A helpful exercise when delegating decision-making authority is to help staff identify and think through potential best-case, worse-case, and most-probable case scenarios of the consequences of the decision.

To delegate decision-making authority and to accomplish work through others, the supervisor also must have excellent communication skills. These skills include communicating the long-range plans and vision of the organization, listening, explaining, and interpreting data and nonverbal cues. A complete listing of communication skills can be found in Chapter 11.

Delegating decision-making requires that staff have a complete understanding of the organization's culture, values, goals, philosophy, and priorities. There is also an implied trust when delegating decision-making authority.

Delegating and Empowerment

Effective delegation empowers employees by contributing to their professional growth, increasing knowledge and decision-making power, and providing increased control over their practices. An empowering environment nurtures staff members to perform to their fullest potential.

The values of the existing work environment exert a powerful influence on professionals who join an organization. Newcomers to an organization progress through a socialization period to become effective members of the group as they learn the culture and digest the values of the organization. In fact, over time, individuals gradually adopt the values of their organization. Consequently, the socialization process of any organization is critical to its success.

An examination of the organization's cultural values and socialization processes can assist a supervisor to evaluate staff learning needs and competencies and to delegate appropriately. This examination can also alert supervisors to potential pitfalls within the organization.

In an empowering environment, nurses are valued as members of the team and not as a source of labor. Empowerment fosters commitment and accountability. Therefore, supervisors should consciously help core staff to develop behaviors that are in the best interest of the organization. A complete discussion of empowerment theory and empowerment models is given in Chapter 4.

According to Benveniste (1994) some professionals seek professional models of governance that allow them control over their work life. These empowerment models or governance structures are appropriate for the 21st century. In these models a group of professionals is headed by a manager who shares responsibilities, such as goal-setting, strategic planning, task-assignments, and coordination with senior staff. Empowerment models occur in decentralized organizations because decentralized decision-making allows managers the authority to delegate decision-making and place far more discretion at the lower levels of the organization.

Delegating to Unlicensed Assistive Personnel

The cost-contained environment and the substitution and reallocation of tasks to unlicensed assistive personnel have made it clear that delegating to less qualified personnel is a primary focus of the future. Current restraints ensure that nurses will lead task groups that encompass increasing numbers of assistive or paraprofessional personnel. Task groups in the health care organizations should identify routinized tasks and tasks that require professional knowledge and skills. Professionals will have responsibility to amass the resources and to organize and assign or distribute tasks in a way that allows the organization to accomplish its goals (Research Box 10–3).

One way to reallocate work is simply to look at the scope of the required tasks and decide which tasks can be assigned to unlicensed assistive personnel. In a technologically advancing field, in which emphasis is on reducing the length of patients' hospitalization, the work of patient care must be organized within a reasonable framework that ensures that competent personnel will provide safe and effective care.

The basic question comes down to deciding what tasks can be delegated to unlicensed assistive personnel. This concern was addressed by the National

---

Research Box 10–3
Practice Partners

The shortage of registered nurses in the high-occupancy, 110-bed critical care unit in the 1527-bed Methodist Hospital in Houston, Texas, prompted an approach in which licensed practical nurses, called practice partners, were selected, trained, and assigned as extenders. Tasks formerly done by registered nurses that could be delegated and those that could not be delegated to licensed vocational nurses were identified. Registered nurses evaluated the program. The mean responses indicated "a moderately positive perception of the role of the licensed vocational nurse in the critical units," with the lowest rating given for the "level of comfort the registered nurses felt in delegating traditional registered nurse tasks to the licensed vocational nurse partner" (p. 34). Although 72% of the registered nurses reported that the quality of nursing care in their units had improved since the advent of the use of practice partners, 23% reported that their workload felt somewhat heavier, and 23% felt that their stress level had increased (p. 35).

Eriksen LR, Quandt B, Teinert D, et al (1992). A registered nurse–licensed vocational nurse partnership model for critical care nursing. *Journal of Nursing Administration* 22(12):28–38.

Council of State Boards of Nursing (1994; p. 11). Its response was as follows:

Delegation involves the transfer of care to a competent individual with authority to do a selected nursing task in situations. If the nurse delegates to a nursing assistant, the nursing assistant is responsible for performing the task; however, the nurse retains responsibility and accountability for the total nursing care of the client.

The National Council of State Board's 1990 Concept Paper on Delegation (1994) states that the decision to delegate should be based on the following:

1. Determination of the task, procedure, or function that is to be delegated
2. Available staff
3. Assessment of client needs
4. Assessment of the potential delegatee's competency
5. Consideration of the level of supervision available and determination of the level and method of supervision required to assure safe performance
6. Avoidance of delegating practice-pervasive functions of assessment, evaluation, and nursing judgment

Supervision of unlicensed assistive personnel and the implications to the supervisory process offer a significant challenge to nursing. Consider the new graduate team leader, unsure of her own skills, who is assigned a complex case involving a seriously ill patient. In her anxiety to get the job done, she reassigns the patient to a nursing assistant who has years of experience. Unfortunately, the nursing assistant lacks the assessment skills and judgment necessary to implement care for the patient. Since the nursing assistant lacks the requisite knowledge and competency to care for the patient, the patient is not assessed properly and dies during the shift.

Although this situation may be uncommon in health care, the seriousness of the situation and the ethical and legal implications cannot be overlooked. The use of job analysis can better differentiate what skills can be delegated to less qualified personnel.

JOB ANALYSIS AND DELEGATION

An analysis of job tasks and work roles will provide the input that will influence supervisory decisions in the future. As organizations adjust to managed care, the complexity of care will increase as the patient population ages, and disease management requires more discerning intervention. Consequently, the redesign of work roles must facilitate a cost-effective mechanism for offering safe care in a variety of health care settings. Monitoring these changes is necessary so that appropriate human resources can be recruited and developed to do the right job.

Supervisors and staff will find themselves reconfiguring job responsibilities to make maximal use of the available professional and assistive resources. As jobs are analyzed and as tasks are identified, supervisors will seek ways to establish an orderly pattern of redistributed tasks.

One way to distribute work is to look at the nature of the tasks performed in the organization and to determine the level of complexity of each task. Then, tasks that are very easy to perform can be organized into jobs that require the simplest level of functioning, and tasks that are highly complex can be organized into jobs that require the highest level of functioning. Mid-level tasks can be combined into mid-level jobs. On the other hand, jobs can be designed that combine tasks that are at varying levels of complexity. Depending on an organization's view of how the use of resources might be maximized, individuals and jobs can be matched. Often, teams can be formed consisting of professional and unlicensed assistive personnel who will be able to handle jobs and tasks at varying levels of complexity. Team members will be responsible to the team leader who will make assignments and report to an appropriate supervisor. Either approach requires restructuring of the human resource management system.

Fine (1992) discusses tasks from the systems approach of functional job analysis (FJA). This approach links an employee's behavior with knowledge, skills, and abilities (KSAs). The questions asked are: Who performs what action to whom or on what? What resources are used? What KSAs and instructions are necessary? and What will be produced or achieved? The systems module for an

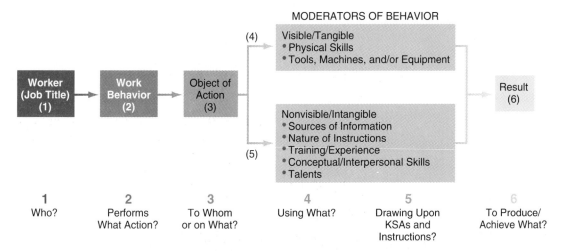

MODERATORS OF BEHAVIOR

Figure 10–1. Functional job analysis task statement: a system module. KSAs, knowledge, skills, and abilities. (From Fine SA [1992]. *The Origin and Nature of Functional Job Analysis.* Presented at the Centennial Convention of the American Psychological Association, Washington, DC, August 15, 1992. ©1992 by Sidney A. Fine.)

FJA task statement is shown in Figure 10–1. It provides a simple way by which supervisors can reconfigure and redesign job tasks and skills.

Knowledge, *skills*, and *abilities* are job content variables. Jobs take place within a context that consists of work conditions, responsibility, and effort. Fine's model (1992), The Holistic Concept of Work Performance, is displayed in Figure 10–2.

Supervisors can use these concepts when assessing performance within a job content and context model. The terms *prescription* and *discretion* within the responsibility component of this figure are especially important. For example, a supervisor may assign the responsibility of diabetic teaching to certain nurses. This task requires a fairly high level of discretion, or judgment, in that the teaching diabetic patients receive should be based on an assessment of their needs and the rapidity with which they master the content. If the appropriate personnel have been assigned to this task, supervisors should not need to prescribe and dictate the steps nurses will use to accomplish this task.

Fine and Getkate (1995) discuss tasks in terms of data, people, and things which, though distributed in different proportions, are common elements of all jobs. For example, an accounting job requires data skills, while nursing positions are primarily involved with people. In a like manner, a machinist job is primarily involved with things. Task analysis

affords the use of a common language with applicability to a wide array of job categories in health care settings.

Task Analysis

To examine tasks systematically, Fine (1992) arranged simple-to-complex hierarchies for functions associated with data, people, and things. Each higher-level task covers the lower-level activities.

Data are defined as information, ideas, facts, statistics, specification of output, knowledge of conditions, techniques, and mental operations (Fine & Getkate, 1995). The lowest level of data-related task is comparing and judging whether observed characteristics are different from prescribed standards. For example, a nurse can be expected to compare a patient's temperature reading with the temperature that generally is accepted as normal to determine whether there is a deviation. The highest level of functioning is synthesizing, which can consist of conceiving new approaches to, or statements of, problems and developing system, operational, or esthetic solutions or resolutions to them.

For example, suppose there is a situation in which a nurse is the only staff member in an underfinanced rural clinic. What action is the nurse to take if the data in the latest research report indicate

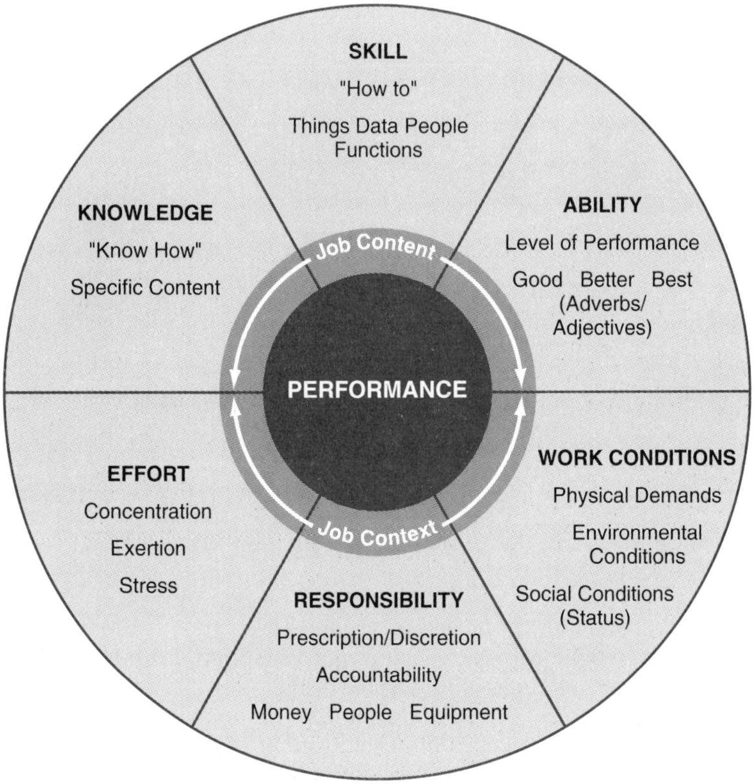

Figure 10–2. The holistic concept of work performance. (From Fine SA [1992]. *The Origin and Nature of Functional Job Analysis.* Presented at the Centennial Convention of the American Psychological Association, Washington, DC, August 15, 1992. ©1992 by Sidney A. Fine.)

that another more expensive medication is much more effective in treating selected illnesses than the medication that is prescribed for patients in this clinic? Most likely, the action selected will be determined by how the nurse synthesizes information while exploring alternative solutions. Fine's model can be used to assess the work of nursing in all health care settings. It helps the nurse determine the complexity of tasks and identify which tasks can be assigned or delegated to nonprofessional staff. This is particularly important in the current era of cost constraints.

Consider the nursing leader who calls her team to a meeting to set goals for the unit for the next year. Three weeks later, the hospital administrator announces that the hospital has been sold and the new owners have decided that the hospital will become a long-term-care facility. Rather than expending useless energy complaining about not being told sooner, the nursing leader calls on her team to develop a contingency plan and short-term goals.

The use of Fine's people scale to examine live interactions will facilitate reassigning jobs and tasks as the organization changes its purpose and goals. In order of complexity, tasks on the people scale include serving, exchanging information, sourcing information, persuading, coaching, diverting, consulting, instructing, treating, supervising, negotiating, and mentoring (Fine & Getkate, 1995). The people scale is especially important to personnel who are involved with the direct delivery of services to patients. This summary is displayed in Figure 10–3.

Job Restructuring and Unlicensed Assistive Personnel

As increasing numbers of unlicensed assistive personnel enter the health care workforce, programs that introduce them to the setting and monitor their progress may become less rigorous. Supervisors must provide adequate job training. Without a systematic way of thinking about redistributing tasks, health care managers may begin to ask "Can an assistive person do this task?" rather than "What is the complexity of the task and the required level of training or education that a worker should have to perform this task safely and effectively?" Even with all the systematic reallocation of tasks, without the appropriate supervisory personnel, there can be a lack of coordination in the delivery of patient care.

Delegation of some of the current tasks from registered nurses to various categories of unlicensed

THINGS	DATA	PEOPLE
4a. Precision Working b. Setting Up c. Operating-Controlling II	6. Synthesizing 5a. Innovating b. Coordinating	7. Mentoring 6. Negotiating 5. Supervising
3a. Manipulating b. Operating-Controlling I c. Driving-Controlling d. Starting Up	4. Analyzing 3a. Computing b. Compiling	4a. Consulting b. Instructing c. Treating 3a. Sourcing Information b. Persuading c. Coaching d. Diverting
2a. Machine Tending I b. Machine Tending II 1a. Handling b. Feeding-Offbearing	2. Copying 1. Comparing	2. Exchanging Information 1a. Taking Instructions-Helping b. Serving

NOTES:

1. Each hierarchy is independent of the others. It would be incorrect to read the functions across the three hierarchies as related although they appear to be on the same level. The definitive relationship among functions is within each hierarchy, not across hierarchies. Some broad exceptions are made in the next note.

2. **Data** is central because a worker can be assigned higher **Data** functions even though **Things** and **People** functions remain at the lowest level of their respective scales. This is not so for **Things** and **People** functions. When a **Things** function is at the third level (eg, Precision Working), the **Data** function is likely to be at least Compiling or Computing. When a **People** function is at the fourth level (eg, Consulting), the **Data** function is likely to be at least Analyzing and possibly Innovating or Coordinating. Similarly for Supervising and Negotiating. Mentoring in some instances can call for Synthesizing.

3. Each function in its hierarchy is defined to include the lower numbered functions. This is more or less the way it was found to occur in reality. It was most clear-cut for **Things** and **Data** and only a rough approximation in the case of **People**.

4. The lettered functions are separate functions on the same level, separately defined. The empirical evidence did not support a hierarchical distinction.

5. The hyphenated functions, Taking Instructions-Helping, Operating-Controlling, and so on, are single functions.

6. The **Things** hierarchy consists of two intertwined scales: Handling/Manipulating/Precision Working is a scale for tasks involving hands and hand tools; the remainder of the functions apply to tasks involving machines, equipment, and vehicles.

Figure 10–3. Summary chart of worker function scales. (From Fine SA, Getkate M [1995]. *Benchmark Tasks for Job Analysis.* Mahwah, NJ: Lawrence Erlbaum Associates. ©1995 by Lawrence Erlbaum Associates, Inc.)

assistive personnel and training them for those tasks seems to have resulted in a manageable workload for registered nurses in a number of institutions. With the transfer of less complex tasks to unlicensed assistive personnel, registered nurses will find themselves in a new workforce performance model. In this model, the personnel configuration requires performance of highly complex clinical tasks and mastery of management skills, especially the supervision and delegation functions.

The results of research on unlicensed assistive personnel suggest that considerable attention must be directed toward the proper use of these staff members. The burden is on the nurse supervisor to be sure that appropriate assignments are made and to see that the work is configured so that patients benefit from the appropriate utilization of available personnel. The use of unlicensed assistive personnel results in a greater accountability of registered nurses for patient care.

LEGAL ASPECTS OF DELEGATION

The legal ramifications of delegation in nursing practice cannot be ignored. According to Mantel (1990), supervisors can be held liable for the acts of their subordinates as well as for their own acts. The law holds the supervisor responsible for knowing the background and experience of a directly reporting subordinate and for making reasonable efforts to discover the same before giving assignments. According to Barter and Furmidge (1994), inappropriate work assignment and inadequate supervision is a breach of duty and could be grounds for charges of negligence. If an injury occurs, the question becomes "Could the injury have been avoided if the person who performed the act had not been assigned or had been supervised adequately?" If an injury occurs that could have been avoided, the nurse would not be held liable for the negligent act of a subordinate, but for a lack of competence in delegating appropriately. Registered nurses must be aware of their legal responsibility when making work assignments, particularly when delegating tasks to unlicensed assistive personnel. Barter and Furmidge (1994) clearly state:

The registered nurse is always responsible for patient assessment, diagnosis, care planning, and

evaluation. **Although assistive personnel may measure vital signs, intake and output or other indicators, it is the registered nurse who analyzes this data for comprehensive assessment, nursing diagnosis and the plan of care. Assistive personnel may perform simple nursing interventions related to hygiene, nutrition, elimination, or activity, but the registered nurse remains responsible for patient outcome.**

A complete discussion of legal aspects in nursing care is given in Chapter 14.

Changing Patterns of Staffing

An examination of personnel systems forces attention to the principle that any change in one part of the system requires a change in another part of the system. Many institutions already have added unlicensed assistive personnel to alleviate the demands on nurses who were in short supply. For example, during the most recent nursing shortage, a hospital that had too few nurses might have resorted to closing beds. In today's environment, such an action is less likely and unlicensed assistive personnel are readily used to provide patient care.

Now, in the interest in controlling the costs of health care and meeting the demands of managed care, supervisors must look at strategies for meeting the health care needs of patients while reducing the cost of delivering health care services. The staffing model that includes the use of unlicensed assistive personnel with various levels of training and a variety of titles is one strategy that is expected to help keep costs down (Research Box 10–4).

As nurses in these situations retain the responsibility for delivering nursing care, they are receiving increased responsibility for the performance of the unlicensed assistive personnel in inpatient and outpatient settings. As new configurations of personnel resources emerge, nurses must remember that the ultimate goal is to deliver safe, efficient, and effective nursing care to those who are in need of such care.

One way to achieve this end is to assemble a task force of representatives of groups of employees whose positions can be affected by the presence of unlicensed assistive personnel. This group can, by working through organizational channels, help to identify, analyze, and determine the levels of com-

Research Box 10–4
Increase in the Use of Unlicensed Assistive Personnel

To examine the magnitude of the movement to increase the use of unlicensed assistive personnel, a survey of approximately 1000 hospitals was conducted by the American Nurses' Association and the American Organization of Nurse Executives. The survey found that 85% of the responding institutions had begun nurse extender programs.

McKibbon RC, Boston C (1990). *An Overview: Characteristics, Impact, and Solutions.* Chicago, IL: American Organization of Nurse Executives and the American Nurses' Association.

plexity of component tasks of current job descriptions. Then, the task force can take the leadership in creating jobs for unlicensed assistive personnel and restructuring or reconfiguring tasks to create job descriptions for professional personnel. Persons who understand the supervisory process are crucial to this mix. Training of unlicensed assistive personnel can then be prescriptive and designed so that personnel can achieve mastery of tasks that make up a certain job (Research Box 10–5).

SUPERVISOR EDUCATION AND TRAINING

Training programs for unlicensed assistive personnel should be designed for adult learners. Knowles (1984) provides the reminder that adult learners respond with resentment and resistance when they are treated as though they are incapable of taking responsibility for themselves. Unlicensed assistive personnel are likely to be heterogeneous groups with a variety of experiences. Knowles (1984) suggests that an adult's identity is derived from life experiences and that these experiences become a rich resource for learning.

Adults approach training or orientation programs with a readiness to learn to perform more effectively in some aspect of their lives. Their orientations to learning are life-centered, task-centered, or problem-centered, and among their most potent motivators are self-esteem and a better quality of life (Knowles, 1984). Given this framework, the training design for unlicensed assistive personnel must be

related to the tasks that are a part of their assigned jobs. The learner should be expected to recognize and understand the competency required, to learn the content related to each competency, to demonstrate and practice using the competency in a simulated situation (whether taking a temperature or bathing a patient), and then to use the competency in the job role. If the learners are heterogeneous, they are likely to accomplish the learning objectives at different times, but they should begin to function in the described role when their competencies have been confirmed. Supervisors involved in the planning and development of educational programs for unlicensed assistive personnel should be responsible for monitoring and reinforcing the achieved competencies. Supervisors should also see that registered nurses develop skills in delegation and supervision (Research Box 10–6).

HIGH POINTS IN DELEGATION

The registered nurse is legally accountable. It is important to remember that the registered nurse is

Research Box 10–5
Hiring Unlicensed Personnel

Barter, McLaughlin, and Thomas received 102 responses from a survey of acute-care hospitals in California. In terms of hiring unlicensed assistive personnel, only 20% of the hospitals required a high school diploma, 26% preferred previous clinical bedside experience, 29% preferred certified unlicensed assistive personnel, and 18% preferred an LPN or LVN. Although the instruction provided was not outlined for each category of personnel, 59% of hospitals provided less than 20 hours of instruction time, and 88% of the hospitals provided 40 hours or less. Ninety-nine percent of the hospitals reported less than 120 hours of on-the-job training. This study indicated that most unlicensed assistive personnel were used in simple bedside care (84%), documented care only on graphic and flow sheets (75%), and were not consistently supervised by the same RN (97%). Most hospitals were not measuring the cost-effectiveness of using unlicensed personnel or the patient outcomes.

Barter M, McLaughlin FE, Thomas SA (1994). Unlicensed assistive personnel by hospitals. *Nursing Economics* 12(2):82–87.

Research Box 10–6
Attention to Delegation

In a 560-bed, unionized, university medical center where the registered nurse vacancy rate averaged 68 per month throughout the hospital in 1989–1990, a project team undertook the task of alleviating the shortage while preserving the institution's professional practice model. In this instance, six assistive personnel with a high school education but no previous training or experience in an assistive position were hired for two experimental units. Although their assignments increased after 10 weeks, "idle" accounted for 21.4% of work activity. In this instance, the conclusions were that:

1. Registered nurses did not alter their work patterns to incorporate the assistive personnel over the course of the study.
2. Patient satisfaction with nursing care was consistently strong and underwent slight improvement over time.
3. Registered nurse satisfaction with staffing held constant while work satisfaction decreased in experimental units.
4. For undetermined reasons, unit personnel patient care costs increased in the experimental units (p. 37).

Outcomes showed that more training was needed "for registered nurses to learn how to delegate tasks and supervise unlicensed assistive personnel hired to fill various roles and job descriptions" (p. 36).

Neidlinger SH, Bostrom J, Stricker A, Hild J, Zhang JQ (1993). Incorporating nursing assistive personnel into a nursing professional practice model. *Journal of Nursing Administration* 23(3):29–37.

always responsible for patient assessment, diagnosis, care planning, and evaluation of patient care. Biester (1993) suggests that Boards of Nursing are responsible for developing clear guidelines about delegation. In this era of fiscal reform, employers will be urging nurses to delegate an increasing number of their tasks and functions to nonlicensed personnel for the benefit of cost containment and it is important to look to the health regulatory boards for direction.

Delegation does not mean abdicating managerial responsibilities for monitoring and supporting patient care. Delegation suggests a transfer of nursing activity and responsibility for completion of that activity to another person. The delegator does not transfer oversight and retains accountability for the activity.

Delegation differs from assignment. According to Milstead (1993), assignment is a lateral shift of nursing activity to someone with the same level of responsibility and accountability. Assignment-making assumes that both caregivers have similar knowledge and skills and, therefore, that the obligations are transferable. The supervisor of professional and unlicensed assistive personnel must remember this distinction.

Milstead (1993) states that every state has a Nurse Practice Act (NPA) that defines nursing and the scope of practice. Each state's laws may allow a different range of nursing accountability, suggesting that nurses must be knowledgeable of the NPAs in their states.

Failure to delegate effectively can result in higher management costs if inappropriate staff are assigned. It can result in a lack of time for adequate supervisory planning and increased stress and burnout for supervisors and staff. Failure to delegate appropriately does not allow staff to grow and develop professionally.

Some supervisors under-delegate because of time factors, risk factors, personal feelings, and an unwillingness to give up part of a former role. Often the attitude is that it takes too long to tell someone else how to do a job or that there could be too much legal risk if the job is not done correctly. Oftentimes, supervisors in nursing are unwilling to take a chance on less qualified staff and are reluctant to give up tasks they like to do themselves.

Delegating to others requires planning with them, and does not provide satisfaction for the action-oriented supervisor.

Washburn (1992; p. 71) says that to be a successful delegator, the "Four Rights" must be considered by the supervisor:

1. The *right task* (the one that can be delegated)
2. The *right person* (the one qualified to do the job)
3. The *right communication* (clear, concise description of the objective and the supervisor's expectations)
4. The *right feedback* (evaluation in a timely manner, during and after the task is completed)

Whether the delegatee is another professional or

an unlicensed assistive staff member, the supervisor must provide the information that person needs to complete the task, the time frame for completion, opportunities for clarification, and opportunities for validating the standards of accountability. Effective delegation as part of the supervisory process will result in maximal utilization of appropriate resources without reducing nursing care outcomes. Professional nurses must now turn their attention to demonstrating mastery of the art and theory related to delegation and supervision.

SUMMARY

Effective supervision and delegation are critical to the changing health care environment. The supervisory process has been defined and applied in clinical practice. Because managed care and cost constraints support and encourage the use of unlicensed assistive personnel, this chapter has suggested a model to assist in the redesign of roles to meet the expectations of the changing health care environment.

■ DISCUSSION QUESTIONS ■

1. Differentiate between supervision and delegation.
2. How does the role of supervision fit into the changing health care environment?
3. Discuss the concept of supervisory power and its potential impact on clinical nursing.
4. Why are supervisory relationships and networking critical in managed care?
5. Discuss the work tasks of supervisors. What impact does the failure to do these tasks have on clinical leadership?
6. Discuss the concepts of standards and supervision.
7. Discuss how tasks should be delegated to assistive personnel.
8. What should the delegator assess before assigning tasks?
9. Discuss how Fine's model can be used to help restructure and decide what nursing tasks can be delegated.
10. What are the supervision and delegation requirements when working with unlicensed assistive personnel?

■ LEARNING ACTIVITIES ■

1. As the regular team leader on the evening shift, you are distressed to learn that you are losing one full-time RN and one full-time LPN. What considerations are necessary as you restructure work roles and consider delegation of responsibilities?
2. As the clinical supervisor of three nursing units, you feel that your stress level and inability to delegate tasks to the nursing managers of these units is causing discontent and a lack of motivation and empowerment among the staff and clinical leadership. How can you approach this problem?
3. You have just received word that you must restructure the busy medical-surgical unit where you have been a staff nurse and leader for 3 years. Your professional staff has been cut from 50% to 35%. Using Fine's model, how would you redesign and delegate work to the increasing numbers of unlicensed assistive personnel that you will be hiring?

■ BIBLIOGRAPHY ■

American Nurses' Association (1991). *Standards for Organized Nursing Services and Responsibilities Across All Settings.* Kansas City, MO: Author.

Barter M, Furmidge ML (1994). Unlicensed assistive personnel: Issues relating to delegation and supervision. *Journal of Nursing Administration* 24(4):36–40.

Barter M, McLaughlin FE, Thomas SA (1994). Use of unlicensed assistive personnel by hospitals. *Nursing Economics* 12(2):82–87.

Beach DS (1985). *The Management of People at Work.* New York: Macmillan Publishing Company.

Benveniste G (1994). *The Twenty-First Century Organization: Analyzing Current Trends—Imagining the Future.* San Francisco: Jossey-Bass Publishers.

Bidwell A, Brasler M (1989). Role modeling versus mentoring in nursing. *Image* 21(1):23–25.

Biester DJ (1993). Delegation: Professional judgement or economic necessity? *Journal of Pediatric Nursing* 8(1):51–54.

Bolman LG, Deal LG (1991). *Reframing Organizations: Artistry, Choice, and Leadership.* San Francisco: Jossey-Bass Publishers.

Chase L (1994). Nurse manager competencies. *Journal of Nursing Administration* 24(4S):56–64.

Darling LAW (1985). Becoming a mentoring manager. *Journal of Nursing Administration* 15(6):43–44.

Dewhirst HD (1970). The socialization of young professionals: A study of changes in the career values of engineers and scientists during the first five years of employment. *In* Shapero A (1985). *Managing Professional People: Understanding Creative Performance.* New York: Collier Macmillan Publishers.

Eriksen LR, Quandt B, Teinert D, Look DS, Loosle R, Mackey G, Strout B (1992). A registered nurse-licensed vocational nurse partnership model for critical care nursing. *Journal of Nursing Administration* 22(12):28–38.

Fields WL (1991). Mentoring in nursing: A historical approach. *Nursing Outlook* 39(6):257–261.

Fine SA (1992). *The Origin and Nature of Functional Job Analysis.* Paper presented at the centennial of the American Psychological Association, Washington Hilton Hotel, August 15.

Fine SA, Getkate M (1995). *Benchmark Tasks for Job Analysis.* Mahwah, NJ: Lawrence Erlbaum Associates.

Hayes PM (1987). Accountability: The supervisors and the system. *Nursing Management* 18(4):81.

Joint Commission for the Accreditation of Health Care Organizations (1994). *Accreditation Manual for Hospitals. Volume 1: Standards.* Oakbrook Terrace, IL: Author.

Kirby KK, Garfink C (1991). The university hospital nurse extender model: Part I, An overview and conceptual framework. *Journal of Nursing Administration* 21(1):25–30.

Knowles MS (1984). *Andragogy in Action.* San Francisco: Jossey-Bass Publishers.

Koontz H, Weihrich H (1988). *Management.* New York: McGraw Hill.

Levey S, Loomba NP (1984). *Health Care Administration: A Managerial Perspective.* Philadelphia: JB Lippincott.

Mantel DL (1990). The double risk of delegating. *RN* 53:67–74.

Marquis BL, Huston CJ (1992). *Leadership Roles and Management Functions in Nursing: Theory and Application.* Philadelphia: JB Lippincott.

Mayer GG (1992). Work sampling in ambulatory care nursing. *Nursing Management* 23(9):52–56.

McKibbin RC, Boston C (1990). *An Overview : Characteristics, Impact, and Solutions.* Chicago IL: American Organization of Nurse Executives and the American Nurses' Association.

Milstead JA (1993). Delegation: A critical skill for the orthopaedic nurse. *Orthopaedic Nursing* 12(2):46.

Mintzberg H (1975). The manager's job: Folklore and fact. *Harvard Business Review* 16(2):49–61.

Minyard K, Wall J, Turner R (1986). RNs may cost less than you think. *Journal of Nursing Administration* 16(5):28–34.

Moore-Greenlaw RC, Decker PJ, Strader M (1994). Accreditation and leadership. *Journal of Nursing Administration* 24(10):6–8.

National Council of State Boards of Nursing (1994). Letters. *Issues: A Newsletter of the National Council* 15(2):11.

Neidlinger SH, Bostrom J, Stricker A, Hild J, Zhang JQ (1993). Incorporating nursing assistive personnel into a nursing professional practice model. *Journal of Nursing Administration* 23(3):29–37.

Quist BD (1992). Work sampling nursing units. *Nursing Management* 23(9):50–51.

Stevens BJ (1985). *The Nurse as Executive.* Wakefield, MA: Nursing Resources.

Swansburg RC (1990). *Management and Leadership for Nurse Managers.* Boston: Jones & Bartlett Publishers.

Thompson JD, Jacobs JE, Pachin NR, et al (1968). Age a factor in the amount of nursing care given, AHA study shows. *Hospitals* 42(5):33–36.

Volante EM (1974). Mastering the managerial skill of delegation. *Journal of Nursing Administration* 4:20.

Washburn M (1991). Delegation: The art of getting things done through others. *Arizona Nursing Times.* Jan., Phoenix, AZ.

Communication, Conflict Management, and Negotiation

Anne Fortenberry, DNS, RN

LEARNING OBJECTIVES

This chapter will enable the learner to:
1. Identify and explore major portions of the communication process.
2. Increase skills in effective and assertive communication.
3. Explore the role of communication in transdisciplinary communication and organizational relationships.
4. Identify causes, approaches, guidelines, tactics, and strategies for managing conflict.
5. Recognize the major phases, characteristics, and tactics in the process of negotiation.

INTRODUCTION

The ability to be an effective communicator is mandatory in the current marketplace. Conflict results from a lack of communication or misinterpreted communication. Success depends on the ability to communicate effectively, manage conflict appropriately, and negotiate productively. The purpose of this chapter is to discuss communication, conflict management, and negotiation as they relate to clinical leadership.

COMMUNICATION

Communication Defined

According to George Miller, the former president of the American Psychology Association, communication is the glue that holds individuals together in society (Littlejohn, 1989). However, to define communication is not simple. Communication experts cannot agree on a common definition and have identified 126 different definitions of communication from the literature (Dance & Larson, 1976). Frank Dance discovered 15 concepts that have become the basic components to distinguish communication from other things (Dance & Larson, 1976), including understanding, process, power, symbols, verbal, speech, channel, carrier, means, and route. The Latin word for communication is *communitas*, which means *commonness*; it would be important to develop a commonness of meaning between two individuals when defining communication. For the purpose of this chapter, communication is defined as the transfer of information and understanding from one person to another (Davis & Newstrom, 1985).

A unique fact about communication is that it requires at least two people: one who sends a message and one who receives a message. Communication is the way in which people share thoughts, ideas, facts, beliefs, and values. Because every individual comes from a different background, communication is influenced from that perspective as well as by understanding and perception. (See Chapter 12 for a discussion of how different cultural backgrounds may affect the communication background.)

Communication Process

The process of communication has been identified as a sequence of activities that are in some way connected (Hawkins & Preston, 1981). Each activity is required, whether it is face-to-face communication between two individuals or person-to-group communication in a seminar or by way of computerized electronic mail. The communication process can be visualized as a circle moving in a clock-like fashion (Fig. 11–1).

The process of communication begins at the 12 o'clock position with an idea or intended message in the mind of the sender. The idea or message is individualized and affected by the perception of the sender. This perception is a reflection of the sender's background and his or her ability to understand. To be able to communicate, the sender must now decide how to pass this idea or message along to someone else; thus, encoding begins.

To encode a message (2 o'clock position in Fig. 11–1), the sender must interpret the internal idea or message into a language the intended receiver will understand. This language can be in the form of words, symbols, pictures, charts, gestures, or some other form of transmission. Encoding can be as simple as ordering from a picture of a salad in a fast food restaurant or as difficult as finding the right words to terminate an employee. Sometimes a mere look from the nurse leader can communicate unfavorable behavior.

When the sender encodes a message, a decision must be made regarding what the intended purpose of the message is and what the message needs to accomplish (Kreitner, 1995). If the purpose is, for example, to persuade the registered nurse to begin a new program, then a detailed technical report would not have the impact that a more motivational, emotional approach would have.

Another significant decision that must be made when encoding a message is what physical form is needed for transmission. Kreitner (1995) identifies the importance of looking at the number of receivers involved and their individual characteristics. A nurse leader can be more informal when speaking face to face with one individual than with a group of nurses at a seminar. The nurse leader would also speak differently to a unit secretary who is familiar with the unit's activities than with an angry physician. Thus, selecting the method by which the message is delivered is the next step.

The method (4 o'clock position in Fig. 11–1) chosen to send the intended idea or message is the pathway of physical transmission. Numerous methods are available for transmission, and they must be considered in much the same way that various forms of encoding are received. The sender must consider the idea or intended message, purpose, number of receivers, and characteristics of the receivers. Some communication methods to choose from include face to face, memorandum, letter, telephone, electronic mail, facsimile (fax), voice mail, photograph, conference, committee, seminar, bulletin board, software, publication, video, news media, radio, and television. It is important to recognize that each method has advantages and disadvantages that need to be identified before a choice can be made. For example, enthusiasm is difficult to transmit over electronic mail, even though large amounts of information can be sent to numerous employees by this means. Telephones may be quick and easy to use, but nonverbal communication cannot be interpreted as when communicating face to

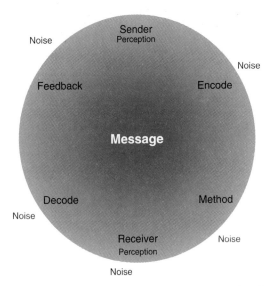

Figure 11–1. Communication process, originating and ending with the sender (read in a clockwise fashion beginning with the 12 o'clock position).

face. It also can be beneficial to have a permanent record of communication readily available, as when using letters and memos. Once the method is selected, the message goes to a receiver.

The receiver (6 o'clock position in Fig. 11–1) is the person who receives the idea or intended message and must interpret the transmission. Interpretation of the message depends on the perception, background, and understanding of the receiver; thus, decoding begins.

When the receiver decodes the message (8 o'clock position in Fig. 11–1), the purpose is to understand exactly what the sender meant when the message was sent. However, because the perceptions of two people are often different, it is sometimes difficult to fully understand the intent of the sender. After the receiver obtains the message, symbols, language, and meaning must be processed for understanding to take place. Decoding is enhanced when the receiver is willing to receive the message, knowledgeable about the language, understanding of the use of terminology, and knowledgeable about the sender's background and purpose. Therefore, feedback is helpful in determining whether the message has been decoded properly.

To complete the communication process, feedback (10 o'clock in Fig. 11–1) from the receiver allows the sender to know whether the idea or intended message has been interpreted correctly. Feedback indicates the effectiveness of the communication and is most desirable in determining whether the initial message was communicated accurately or should be repeated (Cherrington, 1994). Succeeding messages may actually need modification because of feedback. Appropriate methods of feedback may be determined by the same decisions that regulate the sender's encoding. After all, this is how the sender knows whether his or her idea or intended message has been understood by the receiver.

Several factors in the form of noise can disrupt the transmission, receipt of the idea, or intended message from the sender to the receiver. Noise can influence the process of communication at any point (see Fig. 11–1). Kreitner (1995, p. 349) defines noise as "any interference with the normal flow of understanding from one person to another." Noise can be anything from ambiguous wording to static on a telephone line. Noise can manifest itself in the form of poor hearing or listening, poor eyesight,

negative attitudes, misperception, illegible print, garbled transmission, speech impediments, and the like. Therefore, steps must be taken to minimize all forms of noise and maximize understanding of verbal and written messages.

Behavioral Components of Communication

Several behavioral components of communication are identified throughout the literature, such as perception, "management by walking around," nonverbal communication, and informal communication. However, for the purposes of this chapter, the two predominant behavioral components discussed are *perception* and *nonverbal communication*. Both of these components are essential to an understanding of and participation in the process of communication.

Perception

If 20 college students listened to the same lecture, each of the 20 students would have a different perception about the lecture. If three registered nurses witnessed a cardiac arrest, all three would give different renditions of what occurred. For example, one of the things a judge watches for in an eyewitness account is a slight variation in the witnessed episode. If repeated recounting of the episode brought no variation into the eyewitness account, the judge would listen more intently to determine the reliability of the testimony.

What is perception? Is what you see always what you get? If perception is an individual's own view of the world (Davis & Newstrom, 1985), then there should be as many views of the same situation as there are observers. One's perception is strongly influenced by background, interests, beliefs, and values as well as by physiological, cultural, social, and psychological influences (Adler & Towne, 1990). Because perception is essential to communication, it is important not only to understand one's own perception but also to try to understand other people's perceptions.

One of the main characteristics of perception is *perceptual set*, which means that individuals perceive what they expect to perceive (Davis & Newstrom, 1985). For example, if a beginning clinician is told that the nurse leader is friendly, the beginning clinician will be more likely to expect to see a friendly nurse leader and will respond in a friendly manner. Consequently, perceptual set can cause an individual to misread a situation because of what is expected to be seen.

Sometimes optical illusions can cause problems with perception. An individual tends to select things from the environment and arrange or organize these things in a meaningful way. Look at image A in Figure 11–2 *right now*, before reading on any further, and follow the instructions.

Look at the sentence closely; you will see that the sentence contains the word *the* twice. Normally, words are grouped line by line; therefore, a duplicated word tends to be overlooked. This is also true with nurse managers; they may overlook subtle differences among individual registered nurses by grouping them together. However, grouping can also be helpful in quickly sorting out stimuli that may be unusual, such as a defective bottle of intravenous fluids.

Now take a *quick look* at image B (Fig. 11–2). What do you see? Did you see a star burst? Or did you see a sun? Or did you see a sunflower? What

Read this sentence out loud:

A A MOUSE IN THE THE HAND IS USELESS

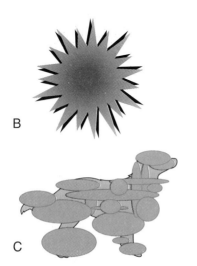

B

C

Figure 11–2. Images used to illustrate optical illusions in perceptions as related to nursing.

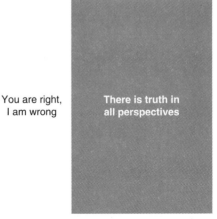

I am right, you are wrong

You are right,
I am wrong

There is truth in all perspectives

The matter is not important

Both are right, both are wrong

Figure 11–3. Perceptual views to increase understanding and empathy for other's beliefs (five different ways to look at a situation).

you saw depends on how you perceived the figure. Individuals often see different objects when looking at the same picture. This can also be true of registered nurses in that one may see a situation or problem differently from another because of his or her individual perspectives. For example, one registered nurse may believe her work hours are flexible because she gets to choose the hours she works. Conversely, another registered nurse may believe his work hours are not flexible because of the time restraints imposed by the children getting home from school.

Now take a *fast glance* at image C (Fig. 11–2). If you see a large dog standing up facing toward the right, you have relied on the perceptual process of *closure*. Closure, in this context, means to mentally fill in the blanks of an incomplete whole. Because you are accustomed to seeing complete pictures of dogs, you completed the incomplete picture. This perceptual process can lead to inaccurate communication and rumors when individuals fill in the blanks after hearing only part of a story. However, closure can be helpful when trying to solve a complex problem with limited information.

Obviously, situations and problems can be interpreted differently. What may appear to be an opportunity for the registered nurse could be a problem for the nurse leader. For example, a registered nurse may have the opportunity to go back to school to pursue a master's degree; however, her return to school may present a problem for the nurse leader when trying to adequately staff the unit.

In trying to understand another person's perspective, Paul Reps (1967) identified five views that a person can take: (1) I am right, you are wrong, (2) you are right, I am wrong, (3) both are right, both are wrong, (4) the matter is not important, and (5) there is truth in all perspectives (Fig. 11–3). An individual can increase understanding and empathy for another person's view by taking the time to work through each of these views.

The following is an example of how these views can be used to defuse misunderstandings and promote empathy.

CASE STUDY ◆ 11–1

When the registered nurse reported to work on her unit, she was told to go to a sister unit on another floor. After reporting to this unit, the nurse leader made assignments that caused a dispute between the registered nurse and the nurse leader. The registered nurse became angry because she believed she had been assigned the more difficult patients on that unit. The registered nurse tried to explain her position, but the nurse leader refused to listen. The registered nurse decided to try and work through the views and then re-approach the nurse leader if necessary.

VIEW 1: I AM RIGHT, AND SHE IS WRONG

The assignment was too heavy. The acuity of the patient's case should be considered before making assignments. I am right to feel dumped on; she is wrong to give me the patients requiring the most care.

VIEW 2: SHE IS RIGHT, AND I AM WRONG

Just because I was "pulled" to another unit does not give me the right to expect special treatment. She actually assigned patients by room number to decrease my steps and make the load easier.

VIEW 3: WE ARE BOTH RIGHT, AND WE ARE BOTH WRONG

I was right to believe I had the hardest patients; however, I do not believe she made the assign-

ment to be unfair. Someone had to have these patients, and I am a very good registered nurse. She was right to refuse to listen to my angry outburst; but I was right in saying the acuity of the patient's case needed to be considered.

VIEW 4: IT REALLY IS NOT IMPORTANT WHO WAS RIGHT OR WRONG

I have to work on this unit for only 1 day and maybe not again for a long time. The incident is not worth my effort in worrying. I have had to face worse difficulties than this. After all, most of my assignments are reasonable.

VIEW 5: THERE IS TRUTH IN ALL PERSPECTIVES

This exercise was helpful to work through because there is some truth in all perspectives. I was angry and indignant about this situation at first. After working through all views, I could actually put myself in the nurse leader's place and understand why she acted the way she did. When we sat down to discuss the matter in a more civilized manner, I was able to listen without becoming defensive, angry, or indignant. I could understand the nurse leader's position, and we both felt good about each other. I probably could not have done this without looking at this situation from all perspectives.

Nonverbal Communication

Ralph Waldo Emerson stated, "What you are speaks so loudly I cannot hear what you say." Sometimes the facial expressions and body movements that accompany verbal communication tend to complicate and cause problems. Nonverbal communication is defined as "the process by which nonverbal behaviors are used, either singly or in combination with verbal behaviors, in the exchange and interpretation of messages within a given situation or context" (Malandro et al, 1989, p. 5). These authors categorized nonverbal communication into several classes: body types, shapes, and sizes; clothing and personal artifacts; body movements and gestures; facial expressions and eye behavior; environment; spatial arrangements; personal space, territory, and crowding; touching behavior; voice characteristics and qualities; smell and taste; and culture and time. All of this nonverbal communication has an important part in the process of communication. Mehrabian (1981) reported that only 7% of communication comes from uttered words, whereas the remaining 93% is nonverbal.

Body Types, Shapes, and Sizes. These give out mixed signs of nonverbal communication. Whether a person is short or tall, skinny or fat, or attractive or ugly sends out powerful messages to other people as well as to oneself. Messages may be positive or negative. Feelings of inadequacy and dissatisfaction affect a person's self-concept and communication behavior. For example, a person who is grossly overweight may believe everyone is staring at him when he ventures out, so he decides to stay at home.

Clothing and Personal Artifacts. Sometimes these can communicate unintentional messages such as status, authority, age, and even sexuality. What one wears—whether it is a navy blue suit to impress the manager in a job interview or a swimsuit to enjoy a day in the sun—sends out either positive or negative impressions. Research has indicated that the person who gets the job is often the one who not only has the qualifications for the job but also has outwardly impressed those around him or her. *Artifact* also contributes to perceptions of people. Slogan T-shirts, briefcases, and eye glasses, to name a few, send out powerful messages.

Body Movements and Gestures. Martha Graham was quoted as saying, "The body says what words cannot." Body movements, or *kinesics*, and *gestures* have been a major concern of research in psychology, communication, and nursing. Sometimes referred to as *body language*, kinesics is an important part of the behavioral component of nonverbal communication. How a person postures herself may influence the recipient of the intended message. For example, if the recipient is sitting or lying down rather than standing, this may actually allow the sender to be more persuasive. If a person stands up straighter, he or she can often look 10 years younger or 10 pounds lighter. Even a person's walk reflects that person's emotional state, attitude, or cultural/ethnic background. In observations of gender differences in body language, women tend to blink and smile more, whereas men tend to point and stare. Hand gestures, nods of the head, and shifts in posture are body movements that also help us interact with others.

Facial Expressions and Eye Behavior. These do provide an enormous amount of information. Malandro et al (1989) reported that facial expressions help to recognize others, predict personalities, and interpret situations. Emotions are also associated with facial expressions, such as the sadness caused by the death of a loved one. Eye movements convey nonverbal information and are influenced by differences in personality, culture, and gender. For example, an intense harsh look from a mother can stop a child in his or her tracks. Some people may perceive individuals who have large, light eyes to be more attractive than people with small, dark eyes. However, other people may see the reverse.

Environment. The *environment* plays an important part in nonverbal communication. Were you comfortable when you entered a particular structure, or were you anxious to leave? Was the structure formal or informal, for example, a government building or a country church? In which type of structure do you feel more at home? Did you have a feeling of warmth, or did the environment give you a chill? While at the physician's office, did you experience a feeling of privacy? Were the surroundings familiar, such as a McDonald's or a Marriott Hotel? Were you in a strange new place and feeling awkward? Did it take a long time to get to your destination, or was it right across town? Did you feel constrained, as in a car on a long trip, or did you have the freedom to move around, as on a train?

Spatial Arrangements. The environment can also be affected by *spatial arrangements*. How were the seating arrangements? Were they conducive to interaction? Because interaction with other members of the class is so important, students usually prefer a seating arrangement that allows for the most interaction, such as the semicircle or U shape, rather than traditional straight-row seating arrangements.

Personal Space, Territory, and Crowding. *Personal space, territory,* and *crowding* are other components of nonverbal communication. When a person thinks of *territory*, his first thoughts may be of an invasion of exclusive property (Malandro et al, 1989). However, territory may refer to personal belongings, a classroom desk, the parking lot, or the immediate space around your body. *Violation* occurs when the territory belonging to someone else is used without permission. *Invasion* occurs when someone crosses the boundaries and seizes another person's territory. Factors influencing territory include gender, intensity of the invasion, and how badly the territory is desired.

Personal space is the territory surrounding us that we carry around as we interact with other persons. Personal space varies depending on gender, age, culture, and relationship with the people with whom we are interacting. When someone gets too close, we have the tendency to push away or flee. According to Malandro et al (1989), *crowding* occurs when people become aware of spatial restriction. Crowding is a psychological experience (eg, stimulus overload), whereas *density* is a physical condition (eg, rush-hour traffic).

Touching Behavior. *Touching behavior* is a functional component of nonverbal communication. Taking someone's blood pressure may be a functional or professional form of touch. Other forms of touch communicate specific information about a relationship between two individuals. These touches may be friendly, social, sexual, or expressions of love. Some researchers state that humans suffer from deprivation if not touched. Humans react to being held, rocked, or stroked like a baby. In nursing, the importance of therapeutic touch with patients of all ages is emphasized. Note the following incident:

A young girl expressed how unhappy she was because her parents never hugged, kissed, or touched her. She felt so unloved and sought solace in the arms of one boy after the other. Her promiscuousness resulted in an unwanted pregnancy. However, due to religious beliefs, she decided not to have an abortion and to have her baby. After the baby was born she said, "At least now I will have someone who can really love me."

Voice Characteristics and Qualities. These also influence how a person is perceived and interpreted. These evaluations are often based on the pitch, volume, or rate of the speaker. Voice is often seen as a verbal fingerprint, and it is not surprising that an individual can be falsely accused just because of voice characteristics. An example of this occurred

with a student who had arrived in the South from the Northwest.

Sarah needed to obtain a preceptor for a leadership clinical experience. She had built up her hopes of working with a particular nurse manager whom she respected on the basis of a past experience. After several telephone calls to set up an appointment, Sarah was unable to finalize a meeting time and felt she was getting the runaround.

The nurse manager's secretary called Sarah's professor to discuss the situation. The secretary and nurse manager had perceived Sarah as coming on too strong and being rude and insensitive; they did not like the sound of the student's voice. Because Sarah was from the Northwest, her voice intonations were blunt, she spoke rapidly, and she had an accent different from the typical southern drawl.

The professor spoke with the student, explained the situation, and advised her to obtain a different preceptor. The student took the professor's advice and found another preceptor. It happened that this new nurse leader was from similar surroundings, and the experience turned out to be positive and successful.

Smell and Taste. *Smell* and *taste* are other components of nonverbal communication. The sense of smell provides information about the environment and the individuals in it. Smell can communicate both positive and negative images. Some smells make a person want to leave the environment immediately, for example, an abdominal bleed out. Other smells, such as freshly cut roses, are pleasant and make a person wish to stay longer. Some odors arouse fear, for example, the smell of natural gas. Smell is also important to taste. Without the sense of smell, it is difficult to distinguish among sourness, sweetness, bitterness, and saltiness (Malandro et al, 1989). Sensitivity to taste also decreases with age because the taste buds have a tendency to diminish as one gets older.

Culture. *Culture* is an important component of nonverbal communication. Because others are often judged according to one's own values and beliefs, people from other countries have a need to understand American culture just as Americans have that same need when traveling abroad. Different countries can have different meanings for the same behavior. Consider the following example:

In one country, it is taboo to extend the left hand to shake hands with another individual; therefore, if a person from another culture extends his or her left hand to a native of this country, the native become defensive, turns away in disgust, and refuses to communicate. The reason is that in this particular country, toilet paper is not used; consequently, the left hand must be used as a substitute. Obviously, it is important to have a basic understanding of an individual's culture. (A more comprehensive discussion of cultural implication is found in Chapter 12.)

A sensitivity to perception and nonverbal communication can be learned. Knowing how to interpret nonverbal cues, such as a nod or grimace, is vital for a nurse leader. A well-timed pat on the back is invaluable to let subordinates know they are doing a good job or are on the right track.

Flow of Communication

In an organization, the three directions of formal communication are downward, upward, and horizontal (Fig. 11–4). Informal communication is circulated through the grapevine. Knowing who communicates with whom is vital to the survival of any new employee.

Downward Communication

Downward communication takes place when information flows from people in higher levels to people

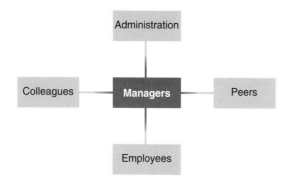

Figure 11–4. Flow chart illustrating three formal types of communication: downward, upward, and horizontal. The center of the flow chart is the manager.

in lower levels. This is the traditional hierarchy of communication. Hawkins and Preston (1981) identify five types of information common to downward communication: (1) specific directives, (2) rationale for understanding tasks, (3) organizational policies and procedures, (4) feedback to employees about performance, and (5) education in the goals and mission of the organization. Some traditional *methods* of downward communication include employee handbooks, policy and procedure manuals, job descriptions, performance evaluations, memoranda, and bulletin boards. Accurate information can be lost if it is passed through multiple levels of the organization; this can happen because information is usually generated for the next immediate level rather than for several lower levels. Serious distortions can occur as people try to interpret and then redefine information (Cherrington, 1994).

Upward Communication

Upward communication takes place when the information flows from people in lower levels (employees) to people in higher levels (employers). This flow of communication provides feedback on how well an organization is functioning, the organization's policies and practices, and the employees' performance. Upward communication that is effective not only provides information but also maintains employee morale. Some common methods of upward communication include written memoranda, suggestion boxes, written reports, group meetings, face-to-face discussions, and employees' grievances. According to Cherrington (1994), one of the problems with upward communication is that it can be biased or filtered. Employees are not likely to give their nurse leader information that will adversely reflect on them. Another problem is caused when, instead of obtaining information from an employee, the nurse leader waits until the employee initiates the information. Even when the nurse manager adopts an open-door policy, this does not mean that employees will volunteer information.

Horizontal Communication

Horizontal communication, often called *lateral communication*, occurs between peers and colleagues at the same level of the organization. This flow of communication can also occur between departments and is more common among managers than among employees in the organization. Horizontal communication furnishes social and emotional support to people. It contributes to the development of friendships and work groups; however, increased horizontal communication has the potential to detract from maximum efficiency (Cherrington, 1994). A form of horizontal communication, *transdisciplinary communication*, is discussed later.

Grapevine Communication

Grapevine communication exists in every organization and is the informal flow of information. Grapevines cut across formal lines of communication and are created by an informal association with individuals. Cherrington (1994) identified some major *characteristics* of the grapevine:

- Grapevines are impossible to eliminate.
- Grapevine information travels more rapidly than other forms of communication.
- Grapevines have a spontaneous form of expression.
- Grapevine information is more informative.
- Seventy-five percent of the grapevine information is correct.
- The number of people serving as links in the grapevine is small.

Wise leaders are able to use the grapevine to their advantage. Nurse managers and leaders can use the grapevine as a substitute for formal communication. For example, the grapevine can be used to leak ideas to other employees and get their reactions to a planned change without making a formal commitment. The leader can also correct distorted information and pass on correct information through the grapevine.

Barriers to Communication

There are several barriers that may disrupt the effectiveness of the communication process. Kreitner (1995) categorized these barriers into four major types: (1) process barriers, (2) physical barriers, (3) semantic barriers, and (4) psychosocial barriers.

Process Barriers

Process barriers can take place at any point during the communication process (see Fig. 11–1). There can be process barriers to the message with the sender or receiver, method, encoding or decoding, and feedback. Most of these barriers are generated by varying degrees of noise. There can be conflicting or inconsistent signals, credibility problems, reluctance to communicate, poor listening, predispositioning, or perceptual differences.

Physical Barriers

Physical barriers can block communication. Distance can be a physical barrier, as can an inconveniently positioned wall within an office. Choosing an appropriate method to transmit the message is important in overcoming physical barriers. For example, a leader with a soft voice may need to use a sound system or electronic mail to reach hundreds of people.

Semantic Barriers

Semantic barriers refer to problems that arise from not having a common understanding of the words in the message. These barriers can cause problems in everyday life because words have different meanings to people with different educational backgrounds. It is important that a person understand the meaning of words in reference to the information being shared. For example, the hospital administrator must be familiar with medical terminology to better understand the medical staff.

Psychosocial Barriers

Psychosocial barriers are the most numerous types of barriers blocking communication. *Psychosocial barriers* refer to differences between the sender and receiver in their backgrounds, perceptions, values, beliefs, needs, biases, and expectations. Included in these barriers are personal and family problems, prejudices, lack of trust, and negative feelings. Sensitivity to the needs of the receiver goes a long way in overcoming psychosocial barriers.

Effective Communication

Because there are so many factors and barriers that can disrupt communication, it is advantageous for leaders to use several techniques to improve effective communication. These techniques include: (1) perception sensitivity, (2) effective listening, (3) effective writing, and (4) effective speaking. All of these techniques can be useful to the sender, receiver, or both.

Perception Sensitivity

For communication to be effective, the leader must be *sensitive* to the *perception* of the employee. For example, the manager who must tell an employee that she has not been given a promotion should recognize the way in which the employee may receive this information. The manager must be aware that the employee may experience feelings of anger or hostility, and the manager should not become defensive in return. The manager should select a method of delivery that is determined by the content of the message and anticipated response of the employee to the message.

Conversely, with the trend in organizational down-sizing, the manager may be the one to receive the news of being laid off. If this should occur, the employees need to be sensitive to the leader's perception and understand his or her disappointment or anger. A special effort should be made by the employees to look for signals that the manager needs to talk about the situation.

Effective Listening

One way to become an effective communicator is to become an *effective listener*. This seems to be the most forgotten aspect of the communication process. According to Kreitner (1995), the receiver must *listen* to accurately decode and understand the intended message, and the sender must *listen* to decode and understand the feedback from the receiver. Some practical tips for effective listening

are noted throughout the literature (Atwater, 1981; Kreitner, 1995; Swets, 1983):

- Be aware of your own listening habits.
- Learn to tolerate silences.
- Ask open-ended questions.
- Encourage the speaker with eye contact and alert posture.
- Use verbal encouragement, such as "yes" or "I see."
- Paraphrase or repeat the speaker's last few words.
- Reflect emotion through empathic understanding.
- Know and correct your biases and prejudices.
- Avoid premature judgments.
- Summarize to identify misunderstandings.
- Concentrate on what the speaker is saying.

Adler & Towne (1990) and Atwater (1981) report a *pseudolistener* to be one who gives the appearance of being very attentive when she or he is not, in fact, listening to the conversation. Pseudolisteners may have become proficient at looking a person in the eye, nodding, and smiling at the right time. They may even answer occasionally. They ignore the sender because their minds are on other matters than what is being said, or they think they have already heard what is being said and so tune out. Regardless of the reason, pseudolisteners are only falsely communicating. An example of this type of nonlistening follows:

Ben was talking to Sue. However, Sue had mentally wandered off during the conversation and was not truly listening. Sue nodded her head occasionally and smiled at appropriate intervals. When it became Sue's turn to speak, Ben also responded to Sue with nods and smiles. Was Ben actually listening, or did he also wander off during the conversation? Do you really listen?

Effective Writing

One of the biggest complaints in management circles is that college graduates are poor writers. Allred and Clark (1978) reported four areas of writing in which graduates have difficulty: (1) being concise,

(2) making the meaning clear, (3) making the message accomplish the purpose, and (4) spelling. A person must practice to become an effective writer. If students do not get the practice in college, they are at a big disadvantage when they go into the workforce or graduate school. Because effective writing is part of the encoding step in the communication process, it must be performed skillfully to avoid potential barriers. Kreitner (1995) offers four helpful reminders for *effective writing*.

- *Keep the words simple.* Complexity turns readers off.

- *Do not sacrifice communication for rules of composition.* Stop trying to make writing conform to rigid rules without regard to style or purpose of communication.

- *Write concisely.* Express thoughts, opinions, and ideas in as few words as possible. Do not confuse conciseness with brevity.

- *Be specific.* Do not be vague. Vagueness destroys accuracy and clarity; say what you mean.

If you are having trouble with writing skills, seek help whether you are a student or beginning professional. Poor writing may not only cause problems for your employer but also damage your career.

Effective Speaking

One of the most important ingredients of *effective speaking* is the speaker's preparation. *Preparation* is accomplished through a step-by-step process that begins with knowing the purpose of the speech. Preparation includes researching the topic, determining the outline, deciding on the method of delivery, and including pertinent notes.

To be an effective speaker, you must have a clear and definite *purpose* and seek to achieve a particular reaction from the audience. This purpose reflects the goals and objectives of the speech and guides the speaker in all phases of preparation and delivery. Rowland and Rowland (1992) classified all speeches into three categories: informative, persuasive, and entertaining. Once the category is determined, the speaker can decide on the reaction desired from the audience.

With the purpose in mind, the speaker *researches* the literature and gathers information on the chosen topic. You select information from the literature and draw information from your past experiences. After information is collected, you evaluate all of the material gathered and decide what will be used in the speech.

At this time, the speaker will determine an effective *outline*. An outline that lists the main points of the speech helps keep the ideas in proper order. This will ensure you of a smooth progression from the beginning to the end of your speech.

Deciding the *method of delivery* is the next step in the preparation of an effective speech. You and the audience must be on the same wavelength for communication to be achieved. Variation in voice, body movement, and appropriate gesturing add to the effectiveness of the delivery. The speaker must be aware that a monotone voice and stiff delivery can be boring, whereas too much movement and awkward gesturing can be distracting.

The use of *pertinent notes* can help the speaker to be responsive to the needs of the audience. Pertinent notes can prompt your memory, help report complex material, and ensure exactness in delivery.

By following this simple step-by-step process, you can give an effective speech. To be an effective speaker, you must always remember to keep the audience in mind and be *sensitive to their needs*. One way to be sensitive is to be *flexible*. Pay attention to the audience's responses to the speech and take their cues, trimming or expanding the delivery to meet their needs. Remember, speeches are delivered, not read.

Communicating in Groups

Groups are important to individuals and provide a significant channel of communication in organizations. Group communication becomes an instrument for accomplishing tasks as well as a means of group maintenance and cohesion. Littlejohn (1989) reported that *group communication* is a system of inputs, internal processes, and outputs. *Inputs* include information and resources; *processes* include group interaction; and *outputs* include completing tasks and solving problems.

As group members communicate, they accomplish their goals while structuring future interactions. Cherrington (1994) identified three variables that influence communication in groups: opportunity to interact, cohesiveness, and status. Instead of telling people what they should and should not do, communication can be influenced by the opportunity for group members to interact. Because communication is more difficult if people are physically separated, leaders can install an electronic mail system or provide opportunities to interact during lunch time. Status relationships influence communication patterns, whether it is leaders communicating with employees or peers communicating in the presence of a leader. For example, employees might censor their comments in the presence of managers to reflect messages they think the manager wants to hear. When group members develop cohesiveness, communication flows freely and becomes more satisfying.

Communication Networks

A *communication network* is a pattern of communication channels among group members in an organization (Cherrington, 1994). A *network* is a group of individuals who develop and maintain contact to exchange information informally about an interest they all share (Davis & Newstrom, 1985). The most frequently studied networks are the circle, wheel, Y, chain, and all-channel (Fig. 11–5). These networks differ profoundly in their degree of decentralization and centralization. The circle network is the most highly decentralized because each position communicates directly with two other positions and *no* position communicates with every position. Conversely, the wheel network is the most centralized because all communication passes through the center position. According to Cherrington (1994), centralized networks are more efficient in solving tasks that are simple, whereas decentralized networks more efficiently solve complex tasks. Centralized networks require fewer messages to perform tasks, whereas decentralized networks have higher levels of employee group satisfaction.

Trust

Communicating in groups is influenced by the degree of trust that is present. *Trust* is confidence or

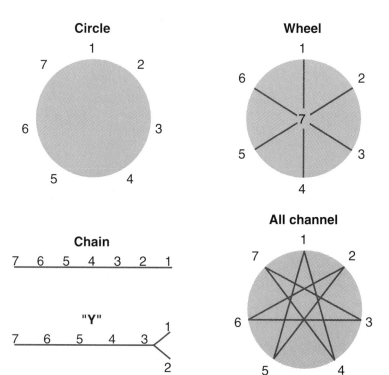

Figure 11–5. Communication networks illustrating five major methods of exchange using seven positions.

faith in another individual. A lack of trust can have damaging effects in an organization. For instance, in situations in which trust is lacking, efficiency can be reduced to the extent that communication is limited or labored (Putnam & Roloff, 1992). Group members may also have a tendency to perform in dysfunctional ways to release their frustrations. On the other hand, when trust is present, group members can enjoy an increased exchange of open communication, interpersonal influence, and self-control (Kreitner, 1995).

Running Meetings

Meetings occupy a major amount of the leader's time in organizational life. Regardless of the purpose for the meeting, the leader must be able to use everyone's talent and time effectively and efficiently. The following are some useful hints for conducting a successful meeting:

- *Make certain the meeting is necessary.* If the same results can be achieved through a memorandum or electronic mail, do not call a meeting.
- *Make an agenda.* Send it out in advance.
- *Keep to the agenda.* Encourage members to express themselves, but keep to the itinerary.
- *Give consideration to those invited to the meeting.* Only invite those who must attend.
- *Give the meeting your total attention.* Avoid distractions and interruptions.
- *Be prepared.* Know what you want to accomplish, do your homework, and anticipate questions.
- *Ask the right questions to stimulate discussion.* Get everyone involved.
- *Summarize the major points of the meeting.* Include actions to be taken, and follow up with minutes.

Effective meetings are important to organizational communication and success. Leaders must practice these guidelines until they become second nature.

Transdisciplinary Communication

Transdisciplinary communication, a form of horizontal communication, is the process of transmitting information across and to several disciplines from

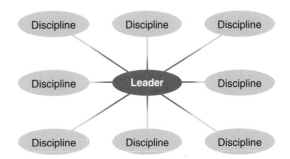

Figure 11–6. Model of transdisciplinary communication depicting the leader as the central focus within all of the various disciplines.

one discipline. A *discipline* consists of a specialty or concentration in one area, such as nursing, respiratory, pharmacy, dietary, and social services. For transdisciplinary communication to be effective, an employee in one discipline (eg, nursing) assumes the leader role and must be able to communicate with personnel in many other disciplines (Fig. 11–6). When transdisciplinary communication is used, groups perform tasks as a team and seek to develop a cooperative attitude. Transdisciplinary communication works best when management creates a supportive environment, there is role clarity within the disciplines, goals are clearly articulated, and a leader is designated from among the disciplines.

An example of transdisciplinary communication occurs within the cardiac rehabilitation team at the hospital. The cardiac rehabilitation team has a nurse leader who coordinates all disciplines that are involved with the patient after a myocardial infarction. Discharge planning is begun with the patient within 24 hours of admission. Each discipline is called in at the appropriate time to encourage the patient to regain his or her optimal level of health. Each discipline meets daily on behalf of the patient, formulates goals and objectives, and follows a designated multidisciplinary plan of care or critical pathway. Transdisciplinary communication provides support for the patient with a much broader scope of discipline involvement.

Role of Communication in Management

Managers and leaders are clearly involved in many types of communication, such as meetings, telephone calls, correspondence, and one-on-one counseling. Griffin (1996) reports 10 different roles:

leader, figurehead, liaison, monitor, disseminator, spokesperson, entrepreneur, disturbance handler, resource allocator, and negotiator. These roles are either interpersonal, requiring an interaction with someone; informational, requiring the dissemination of information; or decisional, requiring decisions to be made and communicated. It would be impossible to fill any of these roles without communication.

Communication also relates directly to the functions of planning, organizing, directing, staffing, and controlling. Communication is necessary to establish standards, monitor performance, and take corrective action. Decision-making, delegation, coordination, and leading all involve communication. It is apparent that most activities require some form of communication through which information can reach employees.

Empowerment Through Communication

Empowerment stems from the structure, practices, and policies that are supported by leaders who have control over others, as well as from the personal choices that are made and expressed by a person's actions (Block, 1987). The communication process is vital for organizations to be successful. Leaders must learn to communicate with *all* levels of the organization as well as build support for their visions if empowerment is to be achieved.

Empowerment in the organization occurs when the leaders communicate assertively. Assertive leaders send direct statements that say what they really mean. They use objective words, send "I" messages, and are honest about their feelings. Assertive leaders are attentive listeners and use appropriate gestures and facial expressions while speaking. Being assertive is the ability of the leader to communicate with others about who they really are and where they are coming from (Cornell, 1993). Assertive communication results in an increase in self-esteem, close relationships, positive emotions, and the ability to meet needs. The following is an example of communicating assertively compared with passive, aggressive, and passive-aggressive communication.

CASE STUDY ♦ 11–2

The manager asked me to work an extra shift and I had planned to take the day off to relax. I did not want to work.

PASSIVE RESPONSE

Leader: Would you please work an extra shift for me today?

Me: I can't today.

Leader: I really need you to work. I cannot find anyone else.

Me: Well, I can't work today.

Leader: Why can't you?

Me: Well, all right. I guess I'll come in and work.

AGGRESSIVE RESPONSE

Leader: Would you please work an extra shift for me today?

Me: You've got to be kidding! You know how I hate to work extra shifts. Go find someone else.

PASSIVE-AGGRESSIVE RESPONSE

Leader: Would you please work an extra shift for me today?

Me: Yes, I will if you really need me. (I then plan to arrive late to prove that I am in control or to take revenge.)

ASSERTIVE RESPONSE

Leader: Would you please work an extra shift for me today?

Me: I have planned to take the day off, and I will not work for you today.

Leader: I really need you to work because I cannot find anyone else.

Me: I understand that you are having trouble finding someone, but I'm not willing to work today.

The best response choice in the above scenario is the assertive response. By handling situations in an assertive manner, you will not only convey positive feelings about yourself but also be better respected by your fellow employees. Remember, communication is a goal and not an end product (Kerfoot, 1996); therefore, empowerment is enhanced with communication, especially assertive communication.

CONFLICT MANAGEMENT

Conflict Defined

Conflict is inevitable when dealing with individuals and groups. Conflict is a natural occurrence in every relationship and can be beneficial. Trying to define conflict is not an easy task. There is no one common definition; however, Hocker & Wilmot (1985, p. 22) defined *conflict* as "an expressed struggle between at least two interdependent parties who perceive incompatible goals, scarce rewards, and interference from the other party in achieving his or her goals."

A conflict exists only when both parties are aware of the disagreement and know that a problem exists. You may be upset for weeks because your colleague made a critical remark about you, but a conflict does not exist between the two of you until the colleague learns of your problem. However, an *expressed struggle*, or an encounter, does not have to be verbalized. You can show displeasure with someone with a dirty look, "the silent treatment," or avoidance of that person.

With *perceived incompatible goals,* all conflicts look as if one person's gain would be another person's loss. However, people may fail to see mutually satisfying answers to their problems, thus causing conflict to exist. Consider the colleague who made the critical remark. If you confront this person, he or she may get angry and make life miserable. On the other hand, you could confront this person, and he or she will appreciate your honesty and explain to you that the remark was merely a matter of misunderstanding or misperception.

Conflict also exists when people *perceive scarce rewards,* such as "not enough to go around." Money can cause many conflicts, especially if an employee wants a raise in pay and the manager does not have the resources to provide it. Conflict can be caused from the scarce commodity of time. With only 24 hours in a day, it is difficult to balance the constant struggle of limited time with families, employers, colleagues, editors, students, and friends, thus causing conflicts. Each wants and needs more time than there is to go around.

Even though one may feel antagonistic toward another, the people in conflict usually are dependent on each other. If this were not so, there would be no need for conflict. *Interdependence* often exists between two conflicting parties, and many conflicts go unresolved because parties fail to understand this interdependence (Adler & Towne, 1990). To resolve a conflict, the parties must realize they are in their situation together.

Conflict refers to any opposition or antagonistic behavior and can be either functional or dysfunctional. *Functional* conflict is a confrontation between two parties that can be constructive and benefit the organization through increased effort, improved performance, enhanced creativity, and personal development (Kreitner, 1995). For example, two hospitals may be in conflict over which will provide women's health services to a specific area in the suburbs. In their attempt to prove that each hospital has the better services, both hospitals create new and improved services that benefit not only that particular population but others as well.

Dysfunctional conflict is any interaction between two parties that hinders or destroys the achievement of the goals of the organization or group and is destructive in nature (Cherrington, 1994). Cherrington (1994) and Kreitner (1995) reported the symptoms of dysfunctional conflict to include indecision, emotional outburst, apathy, resistance to change, chaos, decreased performance, and increased political maneuvering. The most common destructive way in which groups resist conflict is to ignore it and act as if the conflict does not exist (Bormann et al, 1982). Dysfunctional conflict can be resolved through problem-solving, compromise, management goals, forcing, or smoothing. Some of these strategies are discussed later.

Causes of Conflict

Conflict can develop from numerous situations and sources. According to Cherrington (1994), most causes of conflict are derived from task interdependence, goal incompatibility, the use of threats, group identification, and win-lose attitudes. However, conflict can also arise from any situation or source and involve any individual or group. Conflict can stem from sender messages or receiver perceptions. Conflict can arise from roles that the leader or employee must assume. Conflict should not become so great that it prevents the organization or individual from moving toward his or her goals.

Task Interdependence

Task interdependence occurs when two or more groups or individuals depend on each other to accomplish their tasks (Cherrington, 1994). Therefore, as the degree of task interdependence increases, the potential for conflict increases. An example of task interdependence is when a contributor is writing a chapter for an edited book. The editors cannot complete the book until all chapters have been turned in from the contributors. Another example of task interdependence involves how all elements of a health care system work together to provide skilled patient care. Home health care, acute care services, nursing home services, pharmacy, dietary, and nursing must all coordinate their efforts through transdisciplinary and transorganizational communication.

Goal Incompatibility

Goal incompatibility can exist between the organization and the individual as well as between departments and groups. For example, radiology personnel may send for the patient and expect nursing personnel to have the patient ready for transport. However, some arrhythmias may be evident on the patient's electrocardiogram strip, and nursing staff needs to first call the physician. Radiology personnel become frustrated with nursing personnel because they have a schedule to maintain and cannot understand why the nurse did not call the physician sooner. However, nursing staff was busy with other critical patients and did not see the need to contact the radiology department. Thus, a conflict develops.

Conflicts also may arise when resources are scarce, such as when money, space, labor, or materials are limited. If groups are forced to compete for these resources, frequently a dysfunctional conflict will arise due to a *win-lose competition*. Little conflicts usually lead to larger conflicts.

Use of Threats

Conflict increases when one individual has the ability to threaten the other. Studies have indicated that the use of threats decreases productivity (Cherrington, 1994). Individuals tend to stew over the threat rather than get over it quickly. For example, a man-

ager tells an employee that if she accepts scholarship moneys to go back to school, she will have to become part-time in her position. Because the employee cannot afford part-time status, she has to turn down the scholarship. Subsequently, the employee stews over the decision for several months before she is able to get over the leader's decision and become productive again. The quickest resolution to a problem occurs only when neither party has access to a threat. The absence of threats encourages individuals or groups to be more cooperative and compatible (Cherrington, 1994).

Group Identification

Research has shown that assignment of people to different groups allows them to develop a *cohesiveness* that allows intergroup conflict to result (Cherrington, 1994). Conflict between groups is a natural consequence of group cohesiveness. A feeling of solidarity among group members may contribute to an unfavorable attitude toward other groups. As groups become more cohesive, the potential for conflict increases between the groups. An example of this type of conflict occurred between two committees in a school of nursing. As the cohesiveness increased within one of the committees, that committee became judgmental and critical of the other committee, even though they were not in competition with each other.

Win-Lose Situations

It is unfortunate that many situations are perceived as win-lose situations when they are not. Cherrington (1994) identified frequent conditions that exist for *win-lose situations* to occur. These situations occur when someone interprets the situation as win-lose conflict: one group chooses to pursue its own goals while another publicly disguises its needs; one group attempts to increase its power position while another makes threats; one group exaggerates its needs, goals, and position while the other exploits the first group; and one group isolates the other group. When any one of these situations occurs, communication becomes guarded and may even discontinue. Getting two groups or individuals to change this situation to a win-win situation is difficult.

Research has indicated that a person who unconditionally makes cooperative choices does not necessarily lead the group or others to reciprocal cooperation; instead, this may lead to exploitation of the individual (Cherrington, 1994). The most effective strategy for obtaining cooperation seems to be *conditional cooperation* (Swingle, 1970). For example, an individual is willing to cooperate as long as others respond cooperatively.

Conflicting Messages

Conflicts can arise from the *perceptual misunderstanding* of messages by the sender or receiver. This is one reason it is so important to learn to communicate clearly. Sometimes an individual can receive conflicting messages from two or more sources. Many examples of this kind of misunderstanding may occur in a school of nursing; one example is a dean who expects a course coordinator to function as an administrator while the faculty expects the coordinator to act as advocate.

Conflicting Roles

Conflict can arise when individuals belong to more than one group. For example, two committees may be scheduled to meet at the same time. Normally this would not cause a problem, but because you belong to both of these committees, a conflict occurs over which committee meeting to attend. Conflict can also arise when an individual has *unrealistic expectations*. Sometimes individuals may not allow themselves sufficient time to fulfill an obligation, causing increased stress and conflict. This occurs when an individual "wears several hats," such as someone who is wife, mother, employee, student, researcher, and author.

Role conflict can occur when an individual does not know exactly what is expected of him or her (Marriner-Tomey, 1996). This type of conflict stems from *role ambiguity*. Frequently, role ambiguity occurs in organizations that do not have clearly written job descriptions; however, conflict can be caused if the manager has delegated a task to the employee without giving clear guidelines for task completion.

This often happens with beginning clinicians because they tend to hold back and not ask for guidance. A beginning clinician may perceive that the leader will think that the new clinician should know the answer; consequently, he or she will not ask for guidance.

Approaches to Conflict

Adler and Towne (1990) identified three possible courses of action when faced with a conflict: *accepting the status quo* (ie, living with the problem); *using force and mandating change*; or *reaching an agreement by negotiating*. Negotiation is discussed later.

Three types of *outcomes* result from these approaches to conflict management: win-lose approach, lose-lose approach, and win-win approach (Adler & Towne, 1990). Occasionally, a win-lose approach will disintegrate into a lose-lose outcome, causing all persons to agonize over the conflict; however, if the persons involved in the conflict have the proper attitude and skills, win-win outcomes are more possible than people realize.

Win-Lose Approach

A *win-lose approach* can result from a win-lose attitude. In a win-lose approach, one person gets what he or she wants while the other person does not (Adler & Towne, 1990). The most obvious example of this occurs in the field of sports: in baseball, one team must win, and the other must lose. An example closer to nursing occurs when two colleagues are up for the same promotion and only one can be promoted. A characteristic of this type of approach is *power*, real or implied, as when a manager coerces a registered nurse to behave in a certain manner with the threat of termination. Win-lose is sometimes the best approach, especially in a situation of right and wrong. An example of this would be if an individual is out to do someone harm; to restrain this person would be of benefit to all concerned.

Lose-Lose Approach

In a *lose-lose approach,* no one is happy with the outcome (Adler & Towne, 1990). Sometimes, when two parties are both striving to be winners, the struggle ends up with both losing. Compromise is a form of the lose-lose approach that is discussed later; however, because some people are willing to settle for less, a compromise may be agreed on that satisfies neither party completely. A classic case of lose-lose often occurs in the controversy surrounding smoking. For example, if smokers wish to smoke, they must retreat outside to enjoy what they consider a rare cigarette, whereas the nonsmoker feels like a heel for making the smoker go outdoors. Both lose something. The smoker loses comfort, and the nonsmoker loses some good will.

Win-Win Approach

In the *win-win approach* to conflict resolution, the goal is to satisfy both parties involved (Adler & Towne, 1990); therefore, both parties will work together to find a solution that lets everyone reach his or her goal and gain satisfaction, and no one loses. An example is as follows:

The registered nurse is a single parent and has certain needs regarding placement of her children. She cannot leave them at the day care center before 7:15 AM, and she needs to be available to pick the children up before the center closes at 4:00 PM. However, the nurse manager expects the registered nurse to work the entire day shift.

The leader discusses the situation with the registered nurse, and they are able to work out an arrangement to accommodate both the registered nurse and the unit. Because morning report is generally not completed until 8:00 AM, the registered nurse must be at work by 8:00 AM and will be allowed to leave work by 3:30 PM. Working this schedule enables the registered nurse to be available to pick up her children, be on the unit during peak times, and still be considered a full-time employee. Both parties are pleased.

Strategies for Managing Conflict

Leaders and managers often find themselves in the middle of dysfunctional conflict. When this happens, they may choose to do nothing, or they may choose to use a strategy to manage the conflict. The following seven strategies are discussed: avoiding,

compromising, smoothing, forcing, competing, confronting, and collaborating.

Avoiding

Even if leaders choose to do nothing, they are still using a strategy to manage the conflict; this is called *avoiding*. The avoidance approach is to simply ignore the conflict and hope it will go away (Griffin, 1996). Avoiding is often chosen by leaders who feel uncomfortable when they have to deal with conflict. Avoiding may be effective in the short run; however, it does not resolve the problem or conflict in the long run, and the problem may worsen. One positive aspect with this approach is that it enables the parties involved in the conflict to have a cool-down period, a time that may work to defuse a potentially explosive conflict.

Compromising

Compromising involves bargaining or negotiating among parties of equal status over a problem or conflict (Cherrington, 1994) and requires flexibility on both sides. Compromise usually means someone wins and someone loses or both parties may lose something. After the compromise is reached, perhaps the groups or individuals can work together in harmony. Frequently, compromise solutions are inferior, and both sides end up unhappy. Compromising is usually a temporary solution; unless conditions, positions, or people change, the problem often resurfaces.

Smoothing

Smoothing is to minimize the conflict and inform everyone that everything will be all right (Griffin, 1996). Smoothing stresses similarities and common interests and minimizes differences. This strategy usually tones down the conflict in the short run but does not solve the underlying conflict. Smoothing does have its place, especially when there is no time for anything else other than holding things together.

Forcing

Forcing occurs when an influential figure steps in, mandates that the conflict subside, and orders the parties in conflict to handle the situation in a certain manner (Kreitner, 1995). Cherrington (1994) identifies this strategy as *power intervention*. This strategy provides only a short-term solution, with formal authority and power at the core of forcing; however, forcing does not resolve the conflict and may actually serve to make it worse by fostering resentment and mistrust in the involved parties, which creates other problems.

Competing

Competing is a total effort to win regardless of the cost. Competing is power-oriented and aggressive. It is the pursuit of one individual's goals at the expense of another's. This type of strategy is appropriate when a quick or unpopular decision must be made, when an individual is knowledgeable about the situation and able to make a sound decision, or when an individual must protect himself or herself from other aggressive people (Marriner-Tomey, 1996).

Confronting

Confronting, sometimes called *problem-solving*, involves bringing together both parties to confront the conflict (Griffin, 1996). This approach requires maturity on the part of the individuals involved. Confrontation requires a discussion regarding the nature of the conflict with an attempt to reach an agreement or solution. Confrontation is a difficult strategy for many people to master; however, it can be learned and must be as free of emotions as possible. Studies have indicated that groups that use confrontation perform at higher productivity levels than groups that do not (Ward & Price, 1991).

Collaborating

Collaborating is resolving the conflict by talking things over. Both parties should achieve mutual satisfaction in collaboration due to an integration of insights necessary to come up with a consensual solution (Swansburg, 1990). Collaborating is assertive and cooperative—a win-win approach (Marriner-Tomey, 1996). Problems are identified and alternatives explored until a consensus is reached.

The major problem with collaboration is the time-consuming nature of this strategy. Collaboration is paramount in situations in which the loss incurred through compromise will be costly. Collaboration does lead to satisfaction.

Working with Difficult People

Every organization has its share of difficult people. How well you deal with an employer, a colleague, or an employee who may be currently making your life miserable depends on the outcome to be achieved. It is hard not to take other people's behavior personally, especially when the hostility seems to be aimed directly at you. Some people tend to react to difficult people without thinking, thus losing sight of their own interests. According to Ury (1991), there are three natural reactions: *to strike back* (give them a taste of their own medicine); *to give in* (just to be out of the situation and not have to deal with them); or *to break off* (get out of the relationship or resign or dissolve it). However, Lewis-Ford (1993), Righthand (1983), and Solomon (1990) suggested several guidelines that can help leaders and coworkers deal with difficult people.

Guidelines for Dealing with Difficult People

- *Keep difficult people in proper perspective.* Do not take their behavior personally. Remember, you are either an obstacle or an essential ingredient to their getting what they want. Try to break free of their control.

- *Make your choice—you can be positive or negative.* When you cling to negative feelings, it is hard to concentrate on creative alternatives. Retreat to a quiet place, vent your emotions, calm down, and let go of the hurt. Determine the results and take the appropriate action.

- *Do not expect difficult people to change.* Most of the time they will not. However, this may be to your advantage because their behavior will be predictable. Knowing this allows you to plan ahead and decide on the strategy you will use. A proper strategy may change the outcome or allow for a positive resolution of the conflict.

- *Learn how to respond and be a good listener.* Be

assertive and state how you feel about the situation. The offense could be unintentional and therefore easily resolved if allowed to surface. Do not make accusations; instead, ask questions.

- *Give and request frequent and specific feedback.* Know the perceptions of your employer, colleagues, and employees. Ask, do not fret. Allow emotional people to vent their feelings before reasoning with them.

- *Look at the policies and procedures first.* Taking stock of standard operating procedure may place the disagreement on a higher or more professional level. Do not place blame; apologize quickly, and move on. Pay attention to the needs of the other person when looking at options. A simple change in the system may be all that is needed.

- *Deal directly and discreetly.* Choose face-to-face communication rather than a memorandum that can be misconstrued, telephone calls that conceal facial reactions, or ambassadors who do the talking for you. Do not have an audience for personal disagreements. Tactfully put your foot down, and do not let others walk all over you. Get right to the point because excuses or warm-ups rob you of your effectiveness.

- *Document for self-protection.* Get verbal agreements in writing to prevent the other person from backing out. Keep your employer informed with progress reports, especially on projects that may be hazardous to your career. Send copies to all affected in case of a misunderstanding.

- *Be straightforward and unemotional.* By remaining calm and matter-of-fact, you will gain confidence of others. Be straightforward with people so they will trust you. Respect from others begins with self-respect. Do not continue a conversation with anyone who refuses to give you the courtesy you deserve. You have options: ask for politeness or leave the room.

- *Be courteous.* If someone else is rude, this does not give you the right to also be rude. Disarm your offenders; treat them with kindness, share credit, and allow others to feel important. Make friends with your enemies; you never know when you may need them. Show appreciation and give recognition. When your own ego is healthy, you are rich and can afford to be generous.

Tactics Used by Difficult People

There are several unfair tactics that difficult people use to strike out at others. Ury (1991) discusses three categories of tactics that a person needs to be familiar with to defuse and neutralize them: stone walls, attacks, and tricks.

A *stone wall tactic* is a refusal to move. The person tries to convince you that there is absolutely no other choice than his or her position. Nothing can be changed, and all other suggestions on your part meet with a "no." An example of this tactic is when a professor shares with her team a new clinical schedule that she has written. She states that this schedule is the only choice the team has that can handle the number of students involved. All other suggestions meet with resistance along with a final "no."

An *attack tactic* is a pressure tactic that is designed to make another person feel uncomfortable and sufficiently intimidated to give in to the person's demands. Some people actually threaten that things must be done their way "or else." This type of person may attack your credibility, proposal, status, or authority. They may stoop to insulting, badgering, or bullying until they get their way. One example of an attack tactic is when a professor decides that she is unhappy with a colleague who is pursuing her doctoral degree. The professor accuses the colleague of not carrying her teaching load (which is incorrect) and declares that the colleague should either decrease or stop working on her doctoral studies. For several months, the colleague must endure the professor's anger, insults, and bullying behavior.

Trick tactics are tactics that deceive a person into giving in. Individuals who use such tactics take advantage of you while you believe they are acting in good faith and telling the truth. Manipulating the data is one type of trick. Another trick is to mislead a person into believing that he or she has the authority to decide an issue when, in essence, someone else must make the decision. A third trick is the last-minute demand after a person believes an agreement has already been reached. An example of a trick tactic is when a leader draws up a new hospital procedure and submits it to the director for approval. The director, instead of approving the procedure as anticipated, passes it on to administration. Administration makes several changes and sends it back to the director, who sends it back to the leader for revision.

A tactic must be recognized before it can be neutralized. *Keep alert*, *look for clues*, and *watch for mismatching* between words, facial expressions, and body language. Know that difficult people use several tactics, not just one. Remember, if the difficult person perceives that he or she is not able to make you react, then you will probably be left alone, and the bullying will cease.

Dealing with Anger

When an individual encounters an angry person, the normal response is to also become angry because anger begets anger. The individual receiving the anger may feel hurt, confused, frustrated, and even sad. It does no good to respond at this point because judgment will be distorted. The cycle needs to be broken, so you must pause and concentrate on the desired outcome. Some angry people try to intimidate or bully; others are out for revenge. Regardless of the situation, whether the angry person is an employer, colleague, or employee, Solomon (1990) and Ury (1991) suggest a few basic principles on how to deal with an angry person.

- *Control your own behavior.* You may not be able to control the behavior of an angry person, but you can control your own behavior. Buy yourself some time to think. Keep your eyes on the desired outcome.

- *Create a favorable climate.* Resist the person's anger by not attacking back but instead *listening*, acknowledging his or her point, and agreeing when you can. Disarm the person by acknowledging his or her competence and authority. Remember, a word softly spoken defuses anger.

- *Do not reject; instead, reframe.* If you reject the angry person's position, it will only reinforce it; therefore, direct his or her attention to looking at both sides. Reframe whatever the person says in an attempt to deal with the problem. Let the problem be the teacher, not you. Ask questions such as "What would you do if you were in my position?"

- *Build the bridge.* Do not push or insist, but lead the person in the direction you would like him or her to go. Be a mediator. Incorporate the person's ideas and become involved in the process. Help the person to save face, and try to make the outcome appear to be his or her victory. Look at the person's needs, and build a bridge between you.

- *Be firm, forceful, and assertive.* Speak with assurance and confidence. Do not cower; instead, be patient. Educate and use power to bring the person to his or her senses. Treat the person with respect.

By using these principles, the leader or individual will be better able to deal with the person who is angry. By putting your reaction on hold and doing the opposite of what you may feel like doing, you will be able to circumvent the person's anger; you may even make your adversary your friend.

Empowerment Through Conflict Management

The best way for empowerment to be achieved in the organization is for the leader to learn how to manage conflict effectively. Approaches, strategies, and tactics must be learned to be able to resolve conflict. The leader must also be prepared to work with difficult or angry people. All leaders must be able to resolve conflict to provide an environment that stimulates the personal growth of the employees and provides quality care for the patients. Interventions must be directed toward maximizing assertiveness through collaboration and cooperation.

Conflict management requires the leader to have the ability to solve problems, make decisions, view situations with empathy, and focus on problems and issues rather than on persons. It also requires the leader to stay calm and not become reactive when confrontation takes place.

An effective leader may bring together individuals or groups that are in conflict and act as a facilitator. The leader may help conflicting parties identify the problem, sort out ideas and attitudes, and find alternatives to resolve the problem or conflict. Empowerment through conflict management enables the leader to have the ability to listen, instill trust, be open, and be flexible. Empowerment is enhanced through conflict management.

NEGOTIATION

Negotiation Defined

Everyone negotiates; negotiation is a fact of life. However, trying to find a sound definition of negotiation is like trying to find the much-sought-after needle in a haystack. Nierenberg (1973) discusses the broad scope of negotiation. He states that people are negotiating when they exchange ideas with the intent of changing relationships and when they deliberate for an agreement. Because negotiation depends on communication, it occurs between individuals either acting for themselves or as a representative of an organized group. Negotiation is considered an element of human behavior as well as a "role" for the leader. *Negotiation* is often thought of as a situation between individuals or groups in which those involved strive to identify a settlement that is acceptable to all.

It was once believed that there were only two main ways of negotiating: soft and hard. However, Fisher and Ury (1981) identify a third way called *principled negotiation*. *Soft* negotiators want to avoid personal conflict, so they make concessions to reach an agreement quickly, even though they may end up feeling bitter and exploited. *Hard* negotiators look at any situation as a contest of personal wills. They believe that the person who takes the extreme position and holds out the longest does better in negotiating. The hard negotiator wants to win so badly that both the negotiator and his or her resources end up exhausted and relationships are harmed. *Principled negotiation* is the third way to negotiate, and it is both hard and soft. Issues are discussed on their merits rather than through a haggling process focused by what each party says it will and will not do. The method of principled negotiation is hard on the merits yet soft on the people. There are no tricks or posturing. This method allows people to be fair while protecting themselves against others who take advantage of them. Principled negotiation is an all-purpose strategy.

Phases of Negotiation

Negotiation is a behavioral process and should be a cooperative enterprise in which common interests are sought (Nierenberg, 1973). If both parties enter the situation on a *cooperative basis*, there is a greater possibility that mutual satisfaction can be reached. Better results and more lasting solutions can be achieved from a cooperative effort. However, if one party tries to dominate, the spirit of cooperation is dissolved, and true negotiation cannot take place.

The first lesson a negotiator must learn is *when to stop*. A negotiator must learn when he or she is approaching the critical point and stop just before it is reached. All persons should have some needs satisfied when coming out of the process. Everybody should win something in good negotiations.

In preparing for negotiation, you must have *well-established objectives*. Will the process be an individual or a team approach? A *single negotiator* may be able to prevent questions aimed at weaker team members because the responsibility is placed on one person; however, a *team* would use several people with different backgrounds who could pool their judgments. What are the issues to be negotiated, and what positions will be taken? Where will the negotiation take place? Other considerations are how to begin the agenda, what position will be revealed, what long-term strategies should be considered, and how much preparation needs to be done.

Fisher and Ury (1981) identified phases of negotiations to include analysis planning and discussion to reach the desired outcome (Fig. 11–7). The fol-

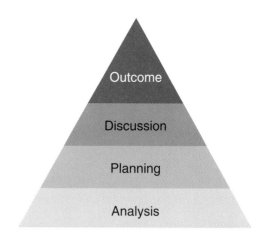

Figure 11–7. Model depicting the phases of negotiation as one strives to reach the desired outcome.

lowing four principles must be considered in each phase of principled negotiations:

- *Keep the people separated from the problem.*
- *Focus on interests and issues, not positions.*
- *Generate a variety of options before making a decision.*
- *Insist on objective criteria or data.*

In the *analysis phase*, a person or team should try to gather and organize the criteria and data to be able to diagnose the situation. In the *planning phase*, all four principles are considered, with special attention given to generating additional options or alternatives before a decision. In the *discussion phase*, perceptual differences and difficulties in communication must be identified and discussed. For a sound agreement and the desired outcome to be reached, negotiations should focus on mutually satisfying options, interests, and clear standards.

Tactics in Negotiation

Effective negotiation is based on communication and persuasion. You must be able to listen, speak clearly, and build relationships; however, some people do not play fair, and tactics on how to deal with these people must be learned. Cohen (1980) recognized the need to build trust, gain commitment, and manage the opposer. Numerous tactics on how to handle the opponent have been identified by Nierenberg (1973). These tactics are categorized into "when" and "how and where" tactics.

"When" Tactics

"When" tactics are separated into the following: *Forbearance* can be referred to as a cooling-off period or a knowing when to stop. For example, when negotiating for the best price, you must have a sense of when to stop pushing the salesperson for a lower price. Therefore, do your homework before negotiating and gather some information on what the company may have paid for the item.

Surprise is a sudden shift or change in positions on an issue. For example, if during the negotiation process one individual starts to act irrational and flies off the handle, he or she is probably using the surprise tactic. This individual believes his or her behavior makes it more difficult for the opposing side to cope with the situation.

Fait accompli (or "now it is up to you") demands that you act to achieve your goal against the opposition and see what the opposition will do. This tactic can be demonstrated by the dismissal of a university president. The board of trustees dismissed the president and then made the announcement to the faculty, students, and alumni. In effect, the board said, "It is done. What are you going to do about it?" Consequently, those affected by the president's dismissal found the situation to be too much trouble to do anything about it.

Bland withdrawal is actual withdrawal in a "Who, me?" type of incident. The story is told of a hotel guest who wrote an irate letter to the manager of the franchise complaining about the bugs in a room. Shortly thereafter, the guest received a letter from the franchise manager discussing at length how delighted they were to hear from their customers, how important communication was, and that the problem would be dealt with immediately. The guest was delighted with the response until he discovered that his original letter had been inadvertently attached to the response. In bold red pencil was printed, "Send bug form letter."

Apparent withdrawal is a tactic in which a person pretends to withdraw. The aim is to convince the opponent you have withdrawn while, in fact, you are still in control. This frequently happens with acquisitions. For example, a company receives word that another company is trying to acquire it. After several retaliatory actions, the acquiring company withdraws. The withdrawal is only apparent because the acquiring company is working behind the scenes to obtain stock options and mutual funds. After a time, the company realizes that the acquiring company has gained control.

In *reversal*, the person acts in the opposite manner of what would be considered the trend or goal. This tactic is difficult to implement. An example is intentionally sending two messages to your opponents so they will choose what they believe is the more advantageous and ignore the other message. In reality, you have embellished on the second message so the first one will be chosen.

Limits can be in the form of communication, time, or geography. A meeting could be called 3 days before Christmas, thus setting a natural limit on the meeting.

Feinting means to look to the right and go to the left (to fake or mislead). It is a distraction strategy and can be used to cover up important elements. An example of this is governmental decisions. Sometimes a "reliable source" releases a decision as a trial balloon before the decision is actually made. This tactic gives the government an opportunity to test the responses that might occur when and if the actual decision is made. If too much opposition develops, a new decision can be made to counteract the adverse responses.

"How and Where" Tactics

"How and where" tactics are as follows:

In *participation*, you enlist other persons on your behalf to act either directly or indirectly. When a large corporation is contemplating acquiring a family-owned business, the corporation will agree to let the family business know it can operate in the same tradition and manner that the business was previously run. After the acquisition, the buyer and seller participate in running the business on a mutually satisfactory basis.

Association is an attempt to get a person associated with a project to take advantage of name recognition. This tactic is used extensively, especially in advertising. For example, a famous person gives a testimonial on television that he or she uses a certain hospital. Many people will believe the hospital is good just because of who uses it. They will identify with the person and begin to use the hospital.

Disassociation is the reverse of association. It is discrediting someone by showing a connection with unsavory characters. In a political race, someone will try to discredit his or her opponent by showing that person with some people of questionable reputation.

With *cross-roads*, a person introduces several matters into discussion so a bargaining position can be staked out. For example, the registered nurse may say, "We want shorter work days." The manager may reply, "In view of the fact that you are now asking for shorter work days, you will have to agree to give up having weekends off, which we previously agreed on."

Blanketing covers as much an area as possible to achieve a breakthrough in one or more places. It can prevent the opposer from knowing where your weaknesses are. An interesting example of this tactic may occur during union negotiations. One employer comes into the designated negotiation room every morning and fills the board with his or her demands, so open spaces on which the union negotiators could write are eliminated. This serves as a visible reminder of the demands of the employer and takes the initiative away from the union to set forth its demands.

Randomizing is outbluffing by chance. Con men are especially proficient in this tactic. The con man randomly chooses a neighborhood and approaches a stranger. For payment in advance he sells them a service to be delivered tomorrow. However, tomorrow arrives, and the con man is long gone.

In *salami*, the negotiator takes concessions bit by bit and eventually wins the entire thing. The national government sometimes uses this tactic to gradually withdraw from purchasing arrangements with certain manufacturers. It phases out the orders to a particular manufacturer until the supply is completely cut off.

The leader should practice and experiment with these tactics, realizing that for every tactic, a set of countertactics must be anticipated.

Effective Negotiation Characteristics

For the leader to obtain what is wanted through negotiation, it is important to know some of the effective characteristics of negotiation. An effective negotiator is familiar with the following characteristics of negotiation (Jandt & Gillette, 1976; Kelley, 1983; Kirk, 1986; Marriner-Tomey, 1996, Nierenberg, 1973; and Sobkowski, 1990):

- *Good communication is essential.* Listen as well as talk.

- *Be well informed through skillful preparation.* Research pertinent information to be prepared.

- *Be positive in your approach.* Optimism goes much further than negativism.

- *Be prepared to take risks.* Maintain credibility and a good reputation for fair play. Examine the consequences of the outcomes.

- *Decide on a mutually satisfying solution.* Remember, for negotiation to be successful, both parties should be satisfied.

- *Have an open mind.* Be flexible in approaches and goals.
- *Achieve harmony during problem-solving.* Select a strategy and use it.
- *Present creative alternatives to meet opponents' needs.*
- *Get it in writing.* Always get the final results in writing—not only for your benefit but also for clarification of the process and solution.
- *Understand the thinking of others.* Discuss each other's perspective. Do not assume the opponent's values are the same as yours.
- *Focus on shared compatible interests,* not just conflicting ones. Know the needs of your opponent.
- *Rank your wants in order of importance.*
- *Identify and know your resources.*
- *Develop positive coalitions quickly.* Begin to network with other leaders, professional colleagues, and employees.
- *Evaluate the effectiveness of the negotiation.* This requires a value judgment. Was it a positive or negative experience?

By focusing on these characteristics, the leader and employee can become effective negotiators. It takes time to develop negotiation skills; however, *practice* and *communication* are the keys to effective negotiation.

Empowerment Through Negotiation

As vision and directions become clear, empowerment will occur through the well-developed negotiation skills of the leader. According to Rowland & Rowland (1992), empowerment requires the ability of the leader to recognize potential and turn control over to those with directions as needed. There are multidimensional opportunities for the leader to use negotiation skills. Kelley (1983) states that effective negotiators never plateau, they just continue to refine their skills and seize every opportunity to develop the technique of negotiation.

To become an empowered leader, agreement and trust must provide the essential elements for negotiation, as does the sharing of vision, purpose, and goals (Block, 1987). During the process of negotia-

tion, the leader becomes able to recognize common communication barriers and has the knowledge, ability, and understanding to select the specific tactic needed. Empowerment through negotiation involves not only the sharing of goals, purpose, and vision but also the resolution of identified issues with proven strategies. Negotiation enhances empowerment in an organization.

SUMMARY

Successful leaders have the ability to communicate effectively, manage conflict appropriately, and negotiate productively. To enable leaders to become effective, assertive communicators, they should understand the process, components, and flow of communication and be able to identify the barriers to communication. They should also understand the causes, approaches, and strategies for appropriately managing conflict. The ability to manage or resolve conflict prepares leaders to work with difficult or angry people. Productive negotiation occurs when leaders are able to recognize communication barriers and have the ability to select specific negotiation tactics to resolve those barriers. Communication, conflict management, and negotiation enhance empowerment.

■ DISCUSSION QUESTIONS ■

1. Discuss the major portions of the communication process. At what level is communication likely to be misunderstood or misconstrued?
2. What is the importance of transdisciplinary communication and organizational relationships in the changing health care environment?
3. Analyze approaches and strategies for managing conflict. When may one approach work when another has not?
4. What are some of the pitfalls of poor communication? How can these pitfalls affect patient care?

■ LEARNING ACTIVITIES ■

1. As a leader in achieving patient outcomes, how would you vary your application of the communication process with the following key players:

physician, dietitian, pharmacist, and social service representative?

2. You have been asked to lead a transdisciplinary team on a cardiac unit. How will you create a supportive environment, clarify roles, meet goals, and establish trust among the other disciplines?

3. Identify and discuss strategies you would use to deal with an aggressive, angry nurse manager.

4. You have been called to interview for the position of nurse leader on an oncology unit. What negotiation tactics and characteristics will you use to meet your needs?

■ BIBLIOGRAPHY ■

Adler RB, Towne N (1990). *Looking Out Looking In Interpersonal Communication*. Fort Worth: Holt, Rinehart & Winston.

Allred HF, Clark JF (1978). Written communication problems and priorities. *Journal of Business Communication* 15:31–35.

Atwater E (1981). *"I Hear You": How to Use Listening Skills for Profit*. Englewood Cliffs, NJ: Prentice-Hall.

Barton A (1991). Conflict resolution by nurse managers. *Nursing Management* 22:83–86.

Block P (1991). *The Empowered Manager: Positive Political Skills at Work*. San Francisco: Jossey-Bass.

Bormann EG, Howell WS, Nichols RG, et al (1982). *Interpersonal Communication in the Modern Organization*, 2nd ed. Englewood Cliffs, NJ: Prentice-Hall.

Cherrington DJ (1994). *Organizational Behavior: The Management of Individual and Organizational Performance*. Boston: Allyn and Bacon.

Cornell D (1993). Say the words: Communication techniques. *Nursing Management* 24:42–44.

Dance FE, Larson CE (1976). *The Functions of Human Communication*. New York: Holt, Rinehart and Winston.

Davis K, Newstrom JW (1985). *Human Behavior at Work: Organizational Behavior*, 7th ed. New York: McGraw-Hill.

Fisher R, Ury W (1981). *Getting to Yes: Negotiating Agreement Without Giving In*. Boston: Houghton-Mifflin.

Griffin RW (1996). *Management*, 5th ed. Boston: Houghton-Mifflin.

Hocker JL, Wilmot WW (1985). *Interpersonal Conflict*, 2nd ed. Dubuque, IA: WC Brown.

Jandt FE, Gillette P (1976). *Win-Win Negotiating: Turning Conflict into Agreement*. New York: John Wiley & Sons.

Kelley JA (1983). Negotiating skills for the nursing service administrator. *Nursing Clinics of North America* 18:427–438.

Kerfoot K (1996). On leadership: The change leader. *Nursing Economics* 14:311–312.

Kirk R (1986). Negotiations: Getting what you want. *Journal of Nursing Administration* 16:6–9.

Kreitner R (1995). *Management*. Boston: Houghton-Mifflin.

Lewis-Ford BK (1993). Management techniques: Coping with difficult people. *Nursing Management* 24:36–38.

Littlejohn SW (1989). *Theories of Human Communication*, 3rd ed. Belmont, CA: Wadsworth Publishing.

Malandro CA, Barker L, Barker DA (1989). *Non-Verbal Communication*, 2nd ed. New York: McGraw-Hill.

Marriner-Tomey A (1996). *Guide to Nursing Management*, 5th ed. St. Louis: Mosby-Year Book.

Mehrabian A (1981). *Silent Messages*, 2nd ed. Belmont, CA: Wadsworth.

Nierenberg GI (1973). *Fundamentals of Negotiating*. New York: Hawthorn Books.

Putnam LL, Roloff MC (1992). *Communication and Negotiation*. Newbury Park, CA: Sage.

Reps P (1967). *Square Sun, Square Moon*. New York: Tuttle.

Righthand P (1983). How to deal with rude demanding unreasonable people. *Nursing Life* 3:28–32.

Rowland HS, Rowland BL (1992). *Nursing Administration Handbook*, 3rd ed. Gaithersburg, MD: Aspen.

Sobkowski A (1990). Everything's negotiable. *Executive Female* 18(8):38–40.

Solomon M (1990). *Working with Difficult People*. Englewood Cliffs, NJ: Prentice-Hall.

Sullivan EJ, Decker PJ (1992). *Effective Management in Nursing*, 3rd ed. Redwood City, CA: Addison-Wesley.

Swansburg RD (1990). *Management and Leadership for Nurse Managers*. Boston: Jones & Bartlett.

Swets PW (1983). *The Art of Talking So That People Will Listen*. Englewood Cliffs, NJ: Prentice-Hall.

Swingle CP (ed) (1970). *The Structure of Conflict*. New York: Academic Press.

Tappen RW (1995). *Nursing Leadership and Management: Concepts and Practice*, 3rd ed. Philadelphia: FA Davis.

Ury W (1991). *Getting Past No: Negotiating with Difficult People*. New York: Bantam.

Ward MJ, Price SA (1991). *Issues in Nursing Administration*. St. Louis: Mosby-Year Book.

12 Group Dynamics and Cultural Diversity

Virginia Kay Rogers, MS, MEd, RNC

. . . .

L E A R N I N G   O B J E C T I V E S

This chapter will enable the learner to:

1. Recognize three essential components involved in group dynamics.
2. Explain the relationship of group dynamics to cultural diversity issues in the health care workplace.
3. Identify strategies that enable a nurse to identify cultural diversity issues as they occur in the workplace.
4. Interpret a model for managing conflict in the health care workplace.

. . . .

INTRODUCTION

The 1990s have revealed major political and socioeconomic changes in the management of health care. Health care reform issues have highlighted the need to examine other methods of delivering nursing care, not only to reflect increased quality but to deliver care more expeditiously and with fewer numbers of nurses. Nursing leaders are having to become more involved with groups of individuals, both internal and external to the organization, to accomplish job responsibilities. In many instances, this involves having to work closely with

_____

This chapter reflects the author's personal views and in no way represents the official view of the Department of Veterans Affairs of the U.S. Government.

individuals in other disciplines for the purpose of sharing information or for solving problems in the workplace. Working with groups of individuals, therefore, requires the basic knowledge of the theory of group dynamics, as well as issues related to cultural diversity within the workplace. Examples of groups commonly seen in health care settings that are led by nurses are focus groups, ad hoc groups, quality improvement teams, project teams, task forces, and process teams. The purpose of this chapter is to examine the theory of group dynamics, explain the relationship of group dynamics to cultural diversity, and suggest strategies and a model useful in meeting the challenges of working in culturally diverse environments.

THEORY OF GROUP DYNAMICS

Group dynamics is a field of study that explains how individuals interact and build unity. A _group_ is a collection of individuals who are attached to one another and held together by a variety of forces. Such forces include three essential dynamics of group process: (1) group membership, (2) social reality, and (3) group development. These components shape the members' attitudes and behaviors within the group (Bettenhausen, 1991). Group membership affects each member's self-identity. No matter how much a person may want to feel comfortable in a group situation, there is a strong tendency to maintain one's self-identity. The component of group membership includes its role, activities, symbols, and rituals. These shape how the members perceive each other, how they feel about themselves, and how each acts within the group. Group expectations may sometimes interfere with the need to maintain self-identity. A common purpose with similar goals, combined with the commitment to and the identification with each group member, ultimately shapes the group's progression and direction (Bettenhausen, 1991).

The norms of the group help guide an individual in developing a social reality. *Norms* are pre-existing standards for behavior that comprise the members' personalities, attitudes, beliefs, communication patterns, and motivation levels. Individuals learn to interpret their world through the social interactions of others. Either through agreement or negotiation, members find out the realities of the group through the visualization and interpretation of group behaviors. When a group meets for the first time, members tend to observe the behavior of others to determine what behaviors will likely be perceived as appropriate. Individuals consider their own experiences and, if some are relevant, will consider whether they might contribute to the success of the group activities. When all the members' visualizations are in agreement about the task to be pursued, work can begin. It is through these interactions that each member learns effective communication patterns. What is being said is referred to as *content* and how the content is being expressed is referred to as the *process* (Bettenhausen & Murnighan, 1991).

The final component in the dynamics of group process is group development. Groups develop through six stages (Bettenhausen, 1991; Smith & Hukill, 1994): (1) orientation, (2) forming, (3) storming, (4) norming, (5) performing, and (6) termination.

Orientation

Orientation is the first stage of the process. In this stage, the group members are exposed to the basic concepts of group dynamics, such as the group's purpose, group rules, and members' role responsibilities. Using a directive style of communication, the group leader outlines the purpose of the group, negotiates each member's schedule, and defines the goals of the group (Smith & Hukill, 1994).

Forming

The second stage of group development is *forming*. Forming is characterized by courtesy, caution, con-

fusion, and commonality (Bettenhausen, 1991). The group's members are learning about each other through verbal and nonverbal communications, decision-making, and problem-solving. A plan is developed with the group primarily focusing on the problem. During this stage, the group leader's style remains directive, to facilitate and foster trust and openness, active participation, and creativity among all members. The leader represents a positive role model by actively encouraging different views, opinions, ideas, and thoughts from each member. The group leader starts to become cognizant of the tone of the group (Smith & Hukill, 1994).

Storming

The third stage is called *storming*. Storming is characterized by concern, criticism, confrontation, and conflict (Bettenhausen, 1991). During this stage, the members are beginning to feel more cohesive and trusting toward one another, yet the ability to be open leads to vulnerabilities, which causes frustration, questioning, and impatience. These may ultimately result in issues of conflict. The group leader begins to become less directive, starts to assign tasks to each member, and refocuses the group toward realistic expectations and goals. The leader may also evaluate the group's dynamics (Smith & Hukill, 1994).

Norming

The fourth stage is *norming*. Norming is characterized by cohesion, commitment, and cooperation (Bettenhausen, 1991). The members of the group have established trusting relationships and are able to identify the roles and responsibilities of one another. The leader's role begins to become less directive and more supportive of the members. Attention is given to content and process. Problem-solving starts to result in recommendations (Smith & Hukill, 1994).

Performing

The fifth stage of group development is called *performing*. This stage is characterized by challenge, consideration, creativity, and consciousness (Bettenhausen, 1991). The members are very active and accepting of their roles and responsibilities. The leader begins to function like the other group members. Each member begins to accept a leadership role. The elements of leadership, which include authority, influence, and power, begin to become more evenly distributed among group members, but the leader continues to give praise for the group's efforts while still reinforcing the goals. When the group leader is able to step back and allow the members meaningful participation in the decision-making process, the members become empowered. As outcomes of the group appear, the leader reviews them with the group. Plans for follow-up are then discussed as a group (Smith & Hukill, 1994).

Termination

The sixth stage of group development is *termination* and is characterized by consensus, compromise, communications, and closure (Bettenhausen, 1991; Smith & Hukill, 1994). The members evaluate the goals and objectives of the completed task or activity. Suggestions for improvements concerning the task, or problems identified during the group process are openly discussed. Closure may even be celebrated by group members in the form of a ritual such as a ceremony or party (Smith & Hukill, 1994).

THE ROLE OF THE GROUP LEADER

We have already reviewed some of the group leader's behaviors during each stage of group development. It has been stated that a person who is not in a position of authority, who is outranked, and is new to the organization can still be a leader. *Managing* and *leading* are action-oriented words that characterize a person's ability to successfully lead a group of individuals (Bellman, 1992). A detailed discussion of managing and leading is given in Chapter 8, and a summary of those differences is given in Table 12–1.

Over the last few years, larger bureaucratic organizations have realized that more leading characteristics are needed to be more competitive in the work world (Bellman, 1992). Therefore, nurse leaders need to examine each individual's unique characteristics and how these characteristics can contrib-

Table 12–1.

Differences Between Managing and Leading

MANAGING IS ...	LEADING IS ...
Working within boundaries	Expanding boundaries
Controlling resources	Influencing others
Planning to reach goals	Creating a vision of a possible future
Contracting how and when work will be done	Committing to get the work done no matter what
Emphasizing reason and logic supported by intuition	Emphasizing intuition and feelings supported by reason
Deciding present actions based on the past and present	Deciding present action on the envisioned future
Waiting for all relevant data before deciding	Pursuing enough data to decide now
Measuring performance against plans	Assessing accomplishment against vision

From Bellman GM (1993). *Getting Things Done When You Are Not in Charge.* New York: Simon & Schuster Trade. Copyright 1992 by G. M. Bellman.

ute to the overall success of the organization and to the success of the individual. This could include mentoring other nurses in obtaining a professional or personal goal, in attaining a leadership role, or in being rewarded for their performance (Bellman, 1992). A nurse leader needs to provide an atmosphere that allows open communication among group members, using communication techniques described in Table 12–2.

When facilitating a group, nurse leaders need to be aware of several other group characteristics that may affect members' attitudes and behaviors. These characteristics include group size, gender composition, race, ethnicity, and age. Group *cohesion,* the degree of attraction and motivation to stay in the group, and group *commitment,* an individual's feelings concerning identification and attachment to the group's goals or activities, are important in meeting group needs (Bettenhausen, 1991).

Table 12–2.
Communication Techniques in Group Process
  Leadership

1. Use open-ended questions to begin discussions.
2. Encourage questions from the group members.
3. Respond with a positive statement or summary each time a participant makes a contribution.
4. Give your full attention to each member's contributions.
5. Refrain from negative comments about the members' contributions.
6. Avoid taking sides on the issues. Instead, summarize differences of opinion. Stress that issues can be viewed from many different perspectives, and emphasize a relevant consensus.
7. Seek equal contribution from each member.
8. Actively listen to all members.
9. Focus discussions on the purpose of the group.
10. Check perceptions of the group.
11. Reflect the ability to convey the meaning of what a team member has shared so that others can see it.
12. Clarify statements by focusing on key underlying issues. Sort out confusing and conflicting feelings and thinking.
13. Summarize by reflecting and restating major ideas and feelings, pulling important ideas together and establishing a basis for further discussion. Summarize points of agreement and disagreement among team members.
14. Encourage the members to openly express their feelings and thoughts.
15. Avoid frequent questioning. Too many questions at one time are annoying.
16. Confirm members' basic ideas by emphasizing the facts and encouraging further discussion.

From Smith GB, Hukill E (1994). Quality work improvement groups: From paper to reality. *Journal of Nursing Care Quality* 8(4):1–12.

CULTURAL DIVERSITY IN HEALTH CARE GROUPS

The use of group process can assist with the challenges of cultural diversity. As we enter the 21st century, there is evidence of major demographic change in the United States. By the year 2000, one in every three Americans will be a member of a non-white ethnic group. A Bureau of Census statistic sketches the picture: 85% of those entering the workforce in the year 2000 will be women, African Americans, Asian Americans, Hispanic Americans, and new immigrants (Grossman & Taylor, 1995). The challenges of revamping policies, redesigning human resource systems, and creating new health care delivery systems will require an understanding of the concepts of group dynamics as well as the concepts of cultural diversity. The nurse leader has the responsibility to apply these concepts in practice to create harmony among culturally diverse employees (Davis, 1995).

Cultural Diversity Defined

As we have already seen, the concepts of group dynamics provide a basic understanding of group membership, social reality, and group development. The concepts of cultural diversity are not only dynamic but complex (Walton, 1994). The definition of *culture* is "a pattern of values and beliefs reflected in outer behavior" (Walton, 1994, p. 6). The definition of *diversity* includes "differences in perspectives, values, and abilities based upon many variables, including gender, age, lifestyles, handicaps, sexual preference, and culture" (Davis, 1995, p. 32A). By combining both definitions, *cultural diversity* is defined as individuals with different perceptions of others based upon their own personal values and beliefs. Since the definitions seem relatively easy to comprehend, why is cultural diversity considered so complex and dynamic? The issues concerning cultural diversity encompass one's values, beliefs, behaviors, perspectives, and abilities. These issues mean something different to each of us, and they change with life experiences. This is part of our uniqueness as human beings. We learn at a very early age the values and the behaviors that shape our future thinking and interactions with others. Consider the new graduate nurse who is caring for a dying Asian female. The dying woman refuses to take her pain medicine, stating that it makes her groggy. Instead, she relies on an herbal treatment native to her country that offers her little relief. The nurse becomes more and more frustrated and leaves her room feeling dissatisfied. This patient's behavior stems from the patient's cultural heritage and experiences. We learn at a very early age the values and the behaviors that shape our future thinking and interactions with others. These values and behaviors stem from birthplace, including the region of the country and town we were raised in, personality make-up, family values, socio-economic status, religious affiliation, race, and gender. When we do not see others behaving or thinking like ourselves, there is a possibility that personal bias may lead to issues of discrimination.

Cultural Diversity in the Workplace

In the working environment, bias leads to breakdowns in communications, greater chances for making errors, and increased complaints from staff concerning job dissatisfaction. Therefore, it is essential that nurse leaders assess their present knowledge and understanding of cultural diversity as they develop their roles. Self-awareness and self-understanding contribute to one person's readiness to learn (Walton, 1994). Completing a self-assessment (Table 12–3) could help nurses who have not been exposed to culturally diverse groups make new self-discoveries in this area.

Davis (1995) has identified 10 actions for nurse leaders that will assist in creating a harmonious working environment. Table 12–4 identifies these actions.

The nurse leader needs to listen closely and work with employees to strengthen group relations because the leader serves as a role model for the group (Davis, 1995).

Conflict Management in Culturally Diverse Health Care Groups

Unmanaged diversity can be harmful to an organization. Because the health care setting comprises physicians, nurses, leaders, clerical workers, immigrants, multi-generation white Americans, and various subcultures, managing conflict within and between groups is paramount to the organization. Society demands that people cooperate with each other to improve our health care system. Pathological issues such as racism and sexism undermine

Table 12–3.
Cultural Diversity Self-Assessment

	Almost always	Sometimes	Almost never
1. I am completely comfortable with cultural diversity in my current organization.			
2. I am familiar with my colleagues' backgrounds and traditions.			
3. I communicate effectively with people from different backgrounds.			
4. I understand the role of gender in relationship to my management style.			
5. I build mentoring relationships at work.			
6. I can work well in diverse groups to solve problems.			
7. I avoid stereotyping my employees or colleagues.			
8. I clearly communicate expectations.			
9. I plan performance evaluations with a sensitivity to diversity.			
10. I understand the interaction between individual culture and organizational culture.			

From Walton SJ (1994). *Cultural Diversity in the Workplace.* Barr Ridge, IL: Mirror Press. Copyright 1994 by R.D. Irwin, Inc.

the effectiveness of the organization (Schwartz & Sullivan, 1993).

Unmanaged diversity in an organization can occur at an individual level, within the same group (intragroup), and between different groups (intergroup). At an *individual* level, there appears to be evidence of physician dominance and nurse submissiveness, verbal abuse of nurses by physicians, and litigation against nurses who are driven to inappropriately obey physicians' orders and against the physicians who are guilty of abusing nurses (Schwartz & Sullivan, 1993, p. 52). These conflicts are perceived by nurses to compromise patient care,

Table 12–4.
Cultural Actions for Nurse Leaders

1. Openly acknowledge and discuss diversity issues.
2. Be educated concerning different cultures.
3. Promote educational programs for individuals from all cultures.
4. Create a socially comfortable environment for culturally diverse staff members so they can experience the uniqueness of each other.
5. Allow for cross-cultural representation in unit activities.
6. Promote equal growth opportunities.
7. Strive to eliminate prejudice, biases, and stereotyping.
8. Monitor standards and norms to assure achievability.
9. Reward those who successfully manage diversity.
10. Openly discuss conflict with group members.

result in increased errors, and contribute to nurses either unionizing or leaving the profession. There is also evidence that nurses mistreat other nurses. If nurses are targeted as a group they may feel oppressed, which contributes to low self-worth. Therefore, they start lashing out at each other. There are issues of gender diversity as well. Specifically, male nurses have been a target of mistreatment in the workplace because they are four times as likely to have substance abuse complaints brought against them to their state's nursing license board as are female nurses (Schwartz & Sullivan, 1993).

Intragroup conflicts result when aggressive leaders enforce uniformity and punish those who do not conform to the group's norms. For example, a nurse leader who feels oppressed by the requests of hospital administrators may redirect that anger toward the staff nurses. The staff nurses in turn may direct their anger toward other members of the treatment team. Unfortunately, this rallies the other group members to become biased in their thinking because they want to belong and feel personally accepted by the staff nurses. This irrational thinking discourages individual thinking, which only causes increased conflict within the group and between other groups (Schwartz & Sullivan, 1993).

Although *intergroup* conflict can move a group in a positive direction to a certain extent, it may also cause conflict resulting in fear, resentment, irrationality, and distrust. This causes further breakdowns in cooperation and problem-solving. Such is the case with nurses who have moved from submissiveness to rebelliousness after receiving misinformation about advanced-practice nurses being given increased decision-making input; professional medical groups challenging nurses about the risks of midwifery; and threats of replacing nurses with nonprofessional personnel (Schwartz & Sullivan, 1993).

Managing Diversity

Managing diversity is a long-term process that occurs in three interrelated phases. These phases are awareness building, discrimination control, and prejudice reduction.

Awareness Building

The first phase of managing cultural diversity is *awareness building.* Awareness building begins with top management's providing personnel with a mission or goal statement that addresses diversity, allowing open communication within the organization, providing the necessary funds to support the process, and involving individuals who truly desire to manage diversity issues. Management efforts include the development and implementation of a culture audit using a combination of research efforts such as focus groups, survey questionnaires, and interviews that target personnel who are interested in exploring a specific diversity issue. Another awareness building approach includes the development of homogeneous groups. These groups provide a safe atmosphere for individuals who feel they have been mistreated. With the assistance of a trained facilitator, group members appropriately resolve the identified problem. Outcomes resulting from the implementation of culture audits and homogeneous groups are the creation of on-going training and orientation programs that address culturally diverse issues.

Discrimination Control

The second phase of managing cultural diversity is *discrimination control.* Discrimination control is a responsibility not only for nurse leaders but for all levels of management supporting diversity initiatives within the organization. *Discrimination,* the mistreatment of people based on factors that are irrelevant, and *prejudice,* the inaccurate perception of others, are sensitive and threatening subjects. All of us at one time or another have either been a target or a perpetrator of discrimination and prejudice, and all of us tend to hold inaccurate perceptions of some other people. Unfortunately, these inaccurate perceptions usually result in some type of mistreatment, referred to as *dispersing blame.* Discriminatory behavior can control the group or undermine group awareness. Nurse leaders should be thoughtful and responsive to the work-related concerns of subordinates by interrupting any reported discriminatory mistreatment. Therefore, the nurse leader should promote healthier interactions among members in the group or between other groups. Serving as a role model for group members decreases the likelihood of intragroup and intergroup pathology.

Management needs to educate nurse leaders concerning the appropriate actions to be taken when confronted with discriminatory behavior of subordinates. It has been suggested that evaluations of leaders by subordinates is a useful human resource management tool. Group management in the form of discussions between influential representatives of conflicting groups may help curtail diversity discrimination. For intergroup interactions to be effective, each group would need to identify its strengths and similarities, yet not deny any uniqueness or differences. The goals of these groups need to be well defined concerning the interventions needed to reach the goal (eg, improved quality of care or effectiveness) versus the differences among the groups (eg, culture or participation).

Reverse discrimination is another component of discrimination control. Despite organizations' trying to maintain fairness within the system, there is always some disagreement as to what is fair. Such are the issues associated with reverse discrimination. In trying to simplify the meaning of reverse discrimination, one could say that there are laws or policies in our society that try to balance discriminatory practices, but these laws or policies may be considered as discriminatory by individuals of certain ethnicity, gender, race, or handicap, such as choosing a person from a particular ethnic group over someone who may have better credentialing or education, or se-

lecting a person of a particular gender over one of another gender. Clearly written policies will help curtail reverse discrimination issues as well as equalize support and resources for career advancement for all employees.

Prejudice Reduction

The last path of managing cultural diversity in the health care setting deals with *prejudice reduction.* Managing prejudices is more difficult and complex than awareness building and discrimination control because prejudice is an abstract, internal, and perceptual phenomenon. Organizations can strive to control the manifestations of prejudice. When racist comments are discouraged, fewer comments are made. Therefore, prejudice reduction is a process that is eventually accomplished by those who complain and those who are truly concerned and sensitive to resolving culturally diverse issues (Sullivan & Schwartz, 1993).

Model of Conflict Resolution

Lowenstein and Glanville (1995) developed a conflict model (Fig. 12–1) to help nurse leaders understand the impact of culturally diverse issues in the health care setting. This model assists nurses in assessing conflict states and consciously selecting a resolution style with subordinates. Four basic transformations occur in this model before a personnel dispute enters the legal system. An unperceived injurious experience is called *UNPIE.* A perceived injurious experience, *PIE,* results in *naming, blaming,* and *claiming.*

UNPIE TO PIE. Disputes first emerge through a process of transformation in which an unperceived injurious experience (UNPIE) transforms into a perceived injurious experience (PIE). This transformation is influenced by an individual's characteristics, including age, experience, socioeconomic status, personality traits, job satisfaction, social position, cultural commitment, and perception of prejudice. The employee's maturity and prior experiences are major determinants in how the workplace will ultimately manage the incident.

The organizational culture or climate establishes

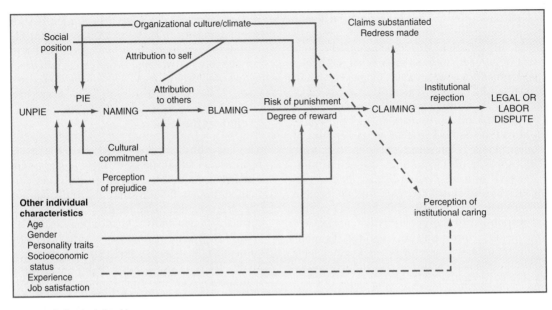

Figure 12–1. Lowenstein-Glanville conflict model. (From Lowenstein AJ, Glanville C [1995]. Cultural diversity and conflict in the health care workplace. *Nursing Economics* 13[4]:207.)

formal or informal norms of expected behaviors and the methods by which grievances are managed. Guidelines are provided for employees to evaluate their own and others' behaviors. Administrators demonstrate either the existence or the lack of caring behavior for the employees. This attitude affects the employee's perceptions of the organization in managing the dispute. Legal action is less likely to occur if the employee perceives the organization as caring.

NAMING. Naming is the second transformation. The specific grievance is described and named.

BLAMING/ATTRIBUTION. Blaming is the third transformation. This stage is also referred to as attribution. Employees blame either themselves or others for the injury. Blaming oneself may end the process; blaming others may result in the fourth transformation of the model, called claiming. Factors affecting this transformation include an indi-

vidual's social position, cultural commitment, and perception of prejudices.

CLAIMING. The fourth transformation is claiming. The individual's social position and awareness of the organization's behavior influence the individual's perception of the risk of punishment or reward surrounding the claim. These perceptions influence either continuance or dismissal of the claim. If the claim is rejected, then it becomes a legal or labor dispute.

Looking at race or culture may not provide enough information for the model, because ethnic groups are generally considered unpure due to mixed racial or ethnic parentage. In addition, individuals willingly change their values to reflect the culture they are living in; therefore, various cultural viewpoints may affect the transformation stages within this model.

When working with individuals from culturally

diverse backgrounds, nurse leaders need to be aware that communication issues, insensitivity, and ignorance of each others' motivations can hinder progress toward conflict resolution. Work ethic, values, and norms of behavior that are culturally and ethnically rooted tend to surface in the workplace. Nurse leaders need to learn to interpret racial feelings even though these subjects are uncomfortable to discuss. Isolated training efforts are not sufficient in managing diverse workforce problems. The entire organization must see the need to change.

Nurse leaders and the entire organization must value each employee's uniqueness and any special attributes he or she brings to the workplace. The nurse leader needs to recognize that the perceptions of others play a major role in working effectively with diversity. Validating perceptions of goals or task assignments helps reduce conflict. All people perceive things differently. Stating one's perceptions and clarifying the perceptions of others by asking for feedback allow others to recognize that there is a clear understanding of what is happening (Lowenstein & Glanville, 1995).

SUMMARY

The major political, economic, and social changes of the 1990s will progress into the 21st century. These changes mandate that leaders in health care be involved with group building processes in the quest of providing quality care with maximal efficiency. This challenge is particularly true for nurses in their pursuit of quality health care delivery. This chapter suggests that nurses need to understand the concepts of group dynamics, to realize new self-discoveries, to implement strategies, and to identify a model relative to managing culturally diverse groups in a health care environment. It is critical that each member clearly understand the group leader's role in this process, for each at some point may assume this role. At some point in any group, there will be a bone of contention because of the inherent and innate cultural diversity of the members. If the process of building a group is properly approached, the end result will be strengthened relationships among group members who will then be able to make better decisions, using problem-solving approaches. Ultimately, the organization, the

nurse leader, the employees, and the patients will benefit from the successful implementation of this process.

■ DISCUSSION QUESTIONS ■

1. Discuss the essential components of group dynamics.
2. Describe the relationship between group dynamics and cultural diversity.
3. Why are group dynamics and cultural diversity issues critically important to health care today?
4. Analyze the strategies nurses can use to identify cultural diversity issues.
5. Discuss methods used to manage conflict in the health care environment.

■ LEARNING ACTIVITIES ■

1. You have just learned that a newly arrived male immigrant from Mexico is refusing his treatment for tuberculosis. The patient is very ill. What culturally specific strategies could you use in working with this man?
2. As a nursing leader on your medical-surgical unit, you are concerned with some of the racial slurs you hear each day from your colleagues about patients and staff members. How can you best approach this problem?
3. As a new nurse in pediatric intensive care, you are overwhelmed because one of your newly delivered patients is a crack-addicted infant. To complete your family assessment, you visit the infant's mother in the post-partum unit, only to have her laugh in your face about your concerns. How would you best handle this situation?
4. A new graduate from the Caribbean has been assigned to your unit. After several weeks, it is clear that she needs an extensive orientation to the unit. You are concerned because you do not have time to do this. You suggest that she be transferred to a less intensive area and she files a discrimination charge against you, alleging prejudice. What cultural actions would you take?

■ BIBLIOGRAPHY ■

Bellman GM (1993). *Getting Things Done When You Are Not in Charge*. New York, NY: Simon & Schuster Trade.

Bettenhausen KL (1991). Five years of group research: What we have learned and what needs to be addressed. *Journal of Management* 17(2):345–381.

Bettenhausen KL, Murnighan JK (1991). The development of an intragroup norm and the effects of interpersonal and structural challenges. *Administrative Science Quarterly* 36:20–35.

Davis PD (1995). Enhancing multicultural harmony: Ten actions for managers. *Nursing Management* 27:32A–32H.

Grossman D, Taylor R (1995). Cultural diversity on the unit. *American Journal of Nursing* 95(2):64–67.

Lowenstein AJ, Glanville C (1995). Cultural diversity and conflict in the health care workplace. *Nursing Economics* 13(4):203–208, 247.

Schwartz RH, Sullivan DB (1993). Managing diversity in hospitals. *Health Care Management Review* 18(2):51–56.

Smith GB, Hukill E (1994). Quality work improvement groups: From paper to reality. *Journal of Nursing Care Quality* 8(4):1–12.

Walton SJ (1994). *Cultural Diversity in the Workplace.* Burr Ridge, IL: Mirror Press.

Planned Change

Kathleen M. White, PhD, RN

. . . .

LEARNING OBJECTIVES

This chapter will enable the learner to:

1. Describe the dynamics of the change process.
2. Compare and contrast selected theories of change.
3. Select appropriate strategies for effecting planned change.
4. Identify sources of resistance to change and steps to deal effectively with resistance to planned change.

. . . .

INTRODUCTION

The health care environment is changing at such a rapid rate that all nurses, and nurse leaders/managers in particular, must be knowledgeable and skilled in the change process. There is a great need for creativity and innovation in health care management to improve efficiency of delivery, stress quality, and maintain cost controls. This need for change in health care is driven by economics and is caused by workplace restructuring, the explosion of technology, the need for efficiency or improved ways of doing business, and the continued rapid growth of new services.

Change itself is neither good nor bad; it is inevitable. There are always forces at work to create or facilitate change. The potential for change is always present. Change will, must, and should occur. Change needs to be viewed as a challenge for man-

agement. The way a group or an organization responds to an attempt to change has an important effect on how the change occurs.

People react to change on the basis of several important factors: their life experiences, knowledge that has come from previous changes or similar encounters, present needs of those involved in the change, norms and values of the group or organization, roles they play in the organization, amount of present stress in the system, and coping abilities of those involved in the change. The nurse leader must plan and control change so that when it occurs, the change happens in the right direction, at the right time, in the right amount, with desired outcomes, and with minimal disruptions. The nurse leader needs to encourage those at all levels desiring or affected by the change to participate, initiate, innovate, and work creatively in the change process.

WHAT IS CHANGE?

To change is defined as "to make different, to alter or vary, to put something in place of something else, to give a completely different form or appearance to, to transform" (*American Heritage Dictionary*, 1991).

Planned change is a conscious, deliberate, and collaborative effort in which a change agent and client system come together to plan to improve the operation and functioning of a system through the use of valid knowledge. The *client system* is the person, group, organization, or community that asks for or receives help and desires or needs some change in performance. The *change agent* is the person or group, inside or outside the client system, that is being used to effect the change and help bring about improved performance (Bennis et al, 1985).

Unplanned change, accidental change, or *change by drift* are all names for a change within a group or organization that occurs by accident without planning, deliberation, or participation of those who usually direct changes or those to whom the change is directed. This type of change just occurs, with no input or feedback about the plan, process, or evaluation of the change.

NURSE AS CHANGE AGENT

A *change agent* is one who plans and works to bring about a change—the individual used by the organization or agency to help bring about improved performance. The change agent initiates the change process and assists others in making the changes or modifications necessary for themselves and the group or organization to change. This person can be an insider, a part of the organization, or an outsider, a consultant to the organization. Nurses are in key positions to be change agents, both as insiders and consultants to health care organizations. Examples of common change agents include clinical nurse specialists, patient care coordinators, clinicians, staff development educators, and nurse managers.

A change agent must develop skill and knowledge in the use of change theory in everyday practice. The change agent plans, guides, encourages, and controls the change through adaptation and facilitation. If the change is mandatory, the agent must develop specific strategies to make the necessary change successful. A change agent can also anticipate a needed change by identifying trends and forces both internal and external, sorting out and evaluating information, and recognizing the need for change (Table 13–1).

TYPES OF CHANGE

Technological Change

The application of new ways and methods to transform organizational resources into products or services is called *technological change*. This is change involving the basic method of doing business or

Table 13–1.
Characteristics/Skills Necessary for a Change Agent

Attributes of a Leader	Attributes of a Manager
Human relations skills	Group process skills
Interpersonal relationship skills	Problem-solving skills
Clear thinking	Planning skills
Articulation	Organizational skills
Flexibility	Coordination skills
Confidence	Controlling and directing skills
Vision	Ability to handle conflict
Trustworthiness	Conflict resolution skills
Expertise	Evaluation skills
Education skills	
Motivation	

operations, often done to correct a deficiency or accomplish greater efficiency in the work of the organization. Resistance to technological change occurs because people sense a disruption to their work patterns or norms and usually attempt to protect routine services and activities, decreasing the uncertainty or complexity of the everyday activities for workers. It is very important to involve the workers and get their input for any technological change to be successful. *Redesign* is the basic method of doing business to improve performance. The use of *quality management* principles examines every aspect of operation and identifies areas for performance improvement.

Product or Service Change

Product or *service change* involves the introduction of new products or services into or by the organization. Health care organizations routinely participate in this type of change to keep pace with the environment and the innovation of new producers or services. This type of change must be carefully thought out and evaluated through pilot testing projects, allowing the participants to have input and provide feedback for the proposed change.

Administrative Change

Administrative change, a change involving policies and procedures, reporting relationships, information systems, philosophy of management, and many other things, deals with the fundamental administrative design of the organization. This type of change is characterized by a down-flow of information and is usually identified by top management. Strategies to facilitate this bureaucratic process of change must be developed. It is important to identify the key players in the change who will be most affected by it, to identify their feelings about the change, and to assess how much power each player has and how each will use it to facilitate or block the change.

Structural Change

A *structural change* is a change involving the organizational structure or strategy of the system that could include departmental relationships, sizes of departments within the organization, viability of various parts of the organization, strategy of the organization, information systems, and other fundamental structures of the organization. This type of change is also characterized by a down-flow of information and communication and is usually implemented to increase efficiency or maintain the viability of the organization to compete or survive.

Attitude or Value Change

Attitude or *value change* involves the changing of attitudes, behaviors, and/or values of the personnel of the organization. This is probably the most difficult type of change to implement and must involve the participants to achieve acceptance. To facilitate an attitudinal/value change, always assess the conditions in the organization, group relations, communication, management, organizational culture, and feelings about work and the organization. The use of the quality management approach is usually the most successful strategy to involve the staff in the change. (Refer to Chapter 16 for a detailed discussion on quality management.) This involves holding meetings to openly discuss the problems of the organization and to generate creative solutions, continuing education for the staff, and encouraging flexibility and acceptance of new ideas, attitudes, approaches, and personalities.

CHANGE THEORY

When attempting to make a planned change, it is necessary to review and be familiar with change theory. By evaluating the basic assumptions presented in these theories, the nurse leader can design a change process that meets the needs of the particular organization and the type of desired change (Table 13–2).

Lewin's Force Field Analysis Model

Classic change theory comes from the work of Kurt Lewin (1951). *Lewin's Force Field Analysis* is a model of change that uses problem-solving and decision-making in the change process and views behavior as a set of forces that are dynamic, in a delicate balance, and working in opposite directions within a "field" or organization. These forces must be assessed and analyzed and dealt with continually through the three-step process of change: unfreezing, moving or changing, and refreezing. Lewin says that change occurs when there is an alteration of certain forces at work in the organization and that it is necessary to identify the forces that will assist and the forces that will act against the change. These forces are driving and restraining forces. *Driving forces* are the forces that assist or help the change to occur. These forces include external pressures to change, internal motivation to change that results from difficulties in the system, or internal motivations to improve. *Restraining forces* are the forces that will prevent the change or will move the organization away from allowing the change to occur. These forces result from fear of failure, fear of loss of current level of satisfaction, or unsuccessful attempts at change in the past.

Lewin's force field analysis is an excellent tool to use in diagnosing the need for change and what specific actions will be necessary to bring about the desired change (Table 13–3). The first step in the analysis involves identification of all of the driving and restraining forces within the organization. These should be listed as forces for or against the change, and a determination should be made of

Table 13–2.
Comparison of Major Theories of Planned Change

Nursing Process	Lewin	Lippitt	Rogers	Havelock
Identification of problem	Unfreezing	Develop need for change	Knowledge	
Assessment	Unfreezing	Establish change relationship		Build a relationship
Diagnosis	Unfreezing	Clarify diagnosis	Persuasion	Diagnose a problem
Goal setting	Moving/changing	Establish goals and intentions for action	Decision	Acquire resources
Planning of implementation	Moving/changing	Examine alternatives		Choose a solution
Implementation	Moving/changing Refreezing	Transform intentions into actual change	Implementation	Gain acceptance
Evaluation	Refreezing	Generalize and stabilize change; achieve terminal relationship	Confirmation	Stabilization

how equal or unequal the forces are that are present within the organization. Then, discussions should follow that analyze the importance and strength of the forces.

As long as the driving forces equal the restraining forces, the status quo is maintained. If a disequilibrium is created with one of the forces gaining strength over the other, a change may occur. To facilitate a change, strategies need to be developed to reduce the restraining forces and strengthen the driving forces.

The benefits of doing a force field analysis include:

- Making a correct assessment of the forces present that are important to the change process.

- Helping to understand how the forces affect one another.

- Allowing identification of what needs to be planned for and manipulated.

- Identifying the forces that could cause resistance, and determining how strong they are.

- Beginning specification of how to meet the goals.

Three Phases of Change

Lewin suggests that there are three phases in the change process. The first phase is called *unfreezing*. Usually, people are very comfortable with what they are familiar with, and the first phase of the change process must introduce doubt or discomfort with the current state of things or how things are being done. People must become uncomfortable enough with the status quo to want to change it. This can be done by providing information or examples of new ways of doing things or getting the job done or by raising everyone's awareness that the goal or goals of the organization are not being met in some way and that a change is necessary to get back on track. While this is all being introduced, however, it is necessary to make those involved in the process feel secure and at ease with the proposed change or changes to reduce threats to the safety and security of those involved and reduce resistance to the proposed change. During unfreezing, the process of developing an awareness to a need or problem is started and change is seen as the only solution. Increasing one or more of the driving forces, remov-

Table 13–3.
Force-Field Analysis Worksheet

Problem specification: Survival of the hospital.

Articulate problem: We must redesign our current system of care delivery to be more responsive to the needs of patients and families and focus efforts on cost controls of doing business.

Who is involved: Administration and staff in all departments.

What type of change is desired? This is an administrative, structural, product/services, and attitudes/values change.

List forces "driving" us toward the change

1. Administration is committed to change.
2. The problem has been studied for 18 months.
3. External economic changes and pressures are present.
4. There is commitment to involve staff in planning the change process.
5. More satisfied patients must be attracted who will come back or recommend the hospital to others.
6. There may be layoffs if there is no change.

List forces "restraining" us from the change

1. The caregivers (nursing/nurse managers, other professionals) have not been involved in selecting the service delivery model change.
2. There is a fear of loss of job as "we know it"; there is security and comfort in the status quo.
3. There is no knowledge of this type of care.
4. Protection of turf and turf battles are involved.
5. Past experiences with change have been resisted and were not particularly successful.
6. There is a fear of the unknown.

Diagram the driving and restraining forces by drawing arrows showing the size of force and a corresponding number to the list:

Driving Forces	1.		3.		5.		
				4.		6.	
		2.					

		2.			5.		
Restraining Forces							
	1.		3.	4.		6.	

Develop strategies to enhance the driving forces

Inform the staff of the commitment by administration, and develop structures such as job descriptions.

Inform the staff of the 18-month study, and bring in consultants to meet with the staff.

Educate the staff about economic and political realities of the current health care market.

Hold regular meetings to involve staff and support their attendance at the meetings.

Develop a marketing plan to inform the public and the community about this new type of patient care delivery system.

Provide for a secure environment, but alert staff that a change is necessary.

Develop strategies to reduce the restraining forces

Inform staff that the roles and responsibilities within the new delivery system would be done by those involved in those responsibilities. Explain to the nursing staff that they will continue as case managers and coordinators of care.

Empower the staff through involvement and decision-making in the process.

Educate the staff about "patient-focused care."

Involve the staff in defining their responsibilities.

Plan for regular evaluation, communication, and feedback to take care of problems in the change process as they arise. Anticipate resistance to the change, and plan strategies to deal with that resistance.

Provide for the continuing education of staff, and have regular and open meetings.

ing an obstacle to change, or increasing or attempting to eliminate a restraining force causes an imbalance in the driving and restraining forces, a disequilibrium in the organization, and allows for an "unfreezing" of the present way of doing business.

The change agent needs to increase pressures toward the change and reduce threats associated with changing. According to Lewin, this is done through three mechanisms. The first mechanism, *disconfirmation*, occurs when the change agent introduces evidence that a need is not being met. This can be done through meeting with the staff in small groups to discuss inadequacies or problems. A second mechanism, *inducing guilt or anxiety*, can be accomplished by introducing a period of uncomfortableness about the way things are and how they are not meeting an important goal or value. *Creation of psychological safety*, the third mechanism, is important to provide sufficient security to minimize risk involved with the change. The change agent can provide time for discussion, involvement, education, and approval to small advances toward the intended change.

The second phase of the change process is called *changing* or *moving*, which is the actual change or implementation phase of the change process. During the moving stage, the driving forces have overcome the restraining forces and the change moves ahead. A new way of behaving or doing business is presented to the group as the "change," and information is presented and group involvement is encouraged to allow the participants to discuss and assimilate the change into their way of doing business. The change is planned in detail and then implementation begins. Time must be allowed for support, group discussion, evaluation, and feedback to deal with resistance as it occurs. Open communication is important.

During *refreezing*, the final phase of the change process, the change has been implemented and needs to be stabilized. The organization must return to its normal level of functioning and the change consolidated into the regular operations of the organization. The change becomes integrated into the whole organization as part of its routine functioning. The change agent must provide guidance and support to ensure that the change will be maintained. However, at this stage, the change agent needs to reduce participation in the functioning of the change and delegate responsibility for the continu-

ance of the change. The integration of the change allows the change process to end and the participants to take on the responsibility for the continuance of operations. This "refreezing" takes place as the group has moved to a new equilibrium of the driving and restraining forces with the change functioning in place.

Lippitt's Model

Lippitt's model of change (1958) expands Lewin's theory to a seven-step change process and concentrates on the role of the leader or change agent in the change process. Lippitt emphasizes the role of planning and problem-solving in the process and adds the dimension of the interpersonal aspects of the helping relationship by the change agent in the change process. The theory discusses the role of the change agent as an outsider with the responsibility to diagnose the nature of the problem, assess the system motivation and capacities to change, assess the change agent's motivations and resources, select appropriate change objectives, choose an appropriate type of helping role and establish and maintain a helping relationship, recognize and guide the phases of the change process, choose the specific techniques and modes of behavior that will be appropriate to each progressive encounter in the change relationship, and contribute to the development of the basic skills and theories of the profession. The seven steps in Lippitt's model for change are the following:

1. The development of a need for change, including problem awareness and a desire for change.
2. Establishment of a change relationship between the change agent and the client system and their mutual decision to work together on the change.
3. Clarification or diagnosis of a client system's problem; a collaborative effort to diagnose the difficulties.
4. Examination of alternative means of action and goals, and the establishment of goals and intentions of action.
5. Transformation of intentions into actual change efforts, in which the active work of changing takes place and success is measured by how well plans are transformed into achievements.
6. Generalization and stabilization of the change. The process of institutionalization occurs.

7. Achieving a terminal relationship to prevent the client system from becoming too dependent on the change agent.

Rogers' Diffusion of Innovations Model

Rogers' Diffusion of Innovations Model (1983) explains change as a result of the introduction of innovation. Innovations is an idea, practice, or material artifact perceived to be new. Diffusion is the process by which an innovation is communicated through certain channels over time among the members of a social system; it is a type of communication concerned with new ideas. The main elements in the diffusion of new ideas are (1) an innovation (2) that is communicated through certain channels (3) over time (4) among members of a social system.

Rogers makes two distinctions between his model and other models. He points out the importance of commitment and maintenance to any change. He says that those involved in making the change happen need to show their commitment and build maintenance into the approach, or the change will be reversed or discontinued if the group is not committed. Rogers stresses the dynamic nature of the change process and that no change is permanent. He suggests that a change that was previously unsuccessful may still be implemented but at a different time or with a modified approach to the change.

Rogers calls his model an *innovation–decision process*. The framework includes information and uncertainty. The information reduces the uncertainty, and communication is the exchange of information. The five steps in this model are as follows:

1. *Knowledge*—Awareness or knowledge is presented to the group, showing that the innovation is available.
2. *Persuasion*—Interest in the innovation begins.
3. *Decision*—The decision to use and evaluate the innovation is made.
4. *Implementation*—Implementation of the innovation occurs.
5. *Confirmation*—The decision to adopt or reject the innovation is made by the group.

Rogers also considers the role of the change agent as important and delineates the responsibilities of the change agent role: to develop a need for change, establish an information-exchange relationship, diagnose the problem, create an intent to change in the client, translate the intent into action, stabilize the adoption and prevent discontinuance, and achieve a terminal relationship. He suggests that the change agent's success is determined by his or her own effort, the orientation of the client in the direction of the change, whether change project is compatible with client needs, and the degree of empathy the change agent has with the client.

Havelock's Model

Havelock (1973) expanded the work of Rogers and Lewin and described a six-step process that discusses how successful innovation takes place and how change agents can organize their work so a successful innovation will take place. Havelock's work focused on innovation in the educational process and emphasized planning and the use of a participatory approach for the group involved. Havelock's theory suggests four ways that a change agent can facilitate the change: as a catalyst, solution giver, process helper, and resource linker. The six-step process for change includes, first, the need to build a good relationship between the change agent and the client. The relationship between the people involved in the change must be carefully developed for success to be achieved. An assessment of the client, his or her norms, the leaders, the gatekeepers, and the larger environment should be completed. Second, the change agent needs to diagnose the problem and make a systematic attempt to understand it. The diagnosis should include details about the symptoms, history, and causes. The change agent should help the client to articulate his or her needs as problem statements. Next, it is important to identify and acquire relevant resources that will help in reaching the solution to the defined problem. Resources are needed for diagnosis, awareness, evaluation before trial, for trial, evaluation after trial, installation, and maintenance. Then, choose a solution to accomplish the change after generating a range of possibilities that follow looking at the implications, testing the feasibility of the alternative solutions, and adapting the preferred one to the needs and circumstances of the client system. The next step involves moving the solution toward acceptance and adoption. Finally, there is the need to stabilize the innovation so that the client system can maintain the change on its own. Gradual termination of the change agent relationship is accomplished.

Planned Change

Bennis et al (1976) described three general types of strategies used by change agents in a planned change.

Empirical–Rational Strategies

Empirical–rational strategies are based on the idea that people are rational and will use self-interest to determine a need for change. It assumes that people are guided by reason and will behave in a rational manner if given knowledge and information about the need for a change and the wisdom of this particular change. It is assumed that people will behave rationally and adopt the proposed change if it can be justified that a new and improved or better way of operating or acting will improve their performance. This strategy assumes that if people will gain from the change, they should welcome the change. It suggests that a leader or change agent has great knowledge and can give this knowledge to the people to be affected by the change and influence them in the direction of the change. This strategy ignores social and emotional responses to change.

Information or knowledge is the primary resource used. This strategy is used when little resistance to the change is expected because a reasoned and logical response to the change is expected. Education, communication, analysis, research, and long-term planning are strategies consistent with empirical–rational strategies. A good example for the use of this strategy is when a new technology becomes available that will save nursing time, improve efficiency, and maintain high-quality care. The communication and education regarding the technology should be sufficient to encourage use of the new technology in practice.

Normative Re-Educative Strategies

Normative re-educative strategies are based on the assumption that people act according to the socio-cultural norms, attitudes, and values of their group or organization. Rationality and intelligence are not ignored, and information is still provided; however, norms, attitudes, feelings, values, roles, relationships, and the group's commitment to these are seen as important and must be taken into account when a change is being planned. These influence the group's readiness for change and its willingness to accept a change when introduced. Some resistance can be expected. This model centers around the change agent's skill in interpersonal relationships. The leader or change agent and those involved in the change want and need to be included as active participants in the assessment, planning, and implementation of the change to gain acceptance, develop a commitment, facilitate the implementation and evaluation of the change, and limit resistance and prevent rejection. The strategy here is to use participation, communication, education, group problem-solving, and collaboration among all those involved with the change. This strategy is more time consuming than the other two; however, resistance can be avoided, and the strategy allows for increased creativity within the group. A good example of the use of this strategy involves the adoption of a new type of nursing care delivery system. The staff would have to be involved in trying out the new arrangement for care delivery and in planning and implementing phases to design a system to the specific needs of that nursing unit.

Power-Coercive Strategies

Power-coercive strategies are strategies based on the application of power, either political or economic. They assume that power is necessary to implement a change and that the less powerful will comply with the direction and leadership of those with more power. The power in this model is authority. The change process involves very little participation by the people affected by the change, and they have no power to modify or stop the change. Their resistance, if any, is handled by power and coercive strategies, such as legal means, threats, or sanctions. This type of strategy is used when there is no consensus on how to handle a problem or need, if great resistance is anticipated to the need for a change, if there is no time to get group participation, or if the need for change is so critical that survival depends on immediate implementation of the change. Examples of the use of this type of model would include the mandate to adopt a new policy or new procedure by the administration of the organization, such as a change in benefits, scheduling, or budget.

THE CHANGE PROCESS

To be successful in any change, it is important to understand the change process and how different factors affect the process, take into account why people resist change, and become familiar with techniques to overcome resistance to the desired change.

The change process is a sequence of steps and stages that is very similar to the nursing process (Table 13–4). There are problem-solving steps to guide the nurse leader through the process. Each of the models of change discussed earlier in the chapter presents key steps that must be followed to be successful when facing different kinds of change situations. It is important to understand the change

that is to be implemented, the type of change, how large or small the change is, the speed at which the change will occur, the organization, its culture, the people involved, and how they view the change. The process is affected by other factors in the organization, such as its degree of complexity, diversity, formalization, communication, coordination, and availability of resources.

To be an effective change agent, the strategies to affect change must be learned. In knowing this information, the change agent can develop a better plan for the change and strategies that will help to implement the change, prevent or overcome resistance, and facilitate a better acceptance and implementation of the change.

When beginning the change process, carefully identify and define the problem or the inefficiency that needs improvement or correction. This important first step can prevent many future problems because if the problem is not correctly identified, a plan for change may be aimed at the wrong problem.

The second step in the process is the assessment step. It is important to identify the forces that will

Table 13–4.
Comparison of the Nursing Process Approach with Planned Change Models

Assessment	Unfreezing
	Identify the need for change or the problem.
	Collect information about the proposed change, organization, people, cost and benefits, winners and losers, and feelings involved in the change.
Diagnosis	Summarize and analyze the data.
Goal Setting	Identify potential solutions and strategies.
	Set goals and priorities.
Planning	Plan strategies to implement the change, including why, where, who, how and with what, when, and for how long.
	Provide information and education.
Implementation	Moving or changing
	Implement the change.
	Implement strategies to overcome resistance.
Evaluation	Refreezing
	Evaluate the change.
	Stabilize and maintain.

work for and against the proposed change. What are the internal and external forces that are at work within the organization? Which ones can or cannot be controlled? How will those involved with the change respond or react to the potential change? A comprehensive assessment step in the change process is crucial to the planning for the proposed change (Table 13–5).

After the organizational assessment is completed, look again at the problem identification and make a careful diagnosis of what change is desired. Develop clearly stated goals and outcomes for the change along with specific and measurable objectives as to how the goals will be met; include time frames and accountability. This should specify the vision and direction along with the outcomes for this particular change. Gradual changes made in clearly defined steps are usually more acceptable than radical sweeping changes that are unpredicted and swift.

Develop a complete plan of action for the implementation of the change. The first step is to increase the readiness of the group for the change by developing awareness and discomfort with the present state of doing business and provide information on other ways of doing the work. This information should provide some interest and motivation to improve the current performance.

The expectations of the organization for the inclusion of the change must be clearly delineated. These should be in some type of written form such as a policy, job description, or evaluation tool format; this shows the organizational support for the change.

Begin the development of a strong working relationship between the change agent and client system to gain trust and acceptance. A strong change agent role increases the coordination of activities and accountability for the implementation of the change plan.

Specify the steps that are needed for this particular change. Again, include time frames and accountability within each step of the plan. Consider all possible solutions and alternative plans. What type of change is really needed? What are the consequences of the proposed change? Where and at what level is the change needed? How will resources be mobilized? Pay attention to the culture of the organization as the plan is implemented and make modifications as necessary. Plan adequate

time for any change to take place—do not shortchange the change process.

Determine where the change will begin, at what level, how small or large the first change should be, whether it will be gradual or complete, and what needs to be in place for the change to be successful. A pilot study or project can be very helpful in deciding on the rate and scope of a change.

Separate from the past, especially comments such as "We've tried this before." Do not allow the past to get in the way of attempting to make a change. Include in the implementation plan a way to deal with those type of comments or the history that the organization has had in making changes or, in particular, trying to meet this need or solve this problem.

Pay close attention to the politics of change (discussed later in this chapter). Anticipate resistance, where will it come from, why, when it will occur during the change process, and what strategies can be put in place to prevent, reduce, or eliminate the resistance. Always expect the unexpected, both internally and externally. Do not push too fast, do not spend too little, and do not stop the process too soon (Table 13–6).

RESISTANCE TO CHANGE

One of the most important strategies to facilitate an effective change is the identification and *neutralization* of resistance during the planning and implementation phases of change. It is critical to expect resistance. Anticipate and look for resistance, use resistance constructively, and overcome resistance to successfully implement the change.

Why do people resist change? The major reason usually given for resisting change is threatened self-interest. The individual or group senses that the personal costs involved with changing are greater than the personal benefits that could be gained from the change. Threatened self-interest involves fear of loss of money, loss of status, loss of freedom, disruptions of relationships, fear of failure, loss or change in work and rewards, and feelings of incompetence (Table 13–7).

Many authors have written about ways to handle and manage resistance to change (New & Couillard, 1981; Hein & Nicholson, 1994; Kotter & Schles-

Table 13–5.
Organizational Assessment for Planned Change

How important is the change to the organization?

How much time is available for the change process?

What are the organization's past experiences or history with changes?

What are the structure and administration of the organization?

Where is this organization now?

What are its mission and philosophy, goals, and scope of work?

What are the lines of communication (formal and informal), patterns of decision-making, lines of authority, authority relationships, division of labor, and type of bureaucracy?

Explore all available written materials, such as the organization's vision statement, mission statement, philosophy statements, long-range or strategic plan, organizational charts, job descriptions, evaluation tools, annual reports, and policy and procedure manuals.

What are the economics of the organization?

What is the environment or culture of the organization?

What is the environment like within the organization; is there trust or mistrust, close relationships/helping relationships among staff, and/or cooperation?

Does the culture of the organization focus on a particular issue, such as effectiveness, efficiency, quality, growth and expansion, decline and reduction, or cost control or cost expansion?

Is it supportive of change?

What are the norms of the organization? Identify and clarify the norms, and explore whether the norms are accepted. Are the norms what the participants want them to be? Identify the culture gaps.

What are the values of the organization?

How are activities coordinated in the organization?

How do departments interact with one another?

How complex is the organization?

Are there social relationships within the organization?

Are there personal freedoms within the organization?

Are participants allowed and supported to be creative?

Is there an adaptive culture? Do they support one another to identify and solve problems? Do they feel they can manage problems, and are they receptive to change?

Consider the individuals within the organization.

Who will be affected by the change? How many people does this include? Do they have power, and what type of power do they have? How do they feel about the change? Will they contribute to the change effort?

Who will resist the change?

Are individuals satisfied with the way things are?

What are the norms and values of the individuals, and are they the same as those of the organization?

Are the individuals committed to the norms and the values of the organization? Are they committed to the organization?

What are the personal characteristics of the individuals/group involved with the change? Is there trust, flexibility, openness, skepticism, resentment, conflict, anger, and so forth?

Table 13–6.
Common Mistakes Made During Implementation of a
Change

Failure to precisely state the objective of the change (not just to "improve things")

Failure to adequately analyze the change, the organization, its environment, and persons involved

Failure to define the intended outcomes, expectations, and goals early in the process

Failure to develop a clear strategy to get to the defined outcome

Failure to assess each change situation as a separate entity and determine the change techniques or processes to be used for that particular situation—no technique can be used in all situations

Not allowing sufficient time for the implementation to take place

Lack of coordination of implementation activities

Distraction or interruption of the change implementation process due to crises or other important activities

Lack of capable leadership to implement the change

Insufficient education of participants in the change process

Failure to win adequate support for the change

Failure to involve all who will be affected by the change

Dismissal of complaints outright instead of taking the time to judge possible validity

several of these techniques may be used during a change.

The first and easiest technique is to *introduce the change gradually*. This is an excellent strategy to minimize resistance to the change by proceeding slowly and introducing the change or changes slowly. This allows everyone to buy into them, accept them, and move on to the next step.

A second technique is *participation*. It allows all involved in the change to be active in the planning and implementation of the change. This can be time-consuming but usually has a high rate of success; people feel as if the change was their idea.

Education during the change process is extremely important. Information should be provided to the participants on a regular basis so everyone understands the change, why it is needed, and the benefits it offers. Constant *communication* and updates will decrease misunderstandings, misconceptions, and rumors, and ensure that all participants in the process have the same information. *Clarification* throughout the process allows the participants to ask questions and seek a better understanding of the change process. It also makes everyone feel that

Table 13–7.
Other Major Causes of Resistance to Change

No felt need for the change

Satisfaction and comfort with the status quo

Disagreement with the change

Threat to safety or security; fear of losing comfort/familiarity

Fear of loss of something of value

Feeling that the costs of change outweigh the benefits

Misunderstanding/inaccurate perception of the change

Lack of information

Poor timing

Lack of resources

Lack of trust

Low tolerance group

Unresponsive group

Fear of the unknown

inger, 1979). They all suggest that resistance should be confronted and used. Discuss openly the negative and positive consequences of the change and the resistance. This forces articulation of what the change is all about, what the expectations are, and what role each participant is expected to play in the implementation process. Listen carefully to what is being said, and look for signs of nonverbal resistance.

There are many techniques that can be used to handle resistance to change during the change process. Depending on the situation, one, two, or they are free to question and seek more education and explanation if they feel uncomfortable with what has been presented.

The *development of trust* during a change is extremely important. This development of a trusting relationship between the change agent and the participants requires that open and honest communication be used from the beginning. A trusting relationship ensures that all of the methods for handling resistance are used openly.

Include the participants in the *revision and modification* step of the change process, and encourage them to be involved in providing feedback for evaluation of the proposed change at regular and periodic intervals. This gives everyone the sense that the change is not a "done deal" and that they do have some say in what will be happening, particularly if it affects the "routine" activities with which most people are very comfortable.

Another often-overlooked technique to decrease the resistance to change is to provide for *extra supports* to the participants during the change. Additional support can facilitate the process and help to allay anxiety and fear of the process and the change. This can come in the form of extra education, counseling, additional staff during training periods, or even a light workload during the change process. *Incentives* can be used during the planning and implementation phases of the change process. The incentives can take any form but should have value for those who are involved in the change or are showing signs of resistance.

Confrontation can be an important strategy to meet resistance head-on. Group or individual face-to-face meetings to confront the issues at hand and to get everything out in the open allow everyone to verbalize their feelings and work to solve the problems and issues identified.

Coercion, another strategy that can be used to decrease resistance, is not always a successful technique for managing resistance. However, if the change agent has the power and authority to use coercion and if timing is critical for the implementation of the change to occur quickly, this may be a way to handle resistance in the short term. Eventually, the coercion and the negative feeling surrounding its use will have to be dealt with.

Another technique to manage resistance to change is *manipulation* of the participants. Manipulation usually involves a covert action, such as leaving out pieces of vital information that the participants might negatively receive. Again, the nurse leader will have to deal with this if the participants find out about the deception.

A final strategy to minimize the resistance to change is to *use an outside change agent*. It can help to facilitate a change by having an objective outside person take responsibility for implementing the change. This is often used when new information or technology is the proposed change. The outside change agent assesses the situation and plans and implements the change, usually with input from the inside manager. Involvement of the participants with the change agent in the implementation of the change is vital to success of the change. The skill and knowledge of this outside expert can help to decrease resistance.

Evaluation is the final but ongoing step in the change process. Regular opportunities for discussion with management and requesting and receiving input, suggestions, and feelings are vital to maintaining trust and commitment to the process. Feedback is important throughout the change process. Plan for and allow ample time for feedback and evaluation at intervals throughout the process. If participants know that there will be time for feedback and modification, they are more apt to support the change.

Communication is vital. Involve participants and be honest. Hold meetings to provide information, explain and discuss, answer questions, build and maintain support, clarify misconceptions, and reduce fears throughout the process. Make sure that there is a plan to maintain and stabilize the change. The maintenance of a change must be ongoing and allow for continuing evaluation of the strengths and

---

Research Box 13–1
The Ten Stages of Change

Perlman and Takacs (1990) found that to cope effectively with change, the organization must go through 10 stages of change and deal with the human reactions, both emotional and intellectual, to the change. The stages of change are: (1) equilibrium, (2) denial, (3) anger, (4) bargaining, (5) chaos, (6) depression, (7) resignation, (8) openness, (9) readiness, and (10) re-emergence.

weaknesses of the change. Management visibility, support, and participation in the change process demonstrate commitment on the part of the organization to making the change process successful.

Monitor the change and the change process, make adjustments and corrections, and evaluate the results according to the specified outcomes and satisfaction with the process. It generally takes a long time to implement a change. Keep the information coming. The timing of communications is important. Keep a sense of humor. Persistence and visibility pay off. Remember that no change is ever final.

POLITICS OF CHANGE

The politics of change involve using all of the leadership and management skills that have been learned and can be applied to change in any group or organization. Analyze the organizational chart and know the lines of communication and lines of authority. Identify the key players and learn about these players—who are the players, what are their roles in the group or organization, how much power do they have, how committed are they to the change, who will be affected by this change, how can they be mobilized to participate in the change, and who is needed for this change to occur.

Take control of the change process. Mobilize a power base through networking and coalition building of key players and supporters to start the change process. Make certain that the support of appropriate people and the necessary material resources are available for the change. Plan and frame the change carefully so that those involved in the change and those affected by the change will participate and be committed and see that this is positive.

Timing is critical for beginning implementation. Is this a good time to introduce a change? How much other change is occurring in the group or organization? How fast or slow should the change happen?

Develop and put in place enabling structures that facilitate and support the change process. Use an oversight committee or a task force with accountability to the change agent and support from management and peers.

FACILITATING AND MANAGING INNOVATIVE CHANGE IN NURSING ORGANIZATIONS

CASE STUDY ◆ 13–1

Hospital XYZ is a 400-bed community hospital located in a large metropolitan area. It is university-affiliated and has nonprofit status for its operations. The hospital has continued to grow and prosper over the years and has always been financially sound. However, over the past 2 years, Hospital XYZ has been facing the same pressures that all the hospitals in the area are experiencing: fewer inpatient admissions, empty hospital beds, decreasing length of stays, some decrease in revenue generation, the pressure to cut costs, the need to attract additional patients, and the need to continue to grow in several services as the only hospital that offers cardiac angioplasty and transplant services.

The hospital administrators are forced to look at the way they conduct business to ensure the hospital's long-term survival as a competitor in the area. The administration, in conjunction with outside consultants, has studied the problem extensively over the past 18 months and has decided that the time is right for a "restructuring" or "redesign" of the care delivery system.

The plan recommends that Hospital XYZ transform its operations into a "patient-focused care" model of delivery of patient care and services. The goal of this type of redesign is to better meet the needs of its patients, improve work performance and quality of care, control costs, reduce waste and inefficiencies, and improve patient outcomes and satisfaction with care at Hospital XYZ. The transformation will redesign the delivery of patient care so the hospital personnel and resources will be organized around the patients rather than through their traditional departments. This will decentralize the standard hospital departments and require cross-training of workers. Pharmacists, physical therapists, housekeeping, respiratory therapists, electrocardiogram technicians, and others may be assigned to units. There may be a pharmacy, laboratory, or radiograph room on the unit. The decentralization of depart-

ments will depend on the needs of the service/
unit.

You, the nurse manager on Unit 200, and eight
inpatient nurse managers are charged with developing a formal plan for how nursing will be included in this change process. The administration
is looking to nursing as a support and leader in
this change process. The nurses would continue
as case managers and coordinators of care.

Engineering the Change Process

It is time to be creative and engineer the change
process. What type of planned change process will
be most effective for this type of change? Which of
the change theories seem to best apply to this situation? What problems are expected? Will there be
resistance to the proposed change? The following is
one way of planning for the restructuring and redesign that will need to take place (Fig. 13–1).

1. *Problem identification*—The problem identified
   by the administration is a need to remain competitive in the current economically constrained
   health care market. The need for change is to
   redesign the delivery system of patient care to
   be more responsive to patient needs and to control costs.
2. *Assessment*—Collect information about the proposed change, the organization, the people, costs
   and benefits, winners and losers, and all the
   feelings involved around the change. Information
   must to be collected and analyzed about the
   current system of patient care delivery. Investigate patient census; patient acuity; staffing patterns; use of personnel, tasks, and functions on
   per-unit, per-service, and per-type of patient
   bases; and who performs these tasks. Monitor
   the use of all support services to determine
   which support services are necessary per unit,
   service, or patient type and which services will
   be cross-trained. Identify driving and restraining
   forces.
3. *Diagnosis*—Are the problem identification and
   the need for change correct? If not, restate the
   problem or change.
4. *Goal Setting*—Begin setting goals with measurable objectives and lines of responsibility, and
   assign the planning function for the change.

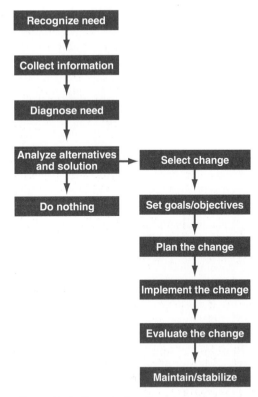

Figure 13–1. Stages in the planned-change model.

5. *Planning*—Plan strategies to implement the
   change, including why, where, who, how and
   with what, when, and for how long.

   - Develop awareness among the staff of the
     forces necessitating the change.
   - Educate staff about the economic, political,
     and social factors.
   - Educate staff about "patient-focused care."
   - Hold regular staff meetings to discuss the
     change and how it will proceed. Present the
     information collected during the assessment
     phase, and discuss how things could be done
     differently.
   - Ensure that the staff feels secure during the
     planning and implementation phases. There
     should be no surprises at this point in the
     process. Plan for regular communication of
     information, allow for a free exchange of in-

formation, encourage idea generation, involve staff in decision-making and planning, and provide a supportive atmosphere for discussions.

- Develop the formal structures necessary to show the commitment to this change. Develop a philosophy of care, standards of care, new job titles, job descriptions, and evaluation tools.

- Anticipate that there still may be some resistance even with a well-developed plan for the change that involves all affected by the change.

- Plan for team building. How will these new groups of people work together? Provide time, support, and education to allow them to develop and grow. Additional education may have to be given on team-building techniques, delegation, supervision, and quality assurance/improvement techniques.

6. *Implementation*—Implement the planned change. Reassign the staff, and begin the new patient care delivery system. Implement strategies to overcome resistance to the changes throughout the process as necessary.

7. *Evaluation*—Evaluate the change at regular time intervals and plan to stabilize the change. There are really two types of evaluation for this case study: an evaluation of the change process and evaluation of whether the changes had the desired effects/outcomes.

■ DISCUSSION QUESTIONS ■

1. Why is the nursing process considered a model for planned change? Apply the nursing process to a clinical as well as an administrative situation. Does it work in both instances? Why or why not?

2. Have you ever resisted a change at work or in your personal life that you later came to accept? Think about the strategies for dealing with resistance that were used on you. Which strategies were successful, and which were not?

3. What are the key characteristics of a change agent? What make some change agents more successful than others? Relate this discussion to a change agent with whom you are acquainted.

4. Why are the culture and politics of an organization important to consider in the change process?

■ LEARNING ACTIVITIES ■

1. Identify a change that is needed in your health care agency. Select one of the change models, and work through the steps of the model to implement the change. Evaluate the model for this type of change.

2. Think of a change that has recently occurred at your agency. Evaluate how the change happened. Was it planned or unplanned? Was a change agent used to implement the change? What do you think would have improved the change process?

3. Use Lewin's Force Field Analysis to make that change. What are the driving and restraining forces that will enable or prevent the change? Develop a plan for the three phases of the planned change. Include any anticipated resistance to the change and strategies to manage the resistance.

■ BIBLIOGRAPHY ■

Beckham JD (1996). Hearing the tidal wave. *Healthcare Forum Journal* 39:68–78.

Bennis WG, Benne K, Chin R (eds) (1985). *The Planning of Change*, 4th ed. New York: Holt, Rinehart and Winston.

Beyers M (1984). Getting on top of organizational change. I. Process and development. *Journal of Nursing Administration* 14(10):32–39.

Beyers M (1984). Getting on top of organizational change. II. Trends in nursing service. *Journal of Nursing Administration* 14(11):31–37.

Beyers M (1984). Getting on top of organizational change. III. The corporate nurse executive. *Journal of Nursing Administration* 14(12):32–37.

Billings CV, Bischoll-Syre R, Durham RK (1986). Growth and change: A nursing organization case study. *Nursing Management* 17:68–75.

Carr C (1994). Seven keys to successful change. *Training* 1:55–60.

Ellis DJ (1987). Change process: A case example. *Nursing Management* 18:14–19.

Haffner A (1986). Facilitating change: Choosing the appropriate strategy. *Journal of Nursing Administration* 16:18–22.

Havelock R (1973). *The Change Agent's Guide to Innovation in Education*. New Jersey: Educational Technology Publications.

Healey TG (1994). Managing the change process. *AANA Journal* 62:106–107.

Hein EC, Nicholson M (1994). *Contemporary Leadership Behavior*. Philadelphia: Lippincott.

Hoffman FM (1985). A finger on the pulse of change. *Journal of Nursing Administration* 15:23–26.

Jenkins JE (1996). Moving beyond a project's implementation phase. *Nursing Management* 27:48B–48D.

Kaplan SM (1991). The nurse as change agent. *Dermatology Nursing* 3:419–422.

Kemp VH (1984). An overview of change and leadership. *Topics in Clinical Nursing* 6:1–9.

King E (1982). Coping with organizational change. *Topics in Clinical Nursing* 4:66–73.

Kotter J, Schlesinger M (1979). Choosing strategies for change. *Harvard Business Review* 57:109–112.

Kotter JP (1995). Leading change: Why transformation efforts fail. *Harvard Business Review* 73:59–67.

Lawrence PR (1969). How to deal with resistance to change. *Harvard Business Review* 47:4–10, 166–174.

Lawry TC (1995). Making culture a forethought: What to do when strategy meets organizational culture. *Health Progress* 76:22–25.

Lewin K (1951). *Field Theory in Social Science: Selected Theoretical Papers*. New York: Harper & Row.

Lippitt T, Watson J, Westley B (1958). *The Dynamics of Planned Change*. New York: Harcourt Brace.

Morris W (1980). *The American Heritage Dictionary of the English Language*. Boston: Houghton Mifflin, p. 180.

New RJ, Couillard NA (1981). Guidelines for introducing change. *Journal of Nursing Administration* 2:17–21.

Perlman D, Takacs G (1990). The ten stages of change. *Nursing Management* 2:33–38.

Rogers E (1983). *Diffusion of Innovations*, 3rd ed. New York: Free Press.

Schaffer RH, Thomson HA (1992). Successful change programs begin with results. *Harvard Business Review* 70:80–89.

Skinner MD (1994). Getting to X . . . The change process. *Nursing Administration Quarterly* 18:58–63.

Spradley BW (1980). Managing change creatively. *Journal of Nursing Administration* 10:32–37.

Tiffany CR (1994). Analysis of planned change theories. *Nursing Management* 25:60–62.

Ward M, Moran S (1984). Resistance to change: Recognize, respond, overcome. *Nursing Management* 15:30–33.

Welch L (1979). Planned change in nursing: The theory. *Nursing Clinics of North America* 14:307–321.

Integrating Systems in Contemporary Nursing Leadership

14 | Legal Considerations of Clinical Nursing Practice

Ruth November, J.D., R.N.

· · · · · · · · · · · · · · · · · · · ·

LEARNING OBJECTIVES

This chapter will enable the learner to:
1. Define the legal scope of nursing practice.
2. Discuss basic laws affecting clinical nursing.
3. Discuss nursing malpractice.
4. Identify the components of a lawsuit.
5. Identify strategies for safe practice.

· · · · · · · · · · · · · · · · · · · ·

INTRODUCTION

This chapter explores basic legal principles of clinical nursing. The changing health care environment requires the nursing leader to have knowledge of this area. Statutory laws, or laws made by Congress and state legislators, are discussed. The board of nursing of each state regulates the practice of nursing; therefore, nurse practice acts are examined. In addition, the changing role and environment of nurses are addressed; expanded roles and different and new settings for patient care and legislation will have an impact. In the 1990s and the 21st century, nurses will have a vastly different set of legal concerns, and the expanded role will bring expanded legal concerns. Current legislation may not be sufficient to address nurses' legal and ethical concerns. Changes in nurse practice acts are being made, and legislative and regulatory changes are necessary to keep up with the changing roles. For definitions of

some legal terms used in this chapter, see Table 14–1.

LEGAL SCOPE OF NURSING PRACTICE

State Board of Nursing Regulations

The legal scope of nursing practice encompasses state boards of nursing regulations, federal legislation, state statutes, and common law. The practice of nursing is governed by the Nurse Practice Act, which was enacted by the state legislature. Nurse practice acts define the scope of legally allowed nursing practice. Although the practice acts may vary in specifics among states, the general scope of laws affecting nursing is the same throughout the country. For further details on the nurse practice acts, see the section Basic Laws Affecting Clinical Nursing.

Federal and State Legislation

The scope of nursing practice is also controlled by federal and state laws. Federal legislation is passed by Congress and signed into law by the president. These federal laws must be followed by all states. State legislation, or laws enacted by the state legislature, affect only those practicing in that state. There is no national nursing practice act or national nursing malpractice act. (The federal laws that affect nursing are discussed in more detail later in this chapter.) These laws generally involve the fundamental rights of all individuals to determine their

Table 14–1.
Definitions of Legal Terms

Causation:	When a failure to provide reasonable care under the circumstances results in an injury
Defendant:	The one against whom a lawsuit is filed
Deposition:	The oral testimony taken of a witness in the period of discovery
Discovery:	A period of time after the filing of the lawsuit, before trial, in which each side discloses what it knows to all other parties
Duty:	A legal obligation. Also see Standard of Care
Interrogatories:	Written questions of a party that are answered under oath; a method of discovery
Malpractice:	Negligence committed by a professional
Negligence:	Failure to exercise reasonable care under the circumstances
Plaintiff:	The one commencing the lawsuit
Statute:	The act of a legislature establishing law
Verdict:	The findings and conclusion of the jury
Voir dire:	The oral questioning of potential jurors to elicit bias and sympathy

health care options and basic rights to safe medical care. State laws address reporting of child and elder abuse, consent for treatment, confidentiality of medical records, malpractice, and other issues.

Common Law

Common law is judge-made law; it is also known as case law. When a judge hears a case and makes a decision, that decision becomes the basis of common law. This opinion is binding in that particular judge's courtroom. Many of the laws that affect nurses stem from actual cases in which the judge interprets statutory law. Statutory law is law that is enacted by legislators at the state or federal level. Case law is binding only on those who appear before that particular court. Of course, a case that is decided by the US Supreme Court is binding on all. In other words, justices of the US Supreme Court write for all citizens; judges of other courts write only for their court and its jurisdiction. Judges, however, may write opinions that might be persuasive on other jurisdictions or other courts; therefore, cases that are discussed later in this chapter should be viewed as illustrations of a point and not an actual law that affects all nurses.

BASIC LAWS AFFECTING CLINICAL NURSING

Nurse Practice Acts: Scope of Practice

Within the Nurse Practice Act are regulations governing the make-up of the board of nursing, licensure requirements, suspension and revocation of nursing licenses, and definitions of nursing. Typically, the definition of professional nursing includes the observation, assessment, diagnosis, planning, intervention, evaluation, rehabilitation, care, counsel, and teaching of persons who are ill, injured, or experiencing changes in normal health processes. The performance of these acts is accomplished by using specialized judgment and skills based on knowledge and application of principles of the sciences learned in nursing school. Many states have expanded the definition of professional nursing to include the maintenance of health, prevention of illness, supervision and teaching of nursing, and evaluation of nursing practices, policies, and procedures (Texas Nurses Association, 1993). Finally, nurse practice acts include in the definition of professional nursing the administration of medications and treatments as prescribed by a physician.

Care must be taken that nurses understand and appreciate the differences between the practice of nursing and the practice of medicine. Often, the acts of a professional nurse overlap with those of a physician. For instance, each of these health care providers may administer medications, take vital signs, or teach a patient about his or her colostomy. Nurses, however, must not administer medications without an order from a physician. Understanding the difference between an independent nursing function and one that requires, by law, a physician's order is paramount to the nurse's ability to avoid crossing the fine line between practicing nursing and practicing medicine. An independent function is one that, by law, a nurse is able to perform without a physician's order. Examples of independent nursing functions are taking vital signs, giving routine morning and evening care, teaching patients, and providing emotional support. A dependent nursing function requires a physician's order, such as administering medication to a patient. As health care reform takes place, this line is apt to move considerably to enlarge the scope of legally allowed nursing functions.

Nurse Practice Acts: Licensure Requirements

Again, although individual state regulations may differ slightly, in general, licensure requirements for the practice of professional nursing are the same. Professional nursing is that practice done by a registered nurse. Fundamentally, to have the "privilege" of practicing nursing, one must first be licensed. Minimum criteria for licensure must be met. The applicant must have attended and graduated from an accredited school of nursing. The applicant must have passed the National Board of Nursing Examination before becoming licensed. States may also require residency in that state, proof of citizenship, or other requirements. Once licensed, there may be continuing education requirements to maintain the license in good standing. These mandates for maintaining education and skills are found in many state nurse practice acts.

Licenses can be suspended or revoked for a variety of reasons. Typically, drug and alcohol abuse, failure to maintain education and skills commensurate with the year in which the nurse practices, conviction of certain misdemeanors and felonies involving moral turpitude, and unprofessional conduct put the nurse's license at grave risk (Va Code Section 54.1-3000 et seq, 1993 supplement). Thus, although the nurse has earned the legal privilege of practicing nursing, he or she also has legal and moral responsibilities.

FEDERAL LEGISLATION AFFECTING CLINICAL CARE

Patient Self-Determination Act

In 1990, Congress passed the Omnibus Budget Reconciliation Act (OBRA), which in part requires institutional health care providers such as hospitals, skilled nursing facilities, home health agencies, hospice programs, and managed care organizations to furnish patients with information about advance directives. The common name of the act is the Patient Self-Determination Act (PSDA) (42 U.S.C. 1395cc, 1990). Before a discussion of what the law requires and how nurses are affected, a few definitions are necessary.

The PSDA is founded on the principle that all adults have the right to accept or refuse health care, including the right to die with dignity. The concept is that *in advance of the need for a health care decision*, a person decides what, if any, health care options he or she wishes. For instance, a competent adult can decide *today* what health care providers are to do if he or she is unable at some point in the future to communicate health care decisions. Advanced directives are documents written before the diagnosis of a terminal condition (living will or, in the event a person is unable to make health care decisions, a health care power of attorney).

The *living will* is a document the competent adult can execute regarding the right to die with dignity. It is a very narrow document in that the living will applies only in a very narrow set of circumstances. Although state laws may differ slightly, the general aspects of a living will are as follows:

■ Definitions as to *when* the provisions of the living will are to become effective must be in place. Typically, the law requires that the individual be diagnosed as having a "terminal condition" before the living will can be effectuated. A general definition of "terminal condition" is a condition in which *without* life support, death is imminent. The fact that life must be sustained mechanically or chemically with medications or in some artificial manner is the crux of the definition of "terminal condition."

■ A provision must be in place for *who* can execute a living will and how it can be done if the person has already been diagnosed with a terminal condition; it would not be an advance directive, but the living will is nevertheless valid.

■ What health care providers are to do in the instance of a living will. A valid living will allows health care providers to *not resuscitate* an individual in cardiac or pulmonary arrest. With an effective living will, a *do not resuscitate* (DNR) order can be validly written by the physician and followed by nurses and other health care providers. A properly executed living will provides for immunity from criminal and civil prosecution.

The second advance directive is called the *health care power of attorney* (HCPOA). This document is much broader than the living will. The HCPOA allows an adult to decide what care decisions are to be made *if at any time the adult is not able to decide for himself or herself.* It is broader than the living will in several ways. First, the HCPOA can apply at any time someone is unable, for any reason, to make health care decisions. Although the living will is limited to a terminal condition, the HCPOA can be used any time the patient is unable to make decisions about care (Meisel, 1989), such as while under anesthesia or unconscious but not because the condition is terminal. Second, the HCPOA requires the adult to appoint another person to make the decisions in his or her behalf; this person is called an *agent.*

The PSDA became effective December 1, 1991; it requires that certain health care providers furnish patients with information about advance directives. These health care providers must maintain written policies and procedures regarding an individual's right to formulate advance directives under that individual's state law. Patients must also be given written information about their state law regarding advance directives. This written information must be given at the time of admission to the facility (in the case of home health agencies and hospices, the decision must be made before the patient comes under the care of the home health agency or hospice). Health care providers must document in the patient's medical record whether or not the patient has executed an advance directive. Patients cannot be discriminated against because they have or have not executed an advance directive.

The nurse's responsibility with the PSDA is to know the state law in which the nurse practices and be sure the patient has been given the required information. Finally, documentation in the patient's medical record must be completed. As nursing roles expand to outside the hospital, the role of the nurse under the PSDA will also expand. Nurses should counsel the patient about options under the state law regarding advance directives. Often, it is the nurse in whom the patient confides; therefore, the nurse must be prepared to discuss *death with dignity* and other health care issues. This means the nurse must be familiar with the PSDA.

Emergency Medical Treatment and Active Labor Act

The Emergency Medical Treatment and Active Labor Act, which is federal legislation, was enacted in 1986 so hospitals would not determine for whom they would or would not care in their emergency departments on the basis of the patient's ability to pay for the care (42 U.S.C. 1395dd, 1986). This law requires that hospitals that have an emergency department provide *any and all* individuals an appropriate medical screening to determine whether an emergency medical condition exists. The law is quite comprehensive and is heavily challenged in courts of law. The nurse is not directly responsible for implementing the provisions of this legislation, but the nurse must have a basic understanding of the law's requirements.

There are three requirements in the Emergency Medical Treatment and Active Labor Act. First, the hospital must provide an appropriate medical screening without regard to the patient's ability to pay. The screening is to determine whether there is an *emergency medical condition*. There are two components to the definition of emergency medical condition. The first part is "a medical condition manifesting itself by acute symptoms of sufficient severity (including severe pain) such that the absence of immediate medical attention could reasonably be expected to result in placing the individual is serious jeopardy, serious impairment of bodily functions, or serious dysfunction of any bodily organ or part" (42 U.S.C. 1395dd, 1986). With respect to a pregnant woman who is having contractions, an emergency medical condition exists if there is "inadequate time to effect a safe transfer to another hospital before delivery, or, the transfer may pose a threat to the health or safety of the woman or her unborn child."

The second requirement is to provide treatment to stabilize the emergency medical condition. The last requirement is to restrict transfer of the patient until stabilized. All three requirements must meet the hospital's capabilities and resources.

Safe Medical Devices Reporting Act

Health care facilities, defined in the act as hospitals, ambulatory surgery centers, nursing homes, and outpatient treatment centers (*not* to include physician offices), have an obligation to report devices that may have caused or contributed to a patient death or injury (21 U.S.C. 361i, 1990). *Devices* include all biomedical equipment, other equipment, and certain instrumentation used in patient care. Because many nurses work with equipment, it often is the responsibility of the nurse to report devices that may have caused or contributed to a patient's injury or death. The law requires health care providers to file a report of equipment-related injuries to the Secretary of Heath and Human Services. In addition, each facility must provide semiannual reports that summarize any and all reports made within the requirements of the act.

STATE LAWS AFFECTING CLINICAL CARE

A variety of laws are enacted at the state level that have a direct impact on the nurse providing clinical care. Again, each state's laws vary, so the discussion below is generalized to principles typically found throughout the United States. As roles change and health care reform escalates, these state laws will change to keep pace with the care the nurse is providing.

Reporting of Abuse

Virtually all states have legislation requiring *health care providers*, including nurses, to report elderly and child abuse. These statutes often allow the nurse to report their suspicions anonymously, and

virtually all provide immunity for those who make reports in good faith. The nurse may be the closest to the patient and his or her family. Often, it is the nurse in whom the patient confides. The nurse's beliefs about any potential abuse of a patient should be communicated with another health care provider, such as the supervisor or attending physician. *Good faith* is difficult to define. For example, suspicions should be supplemented with some medical evidence that makes the "story" of how the patient was injured inconsistent with the mechanics of the injury. Documentation of observations in objective terms is an essential element in reporting of elderly or child abuse.

Consent for Treatment

Every human being of adult years and sound mind has a right to determine what shall be done with his own body.

> *Schoendorf v. Society of N.Y. Hospital;*
> *221 NY 125 @ 129, 105; NE 92 @ 93; 1914.*

These are the words of Justice Cardozo, and they form the foundation of consent laws. Laws regarding consent are based on the idea that each of us has a right to be protected from unwanted intrusion. In actuality, touching someone without their consent is considered a battery, for which there may be legal implications (Keeton, 1984).

There are some general principles of consent. First and foremost, as Justice Cardozo so aptly stated, we each have a right to decide for ourselves what will or will not be done to our bodies. Second, an adult is presumed to be competent to give, or capable of giving, consent. If the court intercedes and declares the patient incompetent, the court will appoint a guardian of the person. The guardian then "steps into the shoes of the patient" for purposes of consent. Without court intervention, the nurse must use assessment skills and judge whether the patient is competent. The third principle is that competency, or capability, is based on whether the individual understands the nature and effect of what he or she is being asked to do (Rozovsky, 1990). If the patient understands the nature and consequences of consenting, then he or she is capable of signing, or competent to sign, a consent form.

State laws vary regarding (1) when consent is

necessary, (2) who may validly give consent, and (3) how consent is withdrawn. Several general rules apply universally. There are two kinds of consent: express and implied. Express consent can be written or verbal. Implied consent is inferred by the health care provider when circumstances make obtaining express consent difficult or impossible. For instance, if the patient has been in an automobile accident and is unconscious, consent will be inferred because the reasonable person would consent under these circumstances to care that is necessary to save life, limb, or health.

Nurses do not generally need to get consent, written or verbal, to give nursing care. The patient has either expressly consented, such as on admission to a hospital, or implied consented, such as admitting a home health nurse into the home. This consent covers routine nursing care. Patients consent to health care in writing or verbally before the health care being given. In the case of an emergency, the consent is implied. Regardless of where you practice, your care requires consent, either expressly or implied.

CONFIDENTIALITY OF MEDICAL RECORDS

The law recognizes the nurse's duty to maintain confidential information revealed by the patient. Possibly as important as the legal duty is the ethical obligation of nurses to maintain confidentiality. One must understand that it is the *privilege of the patient* to reveal medical information to whomever the patient wishes. The legal and ethical *duty of the health care provider* is to keep that information confidential unless certain conditions are met. Generally, the law *allows* you to reveal confidential information when you are speaking with another health care provider who is also taking care of that patient. This discussion, however, must take place in an appropriate place. *Inappropriate* places are anywhere the public is allowed to go; in a hospital, an inappropriate place would be public elevators and public cafeterias. In an ambulatory setting, an inappropriate place would be a driveway or classroom. In a clinic, physician's office, school, or similar setting, an inappropriate place might be a waiting area.

Care must be taken to avoid talking with anyone other than health care providers who are taking care of the patient and their supervisors, and care must be taken to talk in an appropriate place. Last, one needs to always talk in an appropriate manner, that is, a professional tone.

NURSING MALPRACTICE

When a person runs a stop sign and hits another vehicle, he or she is considered negligent. This is called ordinary negligence in the law. When a professional commits ordinary negligence, the law calls it *malpractice*. Either word may be used in this chapter; for our purpose, they are to be considered synonymous.

Elements of Malpractice

There are four elements of malpractice (Keeton, 1990). Each one must be considered separately, and each of the four must be proven by the plaintiff's attorney in the event of a lawsuit. The person who is suing is called the *plaintiff*. The one being sued is called the *defendant*. In a lawsuit against a nurse, the plaintiff's attorney must prove:

1. Duty, or standard of care
2. Breach of duty, or breach of the standard of care
3. Causation
4. Injury

Duty/Standard of Care

What duties do you legally owe the patient? What are the standards of care for nursing? These are best answered by defining *standard of care*. You will be practicing *within the standard of care* if you *do whatever a reasonable, prudent, average nurse would do in the same or similar set of circumstances*. There can be no list of duties, or standards. That is because of the last six words in the definition: *same or similar set of circumstances*. There are no guarantees in health care. Although we know death will occur, we cannot say when it will occur. Each patient is different; even if all the patients you care for are women in labor, each is different. Because each patient is unique, the *circumstances* of their care vary. We can provide *guidelines to practice*. There are many sources of information regarding practice guidelines; nursing textbooks, policy and procedure manuals, and nursing journals are considered guidelines, or parameters, of nursing practice.

Courts have identified three *universal duties* that health care providers, including nurses, have a legal obligation to perform:

1. Provide a safe environment.
2. Maintain education and skills commensurate with the year in which you are practicing.
3. Document the care given to the patient.

What the courts are saying by quoting these three universal duties is that a reasonable, prudent, and average nurse would provide a safe environment for the patient, would maintain education and skills commensurate with the year in which he or she is practicing, and would document care. However, beyond the three universal duties, which are clearly and broadly stated, there is no *list* that can be given to you regarding your legal obligations to care for the patient. The question most nurses ask is: Am I practicing within the standard of care? The answer is to compare your practice with that of other nurses. Ask other nurses if your care is reasonable and prudent. Look at the surrounding circumstances, such as your education and experience and those of nurses around you, the patient acuity level, and available resources. If under all of the surrounding circumstances (or similar circumstances), another reasonable, prudent, average nurse *would* do the same thing you are doing, then you are within the standard of care. If another reasonable nurse *would not* do what you are about to do, then you are not acting within the standard of care and may want to reconsider your plan of action. Unfortunately, we are not able to get a clearer definition of standard of care, or legal duty. The jury will always consider the surrounding circumstances. They will hear what expert nurse witnesses have to say about what should have been done in light of the surrounding circumstances.

Breach of Duty/Breach of the Standard of Care

Simply put, if you fail to do what a reasonable, prudent, average nurse would have done in that set of circumstances, then you have breached the standard of care. Another way to look at breach of standard of care is to view the standard of care as a measuring stick. Do your actions regarding patient care measure up to those of other reasonable nurses? One can consider breach of the standard of care in two ways: Either you failed to do what a reasonable, prudent nurse would have done, or you did something a reasonable, prudent, average nurse would not have done. Either way, you breached the standard of care.

Causation

Causation is the most difficult concept for the plaintiff's attorney to prove, and it is a difficult concept to understand. An (alleged) breach of duty must directly result in, or cause, a patient's injury. Generally, the courts will ask, "But for the act of the defendant (the nurse), would the patient be injured?" If the answer is "no," the patient would not be injured except for what the nurse did (or did not do) to the patient, then the element of causation can be proven. If, however, the answer is "yes," the patient would nevertheless, regardless of what the nurse did or did not do, be injured, then the nurse is not considered to have legally caused the patient's injury. In court, this is called the *but for test*. Another way of looking at causation is to question the nurse's action and ask whether what the nurse did to the patient resulted in an injury to the patient. Of course, there are no guarantees in health care, and patients can become injured through no one's fault. To prove causation in court, the plaintiff's attorney faces a two-pronged test (Keeton, 1984) (Fig. 14–1).

The first prong, or question, that must be answered, is "Did the nurse do something to the patient that resulted in an injury?" The second prong of this test is "Could the injury have been prevented?" The answers to both questions must be in the affirmative for causation to have been proved in the court room. In other words, there may be some injuries to patients that could not have been prevented through reasonable, prudent nursing practice. Sometimes patients are injured through their own fault or through no one's fault.

When considering the prevention aspect of this two-pronged test, one must use policy and proce-

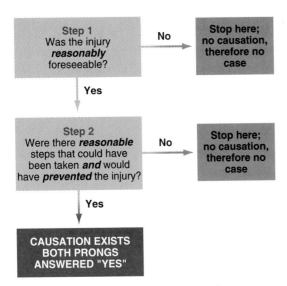

Figure 14–1. Causation two-pronged test.

dure manuals as *guidelines* to whether one is practicing within the standard of care. When considering a policy or procedure, if it can be said that the patient will *not* be injured as long as one follows the policy, then the policy is directed at preventing injuries. If the policy is directed at preventing injuries and the nurse follows the policy, it is unlikely, although not impossible, that the nurse will be found legally liable for causation.

Injury

The last of the concepts that must be proved by the plaintiff's attorney is that the patient received a physical injury. This is the simplest of the four elements to prove; most often, the patient experienced a serious and severe physical injury if the case is in litigation. What is key to this concept is that the plaintiff's attorney must prove that the physical injury *resulted from* the nurse's breech of the standard of care. In other words, the physical injury was not pre-existing or caused by the patient's or someone else's negligence.

This standard of law is sometimes referred to as *tort liability.*

DEFENSES

Statute of Limitations

The statute of limitations is that legal time frame in which a person can be sued. It is a "window of opportunity" for the plaintiff's attorney to file a lawsuit against the defendant. Each state has its own limitation period for personal injury or medical malpractice; however, it is not important for the nurse to understand the exact number of years for a particular statute of limitations. Instead, it is important that the nurse understand the basic concept and, most importantly, the risk management strategy that will help you defend yourself should you be sued.

Generally, the period of time begins with a date of injury. Some states have used date of *discovery* of injury as the beginning of the counting period. Regardless of how your state calculates the number of years, the risk management strategy is the same: *date your notes, every page, every patient.* Dating your notes will enable an attorney to begin with a particular date and calculate accordingly.

Most states allow a different statutory period for minors than for adults. Minors typically have a longer period of time in which to bring a lawsuit. The reasoning is that minors are not adults and therefore have no legal rights. So although an adult in the state may have 2 years from date of injury to bring a lawsuit, a minor in that same state may have until his or her 20th birthday, even if 2 years has long since passed.

Many states are now legislating what is generically termed *foreign objects statute of limitations.* These statutes define a foreign object as something of nontherapeutic or nondiagnostic value that is left in the patient. These statutes of limitations are geared toward operating room nurses and labor and delivery room nurses if the nurses assist in scheduled cesarean sections. However, any nurse who participates in a procedure in which a foreign object could be left in the patient is open to litigation under a foreign objects statute of limitations. These statutes were enacted because often the patient does not discover he or she has been injured by a foreign object until long after the general adult statute of limitations has expired. If you plan to work in an operating room or a labor and delivery room, you must be aware of whether your state has a foreign objects statute of limitations because it will likely add many years to the time in which you could be sued under the normal adult statute.

Some states have enacted the *continuing treatment rule*. Typically, this rule applies to office physicians who see a patient *for the same illness or injury during an uninterrupted period of time*. For instance, an orthopedic surgeon who has seen a patient for postoperative care secondary to a total hip replacement is an example of the continuing treatment rule applied. As long as that orthopedic surgeon continues to see the patient for postoperative care, the statute of limitations will not begin until the day that the patient is discharged from the physician's care. That is because the courts do not want to burden the plaintiff with filing suit against a physician while still under the physician's care. Therefore, in states that have a continuing statute of limitations, even though the actual injury may occur earlier than the date of discharge from the treatment, the date of injury will be considered the date of discharge from care. This author is unaware of any case in the United States that held that a *nurse* could have a continuing treatment statute of limitations applied against him or her.

Contributory or Comparative Negligence

The second defense that is often available in malpractice cases is the defense of contributory or comparative negligence. Although few states still have the defense of *contributory* negligence, we review what contributory negligence is and how it differs from comparative negligence. You are likely to be practicing in a state that has comparative negligence.

Consider the components of contributory negligence. When a *patient* is negligent in that he or she is noncompliant with physician or nursing orders and an injury results owing to the patient's as well as the defendant's negligence, the jury may find that the patient was *contributorily* negligent. A hypothetical case is that of Mr. Jones, who is a newly diagnosed diabetic patient. He has been taught about diabetes, insulin, diet, and exercise. He has been taught and can demonstrate how to calculate the proper dose of insulin and how to give his insulin injections. He has been taught and can verbalize an understanding of the proper diet and exer-

cise regimens that he should be on. You are the nurse in a physician's office, and Mr. Jones is now seeing you for his first follow-up visit. Your physician's office procedure mandates that you take a blood specimen from Mr. Jones. When you test his blood glucose level, you find that it is highly elevated. This, of course, indicates that there is too much sugar in Mr. Jones' blood and could mean that he is not correctly calculating his dosage of insulin. You then ask, "Mr. Jones, have you been giving yourself insulin as we taught you?" Mr. Jones replies, "Well, I really don't like giving myself those shots, so my wife does it when she is in town." Is Mr. Jones intentionally being noncompliant? Contributory negligence (or comparative negligence) requires intentional noncompliance of the patient. First, you must validate that Mr. Jones is contributorily negligent as opposed to uneducated. Often, when the patient appears not to be compliant, it is due to lack of education, not actual noncompliance. You must repeat the entire diabetic teaching process and have Mr. Jones verbalize an understanding of his disease and demonstrate how to give himself the injections before you can validate his educational status. If Mr. Jones is able to verbalize and demonstrate an understanding of his disease and then says, "I'm still not going to give myself that insulin," you have a noncompliant patient. If after reeducating Mr. Jones, he says, "Well, gosh, I know that you taught me that I could go into a diabetic coma, but I forgot about that. I am going to give myself those shots," what you have is a lack of education and understanding, *not* a noncompliant patient. The difference is essential, and the difference will be found in your documentation of:

- The diabetic teaching.
- Mr. Jones' understanding by verbalization of his diabetes.
- Mr. Jones' ability to demonstrate giving himself insulin injections.

When Mr. Jones is able to demonstrate an understanding of his disease process and *still* refuses to give himself insulin injections, then if Mr. Jones does go into diabetic coma, the jury may find that the patient was contributorily negligent.

In states in which the defense attorney can prove contributory negligence, the patient will not be able to recover any money even though the defendant may also be negligent. In states that have *comparative* negligence or comparative responsibility, the jury will hear all of the evidence and apportion a percentage of the responsibility, or a percentage of negligence, to the plaintiff and the defendant. The difference in states that have contributory negligence and states that have comparative negligence is an important one. In states that have contributory negligence, the case is dismissed and the patient is not allowed to recover any money because the patient was negligent and caused the ultimate injury. In states in which there is a form of comparative negligence, the verdict can still be in the plaintiff's favor even though the plaintiff was partially responsible for the injury. The plaintiff will receive only that portion of the verdict for which the jury found the defendant responsible. Reconsider Mr. Jones. If the jury found Mr. Jones was negligent and assigned his percentage of negligence at 30%, in a state with *contributory negligence,* Mr. Jones would not recover any money. In states with *comparative* negligence, he would recover 70% of the verdict.

Risk Management Strategies for Your Defense

Whether you practice in a state with a 2-year statute of limitations or a state with a 1-year date of discovery of injury statute of limitations, the risk management strategy is the same. The risk management strategy remains the same even though your state legislature may change the number of years in the statute of limitations. The risk management strategy for protecting you in a statute of limitations defense is *date your notes, every page, every patient, no exceptions.* If you date your notes, your attorney will be able to argue to the court when the statutory period began and when it should end. Without a date, your attorney has a very difficult standard of proof. If you remember to date every page, every patient, every time, then there will be a date on which a statute of limitations argument can be made.

It does not matter whether you practice nursing in a state that has contributory negligence or comparative negligence; the risk management strategy is the same. Each time you identify a potentially noncompliant patient, you must do the following:

1. Validate the noncompliance through re-education of the patient.

2. Validate the patient's understanding through good patient teaching principles.
3. Document your teaching and the patient's understanding and demonstrations of skills. Elicit from the patient his or her intentions regarding medical and nursing orders. Will the patient continue to be noncompliant, or has your teaching been effective in enlightening the patient on the benefits of compliance?
4. Document the patient's response, as illustrated with Mr. Jones.

In all states, the burden is on the defense attorney to prove the defenses of statute of limitations and comparative responsibility. This means that your attorney must provide evidence that the statutory period for filing a lawsuit has ended or the patient has been intentionally noncompliant and contributed to his or her injury. Therefore, the way to help yourself is to date your notes and identify and validate actual noncompliance versus lack of education. Doing these two simple things may some day prove to be quite valuable should a malpractice case be filed against you.

ANATOMY OF A LAWSUIT

Claim and Filing of Lawsuit

States vary in the name they give to lawsuits—complaints or motions for judgment—and the procedural steps to court (Fig. 14–2). However, typically the lawsuit is begun with a claim by a disgruntled patient or family member. Often, a family member has a limited view of the care of the loved one and becomes angry. An attorney is usually called, and a discussion begins with the family and patient. After the attorney reviews the medical records at issue, he or she decides whether there is a case of merit and a want to proceed. Usually, the institution that is the potential defendant (hospital, home health care agency, hospice, or managed care organization) is also aware of this disgruntled patient or family member and has begun its own investigation. Eventually, an attorney who believes he or she has a meritorious case will file a lawsuit. This lawsuit may be called a *motion for judgment* or *complaint*. What is critical is that you answer the allegations made in a timely fashion, generally

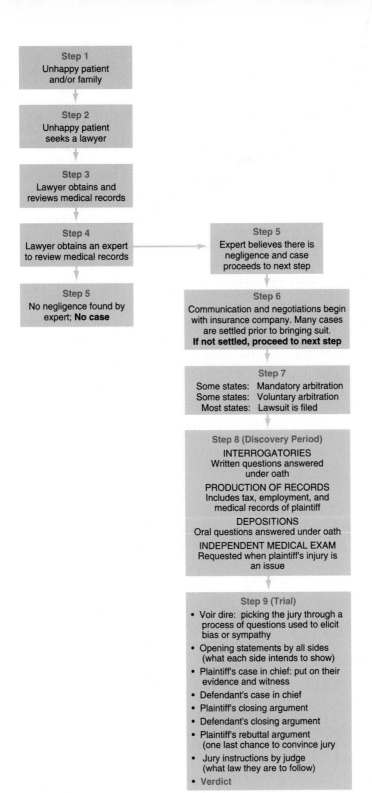

Figure 14–2. Anatomy of a lawsuit.

within 21 days. Consequently, any nurse served with a motion for judgment, a complaint, or other legal paper alleging nursing malpractice must immediately seek legal counsel. In addition, virtually all insurance policies require immediate notification to effectuate coverage, so notify your professional liability insurance company immediately.

Discovery

Once the answer or response is filed, there will be a period of *discovery*. Tools of the discovery allow each side to find out what the other side knows. Such tools may be interrogatories, production of documents, depositions, and an independent medical examination. Interrogatories are written questions that must be answered under oath and are proposed by one party to the party on the other side. The defendant will ask for a production of documents, such as the medical records, proof of wage and salary loss, and tax records. Depositions are questions answered verbally under oath; typically, each side will depose the other party as well as factual and expert witnesses. The independent medical examination may be requested by the defense team if they feel that the plaintiff has not been injured or has not been injured to the extent claimed. The purpose of these discovery tools is to find out what may not be readily apparent by merely reading the medical records.

Settlement Negotiations

Eventually, the discovery period will end, and settlement negotiations may begin. Many malpractice cases, approximately 75%, are settled out of court. If settlement negotiations are unsuccessful, the case will be set for trial.

Trial Begins with Jury Selection

The trial begins with selection of the jury through a process called voir dire. The purpose of voir dire is to elicit bias or sympathy from potential jurors. Questions are asked of the jury panel regarding their potential prejudices, biases, or sympathies. Jurors who have obvious biases or sympathies toward one side or the other are eliminated from the jury panel. Eventually, a jury is selected and sworn in.

Opening Statements and Testimony

The case begins with opening statements by each party. The *opening statement* is the statement of what each party intends to prove at trial. It is not meant to be an argument or considered evidence by the jury. The *case in chief* is the part in which the jury will hear from all of the parties, witnesses, and experts. Since the plaintiff has the burden of proving malpractice, the plaintiff puts on his or her case in chief first. The patient, family members, defendant, and expert witnesses will likely take the stand. The expert witnesses must prove that there was a duty on the behalf of the defendant, that the duty was breached, and that the breach of duty directly caused the plaintiff's injury.

A simple example is the following hypothetical situation: A nurse has just started an intravenous line. The bed was put in high position, with the side rails down to facilitate good body mechanics while performing the nursing function. Once the intravenous line was inserted, the nurse failed to put the bed in low position and failed to put the side rails back up. The patient falls out of bed and fractures a hip. The issue to be addressed by the expert witness is whether the nurse was negligent. The expert for the plaintiff will assert that the nurse failed to provide a safe environment and that the failure to put the bed back in low position and put up the side rails thus caused the patient to fall out of bed, resulting in the fractured hip. In other words, the nurse had a duty to provide a safe environment; the duty was breached; and the breach caused an injury. Further, the plaintiff's expert will testify that the injury was foreseeable and could have been prevented.

Expert witnesses on behalf of the plaintiff have a number of sources that they may use to supplement the expert opinion. For instance, the plaintiff's expert witness may use nursing textbooks, journal articles, or treatises to supplement the opinion that the standard of care was breached. The defense expert witness may use different nursing textbooks, general articles, or treatises or the hospital's policy and procedure manual to supplement the opinion that the nurse did abide by the standard of care.

Sources of the standard of care that can be used to supplement expert witness opinions on both sides are textbooks, general articles, treatises, professional organization statements, policy, procedure, and protocol manuals, and other written guidelines published by nursing organizations. Nurses involved in malpractice actions fare much better when they are active in professional organizations in which they are able to network with other nurses and discuss current practice guidelines, protocols, and parameters. Joining nursing organizations is also helpful because they provide networking, journals, and scholarly publications that include current practice knowledge and research findings.

After the plaintiff puts on the case in chief, the defense does the same. At the end of the case by the defense, the plaintiff and defense attorneys will make their closing arguments. The plaintiff's attorney has a final say in the form of a rebuttal closing argument that finishes the trial. Typically, the first story that the jurors hear is that of the plaintiff in their opening statement; it is also the last thing they hear by the plaintiff's attorney in closing rebuttal arguments. Finally, the judge will instruct the jury, and the jurors will deliberate the case. They will come to a verdict for the plaintiff for money or for the defense. Appeals are allowed only for errors of law. (An exploration of this topic is outside the scope of this chapter.)

PREVENTION TIPS: RISK MANAGEMENT STRATEGIES FOR THE SMART NURSE

Use Good Communication Skills

There are a number of things that a nurse can do on a daily basis to help mitigate the damage of a lawsuit, if not prevent one. Caring communication is your first *offense* to litigation; most people will not sue someone they like and will not sue someone they think likes them. Would you sue a friend? If you make it your custom and habit to have good communication and a good bedside manner with your patients, you will go a long way in preventing a lawsuit being filed against you. Learning and using the patient's name and using good eye contact are two of the best methods of building rapport with your patients. You should make it a point for your

patients to know your name and how to reach you when they need you. Written and verbal communication skills are critical tools in the avoidance of a malpractice case. When you communicate with your patients and allow them the opportunity to communicate with you, you are building rapport and thus are far less likely to be sued. Good communication skills with a physician and other members of the heath care team not only help the patient in terms of patient care continuity but may alert other health care providers to potential problems that could result in a malpractice claim.

Be Familiar with the Policies and Procedures of the Workplace

Another tip is to know your employer's policies, procedures, and protocols. These manuals are evidence of your employer's guidelines or parameters to practice. They are also the standard of care in your organization. It behooves the nurse to review policy, procedure, and protocol manuals on a routine basis, such as your annual anniversary of employment as well as every time you perform a procedure or treatment you are not familiar with or have not performed for a long time.

Use Good Documentation Skills

Good documentation skills are important in defending the health care provider. A brief outline of those principles is provided here and in Table 14–2.

Critical to your documentation should be the skills of documenting only that which is clinically relevant information and of documenting in an objective form. Clinically relevant information is information that another health care provider needs to provide care for purposes of continuity. In fact, the purpose of a medical record is to communicate patient care from one health care provider to another for purposes of continuity. If you communicate what happened to the patient while you were with him or her, you will be, by definition, communicating clinically relevant information. Ask yourself, "Is this information that I am about to write in a medical record information another health care provider *needs to know*?" If the answer is "yes," then it is clinically relevant. If the answer is "no,"

Table 14–2.

Examples of Documentation

Situation 1: Patient found on floor; bed in high position, side rails down.

Risky Charting	**Safe Charting**
Patient fell out of bed.	Found patient lying in prone position on floor. Patient states, "I fell out of bed."
Lesson: This is an assumed conclusion.	Lesson: This is an objective/factual conclusion.

Situation 2: Patient is given Demerol, to which she has an allergy. Vital signs: T 99.6, P 78, R 24, BP 112/64; skin is warm and flushed.

Risky Charting	**Safe Charting**
Patient is given Demerol in error; physician notified; VSS	8/2/94 0900. Demerol 50 mg. IM UOQ lt. hip for c/o pain at incision; VS T 99.6, P 78, R 24, BP 112/64; skin warm and flushed. Dr. Smith notified of same, no orders received.
Lesson: Not the accepted way of documenting a medication; not clear who exactly was notified and what was relayed. "VSS" is a conclusion.	Lesson: Factual; proper method of documenting a medication; more precise.

Situation 3: Patient's vital signs and condition are deteriorating. You have been unsuccessful in notifying the physician.

Risky Charting	**Safe Charting**
Patient unstable; BP 60/0, P102. Dr. Jones called 2/94 1300 at his office, no answer.	R 34 and shallow; color pale, skin cool and clammy; PEERLA; Dr. Jones' office called (567-0987); no answer. Drs. Smith and Jones paged; supervisor Murphy notified of above.
Lesson: Not enough specific information.	Lesson: More detailed and specific.

do not document it. Objective information is factual information. Use your skills of observation in determining what information is factual. Do not jump to conclusions and do not make assumptions, for these are subjective observations and have no place in a permanent medical record.

Consider this situation. You came into a room and found a patient lying on the floor. You may conclude that the patient fell out of bed, but you should not document your conclusion until you can document it with fact. Therefore, in the situation just described, you would document as follows: date/time—Found patient on floor lying in supine position. A & O × 3. Bed rails up, bed in low position. Patient states, "I fell out of bed while trying to go to the bathroom."

Unless you saw the patient fall out of bed, you do not have any facts before you other than those described in the note above to prove whether the patient fell out of bed. It is best, therefore, not to write any conclusions or assumptions in the record but merely the facts you have observed. Your senses of observation are sight, hearing, speech, and smell as well as what you did for the patient. The sample note above is incomplete until you document the patient's vital signs and other assessment information subsequent to the assessment you would do after finding a patient on the floor.

Other documentation principles include putting a date on each page, writing legibly, recording the time of each entry, using employer-approved abbreviations, correcting errors per your employer's policy, and making late or supplemental entries in the medical record in a proper format.

Assess and Monitor Patients

Failure to assess and monitor the patient is a common thread in nursing malpractice cases. Nurses must have an organized and effective method of assessing and monitoring patients. In addition to the *action* you take, your actions *and* the patient's condition *must* be charted in the patient's record. Assessments need to be done as often as the patient's condition requires it. Charting should include the time of assessment along with the findings.

Take Timely and Appropriate Action

A second common thread is failure to take timely and appropriate action. Consequently, the prudent nurse is wise to communicate the assessment of a patient whose condition is deteriorating. The communication must be both verbal and written. Certainly, documenting the patient's condition in the medial record is paramount. Communicating the patient's condition and your nursing actions to the physician is also necessary for the patient's well-being. Documentation of the nurse's telephone call to the physician is essential. When your employer's policies require you to notify a nursing supervisor, documentation of verbal notification should be made. It is not legally improper to document notification activities in the patient's record. For examples of good and poor charting, see Table 14–2.

LEGAL CONSIDERATIONS IN THE HOME SETTING

Health reform and changes in clinical practice have determined that a hospital setting is no longer the major arena for nursing care. It is clear that nursing care is moving out of the hospitals and into the community. The thrust of health care reform is focused on access, cost, and quality. To achieve the "lower cost" aspect of health care reform, it is necessary to rely on professionals such as nurses to provide more of the care that has traditionally been provided by physicians. Traditionally, patients in the hospital setting have a variety of health care practitioners who provide care. This will change as the pressure to reduce cost increases, the length of stay decreases, and care moves into the community. It is abundantly clear that health care will move from high-cost settings such as hospitals to lower-cost settings such as home health and community clinics.

Nursing will be practiced in a more autonomous and isolated environment out of necessity. For instance, home health nurses are generally the only health care provider in the patient's home when they are giving the care. This expanded role brings with it additional clinical responsibilities and legal considerations.

In the home setting, a nurse's ability to assess and monitor a patient is critical; important to this assessment is the nurse's ability to take timely and appropriate action. This will bring new legal considerations. The first consideration will be the definition of nursing itself. Much of nursing practice will be independent as opposed to dependent. Although nurses previously relied on a health care provider *team*, it is unlikely that this entire team will be available in each of the expanding environments. Thus, one of the potential legal considerations will be redefining the practice of nursing to allow nurses to make *preliminary* diagnostic and treatment decisions. Consider the following hypothetical situation of a home health nurse:

You have gone to the home of Mrs. Smith to perform wound care. Mrs. Smith, who lives alone, is a 72-year-old patient with diabetes. She has a history of congestive heart failure, and her diabetes is not always under control. When you arrive at her home, you observe that she is cold and clammy, with a blood pressure of 50/20 mm Hg, a rapid respiratory rate of 32, and a weak, rapid, and thready pulse. Mrs. Smith's color is a dusty gray; however, she states she feels fine. You test her blood sugar level to determine whether this is the cause of the signs and symptoms you are observing. In the hospital setting, you may call a supervisor or even a physician to see this patient. In the home of Mrs. Smith, *out of necessity, you will be required to make a preliminary diagnosis and treatment decision.* Of course, you call a physician and see whether you can consult over the telephone. The situation is further complicated because the physician is not available and Mrs. Smith lives approximately 40 minutes from any medical facility. As a home health nurse, your job is to assess, monitor, and evaluate care for Mrs. Smith in her home. However, your nursing assessment brings you to the conclusion that Mrs. Smith needs more care than you are able to provide. The legal considerations are that you will be diagnosing and treating without a medical license.

In this new environment, independent and dependent nursing functions will also change. Those functions that currently require a physician's order may become independent functions as the nurse's role expands. An example may be in the occupational health setting. In the hospital, a nurse may not administer any medication absent of a physician's order. However, there may not be a physician on site, or even on call, in the occupational health care setting. When an employee comes to the employee health office complaining of a headache, can a nurse administer Tylenol, aspirin, or ibuprofen *without* a physician's order? If the nurse does so, he or she is practicing both medicine and pharmacy. The nurse may be liable for an injury that results from the medication. What if the nurse does not take a history? What if a patient's history would have revealed a contraindication for the medicine dispensed? What if the nurse failed to conduct even a cursory examination? Does the nurse have the necessary resources or equipment available? The legal scope of nursing must be reviewed in light of this new role. As the role expands, however, so will malpractice liability, as the foregoing series of questions illustrate. The answers to these questions depend on what a reasonable, prudent, average nurse would do in the same or similar set of circumstances.

ETHICAL CONSIDERATIONS IN CLINICAL PRACTICE

Often, the law and ethics are blurred. The nurse may want to have a legal answer to a dilemma or question, but the real answer lies in the individual's code of ethics. The legal answer often is insufficient for the nurse's code of ethics. For instance, you are in a hospital setting and are concerned about a particular aspect of the quality of patient care. You have implemented all of the proper policies and procedures regarding quality of care concerns. You have had a "heart-to-heart" discussion with your head nurse and supervisor to no avail. Your employer seems to be unwilling to make patient care changes that you feel are necessary to improve quality. Your question to a lawyer may be "What else can I do legally to make the employer change?" Generally, the answer is "nothing." If you have fol-lowed your employer's policies and procedures regarding quality of care concerns and you are sure there is no law mandating some sort of disclosure (as in child abuse), then the law does not provide you with an outlet. You may well have to quit to "live with yourself." What you have is not a legal question but an ethical dilemma. Does your own code of ethics allow you to sleep at night and continue to work at your place of employment even though no changes in patient care are made? Or does your code of ethics "require" you to change employers so you can live with yourself? A more comprehensive discussion of these ethical issues is found in Chapter 15.

Many of the health care activities in which nurses participate have tremendous ethical responsibilities, such as transplantation, the patient's right to die, and bioethical decisions regarding treatment for very premature infants (20 to 28 weeks). Although the law may address each of these aspects of health care, ethics committees work daily on addressing the moral and ethical responsibilities of health care providers on these and numerous other ethical issues. It is apparent that with the increased technology available to save human lives, nurses and other health care providers will face an increased number of ethical dilemmas. Nurses must be aware of ethical principles and the law and keep pace with the changes and advancements in health care technology. However, even if the law expands and changes, your own set of ethical codes must constantly be re-evaluated.

SUMMARY

This chapter explored the fundamental legal concepts of nursing practice and their implications. The legal scope of nursing practice, laws affecting clinical nursing, and the concepts and principles of nursing malpractice were examined within the context of the changing health care environment.

■ DISCUSSION QUESTIONS ■

1. How has the changing health care environment changed the legal environment for nursing?
2. Discuss the scope of nursing practice and how the practice of nursing is regulated.

3. What are the basic laws affecting clinical nursing?
4. What are some of the basic things to remember when documenting clinical care?
5. What are the common types of nursing malpractice?
6. Suppose you saw another nurse on your unit give a patient the incorrect drug and she did not report it? What should you do?
7. Discuss what you can do to prevent yourself from being sued.
8. Discuss the "reasonable practice" standard and how it relates to clinical practice.
9. Discuss the concepts of contributory and comparative negligence.
10. Name five strategies for prudent practice.

■ LEARNING ACTIVITIES ■

Case Study 1

As a busy new graduate on a head injury unit, you have noticed that Mr. B is becoming increasingly combative and disoriented. The physicians do not want to sedate him because of his respiratory status, but you are afraid he will hurt himself and continue to pull out his IV lines. You are particularly concerned that he is pulling at his chest tube and arterial line. His family *has requested that Mr. B not be restrained under any circumstance.*

1. What are your legal duties and obligations to the patient?

Case Study 2

The vascular surgeon, the medical director of your unit, has asked you repeatedly to obtain signed consents on his surgical patients. You know from nursing school that you're only supposed to *witness* consents, but that surgeon has gotten angry and threatened to report you. In addition, the patients often have received preop medication and narcotics before signing the permit, and you are worried that they do not understand the consent form.

2. How can you handle these incidents legally and protect your license?

Case Study 3

As the charge nurse in a busy emergency department, you are dismayed and frightened to learn that four registered nurses have not shown up for work. Every trauma room is busy, and med flight has just radioed that they are bringing in the victims of a six-car collision on the interstate. You call your supervisor and ask to close the emergency department to incoming traffic. She refuses.

3. What should you do next?

■ BIBLIOGRAPHY ■

Austin S (1996). The legal side: Missed DNR order. *American Journal of Nursing* 2:55–56.

Becker JH (1996). The legal side: When you need to use restraints. *American Journal of Nursing* 4:89.

Calfee BE (1996). Labor law: Working to protect you. *Nursing* 26:34–39.

Collins D (1995). Can't you take a joke? Sexual harassment in health care. *Revolution: The Journal of Empowerment* 3:68–74.

Court case: After the fall (1996). *Nursing* 2:25.

Eggland ET (1995). Charting smarter: Using new mechanisms to organize your paperwork. *Nursing* 25:34–41.

Fiesta J (1995). Legal update 1995: Part 1. *Nursing Management* 27:22–24.

Fiesta J (1996). Legal issues in long-term care: Part 1. *Nursing Management* 27:18–19.

Grane NB (1996). Charting tips: Things that should stay off the record. *Nursing* 26:17.

Guanowsky G (1995). Liability in managed care for the health care provider. *Nursing Management* 10:25–26.

Keeton PW (1984). *Prosser and Keeton: The Law of Torts*, 5th ed. St. Paul, MN: West Publishing.

Lilley LI, Guanci R (1994). Getting back to basics: Med errors. *American Journal of Nursing* 9:15–16.

Meisel A (1989). *The Right to Die*. New York, NY: Wiley Law Publications.

Rozovsky FA (1990). *Consent to Treatment: A Practical Guide*, 2nd ed. Boston, MA: Little, Brown and Co.

Texas Nurses Association (1993). *Texas' Nursing Practice Act Annotated Guide*. Dallas, TX: Texas Nurses Association Publications.

15 Ethical Leadership in Nursing

J. Anne O'Neil, PhD, RN

• •

LEARNING OBJECTIVES

This chapter will enable the learner to:
1. Discuss ethical theories of importance in nursing leadership.
2. Discuss both a patient-centered framework and a policy/organizational framework for resolving moral conflicts.
3. Describe the unique role of nursing in addressing organizational ethical concerns.
4. Describe some of the current ethical concerns of nurse leaders.

• •

INTRODUCTION

CASE STUDY ♦ 15–1

Jane Miller has just become the unit manager of the surgical cardiac care unit. She is excited about this new position. She hopes through this leadership role to have a significant impact on the care provided patients. However, in her first meeting with the vice president of surgical services she is told that one fourth of the nurses on her unit are to be replaced by unlicensed personnel. These technicians have had 6 months of training in a special cardiac care class. Jane is very distressed and is certain that this cost-containment maneuver will result in poorer patient care. In the past, as a staff nurse, Jane has experienced moral conflicts. She has learned how to work with patients, fami-

lies, and other health care providers to discuss and work through ethical problems in patient care. However, the management dilemma that she is now facing as a nurse leader raises questions she feels unprepared to handle.

Jane Miller's concerns are not uncommon. The purpose of this chapter is to explore the world of ethics as it pertains to the nurse leader. To understand the responsibilities of the nurse leader in ethical issues, it is necessary first to discuss basic ethical concepts in terms of the historical roots of ethics, ethical theories, and decision-making frameworks used in clinical ethics. However, the focus of this chapter is on a broader view of ethics, to include institutional, communal, and societal ethics and the responsibilities of nurse leaders in this expanded arena.

HISTORICAL ROOTS OF BIOETHICS

Bioethics is a relatively new discipline within health care. Concerns regarding patient rights, scientific integrity, futility of care, termination of life support, and assisted suicide, among others, were not common topics of discussion 30 to 40 years ago. Parentalistic views of health care predominated. Beneficent care of patients was related to doing what physicians and nurses felt was in the best interests of their patients. Issues of futility and discussions of the morality of turning off a ventilator were not possible in a time when ventilators did not exist. Furthermore, in previous times, members of a community had similar beliefs regarding such issues as when life begins or how to care for the terminally ill. Questions such as these did not arise when most members of a society shared common cultural values.

Today the best interests of patients are more likely defined by the patient and his or her family in conjunction with health care providers. Technology has provided a plethora of new and innovative materials and treatments to cure disease or postpone dying. Health care providers and patients must continually evaluate the appropriateness of the use of technology. Adding to the complexity of these moral questions is the multicultural nature of the communities in which most people live. How are a doctor from India, a nurse from a small rural community, and a Jewish patient able to discuss and evaluate treatment options when they come from such varied backgrounds?

Philosophers and theologians had long discussed questions of what it means to lead a "good" life, but in the last 50 years they began more and more to relate ethical discussions to questions of right and wrong behavior in medical research and patient care. Hospitals and health-care professionals have begun to call on the expertise of a new breed of philosopher-ethicist for assistance in the complex questions they face in the modern practice of medicine.

Several factors were responsible for this growth. The end of World War II uncovered atrocities that had been done to humans in mental institutions, hospitals, and concentration camps. The subsequent Nuremberg trials, and the adoption of the Nuremberg Code, heightened an interest in issues of patient autonomy and the patient's right to refuse treatment or to participate in medical research.

The law has led the way in issues concerning patient rights. As this century began, court cases established the right of patients to give consent to medical procedures and the duty of physicians to obtain patient consent. Further breakthroughs in court cases began in 1957, when the Salgo case put forth that patients must give *informed* consent to treatment plans. In Natanson v Kline, court cases shifted from problems of battery and the resulting physical harm done to patients. Now the emphasis became the totality of medical negligence. This shift provided a strong statement to physicians to understand that they had a *duty* to disclose all pertinent information needed by patients regarding planned treatments before patients gave consent. Failure to disclose could open physicians to possible malpractice liability. They would be held accountable for failure to disclose even when the patient was not physically harmed by the lack of disclosure. Canterbury in 1972 extended physician disclosure to mean providing patients and families with as much information as the average person would be expected to desire in order to make an informed decision about treatment *(reasonable person standard)*. Prior to this, physicians were held to a standard of providing information that was professionally customary in their community *(professional practice standard)*. By this time, in the mid-1970s, the courts had substantially defined patient rights. Court cases also decided issues of privacy and confidentiality standards for patient care. Along with court cases, state and federal legislative initiatives codified informed consent and other health care issues (Beauchamp & Childress, 1994).

Throughout this period, physicians played a more reactive role in the growth of bioethics. Court cases pushed physicians to examine the ethics of their traditional paternalistic practice. Patients who in the past acquiesced to physician decisions on care now demanded dialogue with health care providers and a right to make their own decisions on what they considered to be in their best interests.

Nursing during this period began to find a stronger ethical voice. In the past, nursing ethics had been concerned with questions of obedience to physician orders and issues that related more to matters of etiquette than ethics. With the growth of civil rights and women's rights in the 1960s and 1970s, nurses began to view themselves as patient advocates rather than physician servants. They began to discuss and question their obligations as nurses to patients, hospitals, colleagues, and the communities in which they lived.

The late 1970s brought about The National Commission for the Protection of Human Subjects of Biomedical and Behavioral Research (1978) followed by the President's Commission for the Study of Ethical Problems (1982). Both these commissions were made up of philosopher-ethicists, lawyers, physicians, and theologians. All were brought together to discuss the growing moral concerns regarding the ethics of medical research and the increasing ethical complexity of patient care. The work of these commissions set ethical standards for the conduct of scientific research and protection of human rights, both in research and in clinical medicine. Their recommendations included the protection of research subjects from coercion or harm, the need for informed consent, and the special protection needed for the incompetent patient. During this period, ways in which to organize discussions regarding the appropriate use of technology, when life begins and ends, and access to health care were of prime importance.

The work of Beauchamp and Childress (1979) and others brought various ethical theories and frameworks forward for exploring decisions in patient care. Today participants from philosophy, the law, medicine, nursing, and other health care disciplines work together to enhance the ethical environment of patient care, whether that care is provided in the hospital, outpatient settings, managed care settings, nursing homes, or the patient's own home. More and more, bedside decision-making is viewed as an interdisciplinary concern with input from philosophy on ethical theories, organizational legal departments on legal precedents and laws, clinical knowledge from medicine and nursing, psychosocial information from psychology and social work, and administrative concerns from risk management.

PATIENT CARE DECISION-MAKING

Traditionally, the heart of health care ethics has involved issues of concern to individual patients and health care providers. Broad ethical theories and frameworks have guided decision-making when moral conflicts arise. Is it morally right for Mary Jones to undergo one more course of chemotherapy for metastatic cancer that has little possibility of gaining quality time for her? Does 90-year-old John Andrews have the capacity to decide whether he can care for himself at home or should acquiesce to family concerns for his safety and enter a nursing home? Is it morally right for Dr. Smith to assist Patricia White, who is in the terminal stages of AIDS, with carrying out her plans to terminate her life? What might a nurse do with a conflict between obligations to a patient she cares for and an obligation to the physician she works with? And more recently, how are nurses and physicians to balance the bottom-line issues governing the managed care organization that employs them with the therapeutic needs of their patients?

Traditional Ethical Theories

Several ethical theories have organized discussion on questions of this nature. Traditionally, these theories have discussed ethical questions from perspectives such as: What is my duty in this situation? What will be the consequences of my actions? What kind of person am I?

What Is My Duty?

Theories based on duties and obligations come to us from Kantian philosophy and emphasize principles and rules. These rules and the principles must meet a standard that is universal and applicable to all humans (Beauchamp & Childress, 1994). For instance, nurses have an obligation to care for all in need of their services (American Nurses' Association, 1976/1985). This rule guides nurses in decisions of caring for all patients no matter what their station in life. The criminal, the AIDS patient, the homeless person, or any patient that might be considered "undesirable" is still to be cared for under this nursing obligation.

What Will Be the Consequences of My Actions?

The most well-known consequential theory is based on the philosophies of Bentham and Mill in which actions taken to implement decisions are evaluated on their utility—how well they produce a maximum balance of benefit over harm (Beauchamp & Childress, 1994). For example, nurses desire to assist their patients in a return to good health. Nurses' actions then must maximize reaching this goal and not contribute to patients' remaining in a state of illness. Nurses demonstrate this theory on a daily basis. They make ethical judgments in deciding how to best utilize their time between several patients to provide the maximum benefit to all their patients.

What Kind of Person Am I?

A traditional ethical theory that has recently engendered renewed interest is that of Aristotelian virtue ethics. In this theory it is not the actions of individuals that are of interest, but rather the character of the actor. Virtue theory asks what moral values a person must possess to lead a "good" life, what a virtuous person is, and how we might enhance the inner virtue of the professional (Beauchamp & Childress, 1994). The public usually views nurses as virtuous, possessing a value system that supports virtues such as empathy, compassion, and fairness. Nurses act in accordance with an inner desire to do good and be of help to their patients. Their desires and motivations result in actions that reflect a moral ideal.

These distinct ethical theories all guide health care professionals as they work through the moral conflicts they encounter in their clinical practice. Some nurses and physicians are more strongly guided by their sense of duty and adherence to basic ethical principles, such as autonomy, justice, and beneficence. Others may be more concerned with the overall outcomes of their actions. Still others may place more emphasis on the strength of their own and others' characters and a belief that right actions flow naturally from right motives and desires.

In many cases, moral conflict in health care is so complex that a blending of theories occurs. Over time, however, guidance in ethical decision-making has been highlighted by four ethical principles.

1. Respect for autonomy—wherein the health professional is guided by the inherent respect owed patients to maintain control of their decision-making capacity even when this may differ from what the physician or others may see as in the patient's best interest.
2. Beneficence—by which the health care professional is obligated to act in a manner that is of benefit to the patient, to produce good and not harm.
3. Nonmaleficence—the counter to beneficence, directs the health care professional never to produce harm even during those times when it is not possible to directly benefit the patient.
4. Justice—guides ethical thinking to consider the fairness of actions and to attempt a just distribution of health care goods. This principle will be discussed further when the responsibilities of the nurse leader are explored.

Additional Ethical Perspectives

Recently, other ethical frameworks have been presented for discussion. Care-based ethics, casuistry/ contextual, and communitarian-based perspectives have been brought forward to broaden the discussion of ethical decision-making.

What Are the Needs of This Relationship?

Until recently, ethical theories have been dominated by perspectives from male philosophers. Now a feminist perspective is being heard from the work of Gilligan (1982), Noddings (1984), Carse (1991), Sharpe (1992), Warren (1992), and others. The impetus for this in nursing has come from the work of Leininger (1981), Watson and Ray (1988), and Benner and Wrubel (1989). This care/relationship perspective stresses that what is important in ethical decisions is the strengthening of the relationships of those involved in a moral conflict rather than simply a strict adherence to principles or rules. This perspective has been attractive to nursing because it places the interconnections of humans at its center. Typically nurses faced with a moral conflict ask questions such as: What good is accomplished if a health maintenance organization (HMO) insists Mrs. Hilton be discharged home and no one is there to assist her with her meals? Is it right to turn off the ventilator before Mr. Schultz's brother arrives from Tennessee? Is it good nursing practice to not tell little Christy's parents that further chemotherapy will not delay her death? The care perspective provides a framework for exploring these questions.

What Is the Context of This Situation?

Another line of ethical thinking states that it is the specifics of the situation that are of importance in reaching any ethical decision. Jonsen and Toulmin (1988) put forth a view of ethics that considers it too early in the history of bioethics to establish rigid theories, principles, and rules. Only by exploring more thoroughly the questions that arise from the practice setting will theories relevant to medicine and nursing arise. These casuists ask that ethicists, health care professionals, patients, and their families discuss more fully and deeply the history and narrative of their dilemma, focusing on all possible resolutions rather than a simple commitment to, for example, preserving patient autonomy. Casuists state that it is only from building a foundation of paradigm cases that future guidance in ethical decision-making will come. This contextual approach appeals to nurses because it recognizes the complexity of difficulties and decision-making in health care environments. Nurses realize the importance of obtaining a full "story" of patient lives. With the growth of home care, nurses are even more aware of the full fabric of the patient's own lifeworld. They are intimately aware of how deep-seated values, socioeconomic status, and family interactions all have an impact on the rightness of morally difficult choices that patients and their families make.

What Actions Are in the Common Good?

Another perspective currently being discussed is that of the communitarian. Contemporary communitarians ask questions that broaden our horizons from the individual patient to what is best for a particular community or what the moral principles of the community are, whether the community is a family, a small rural community, a large urban center, or a nation. As cost-containment issues in health care grow, the questions of how to live a good life in the community have taken on more importance in ethical discernment. Nursing has traditionally focused on relationships with individual patients, but has harbored a knowledge that patients exist in community with others and that the needs of the whole community are affected by the decisions of individuals within it. Nurses are asking hard questions related to who is "deserving" of scarce organs for transplantation, whether limited ICU beds should be occupied by the terminally ill, whether it is good for society to invest more dollars in research to the neglect of primary health care needs, and whether it is ethical for those employed by HMOs to accept bonuses for limiting referrals.

As we near the 21st century, approaches to ethical discussion that speak to the complexity of human relationships will play a more important role in health care decisions. We are at an exciting point in the history of bioethics. Rampant technology, runaway costs, and the complexity of a multicultural society have brought to the forefront of ethical thinking how we might live a good life *together*. The history of the United States is that of a nation

that has relied on rugged individualism. The future may alter this history, putting greater emphasis on the needs of the nation as a whole than on the autonomy of the individual. This is a difficult transition to make and many questions remain as to the necessity of a new vision of health care, access to that care, who will gain, and who will suffer. Leaders of health care professions must continually question their own ethical values and obligations in this new environment. Will health care providers take a strong leadership role or a reactive stance to the ongoing changes in health care? Will health care professionals continue to set a high moral standard for their conception of health care in the United States? Will physicians and nurses broaden their ethical thinking from the needs of the patient to include the needs of the institution or agency that employs them? What obligations are asked of nurse leaders by the community they live in?

ETHICAL NURSING LEADERSHIP

Nurses in leadership positions have a broad, more encompassing responsibility in the health care arena, whether that responsibility involves chairing a hospital committee, being a team leader, case manager, union representative, or nurse entrepreneur, or acting as an elected official in the state legislature. Distinctive ethical obligations are shaped by the responsibilities entailed in leadership; however, the nurse in a leadership position will reflect her or his own personal and professional values.

Personal and Professional Values

Personal moral values drive responses to ethical questions. Values reflect what a person considers to be of importance in his or her ability to lead a good life. In the scenario that opened this chapter Jane Miller values her ability to provide patients with good nursing care. She is concerned that altering the ratio of licensed to unlicensed personnel will not allow for the provision of good care.

Of course, not everything that a person values has *moral* value. Cars, wine, a good book or movie, a favorite sweater, or a beloved home may be valued by an individual but have no inherent moral value.

Moral values are associated with the actions of individuals, communities, and nations that are considered worthwhile or set a desirable standard or quality of behavior (Fry, 1994). Moral value is often given to institutions such as churches and charitable organizations or to virtuous characteristics such as honesty, loyalty, and altruism.

Children's moral development is influenced by the environment in which they grow up. They absorb the cultural and religious values their parents believe are important. As they enter the educational system, what children value is augmented and possibly changed. They learn broader societal values as reflected by their teachers. Those who enter a service profession, such as nursing, are called by values that place importance on helping others, a high regard for medicine and science, and challenging work. Through their education, nurses learn the values of their profession. They incorporate into their value system standards of importance to nursing, such as maintaining competence and a sense of compassion (Fry, 1994). Principles of bioethics incorporate values that are of importance to health care providers. For instance, when a nurse states that the principle of respect for patient autonomy is important, she is stating that she values a patient's right to make independent decisions about treatment.

Moral Conflict

Ethical dilemmas arise when two or more moral values or principles come into conflict. Conflict may come between personal and professional values or between conflicting professional values. Nurses with children may feel a conflict between the need to finish their shift and return home and the equally strong need to stay and work extra hours on a short-staffed nursing unit. Or, consider the following quandary.

CASE STUDY ◆ 15–2

Bob Littleton, an excellent adult medical-surgical nurse, is usually the charge nurse on the adult medical unit of a small community hospital. One evening, as he is receiving report from the day charge nurse, he is told to report to the pediatric unit because the charge nurse and one of the two nursing assistants who usually staff the unit at night are out sick. Bob has not worked in pediatrics since he was a student nurse. Bob is concerned that he might harm a child if he accepts this assignment. At the same time, he is concerned about leaving the children in the care of one nursing assistant.

Bob has a moral conflict. He values giving competent care to his patients. He also values not abandoning his patients. He cannot act on both values at the same time. Jane Miller also is conflicted between two professional obligations: her responsibility to provide good patient care and her obligation to control cost. Particularly for nurses in leadership positions, conflict may arise when they know what the "right" thing to do is, but are constrained from acting on their convictions (Jameton, 1984). Jane Miller values the care that registered nurses provide patients. She does not believe unlicensed personnel can provide this level of expertise to patients. However, she does not view herself in a position to set policy on her unit for the ratio of nurses to unlicensed personnel.

Nurses in leadership roles may also feel conflict when there is no best answer to an ethical dilemma. Consider this example.

CASE STUDY ◆ 15–3

John Vargas has owned his own health care agency in a small rural community for 2 years. During a flu epidemic that affects his highly skilled nursing staff, he finds himself having to decide between sending out a critical care nurse to three ventilator-dependent patients for only 2 hours or providing each with a home health aide for a full 8-hour shift. Neither choice seems desirable, but no other solution appears possible until other trained staff return to work.

Solutions to ethical dilemmas typically have no perfect answer that is satisfactory to all involved. More and more, ethical problems involve professionals across disciplines who come together to discuss and work through to what may be the less undesirable of two solutions to patient care situations.

Help with Ethical Dilemmas

As noted, nurses are gaining competency in addressing patient care dilemmas and their own moral conflicts. Numerous ethical decision-making frameworks have been developed to assist both individual practitioners and groups in working through ethical dilemmas they encounter in the clinical setting (Table 15–1).

All frameworks have in common the gathering of as much information about the problem as possible, determining who the appropriate decision makers are, identifying and discussing all possible courses of actions, obtaining guidance from ethical princi-

Table 15–1.
Model for Resolving Ethical Problems

1. Identify the problem
   - What is at issue (values, conflicts, conscience)?
   - What is your relation to the problem?
   - What are the time parameters?
2. Gather data
   - Who are main people involved?
   - What does the patient want?
   - Construct a case story
3. Identify options
   - What courses of action are open?
   - What are possible outcomes?
   - What are the potential impacts of outcomes?
   - What future decisions are likely?
4. Think the ethical problem through
   - Consider basic conventional principles
   - Consider universal principles or basic human values
5. Make a decision
   - Choose a course of action that best reflects your judgment
6. Act and assess
   - Compare the actual outcome with the projected outcome
   - How would you improve the process next time?
   - Would you generalize this decision to future situations having similar characteristics?

From Jameton A (1984). Nursing practice: The ethical issues, Englewood Cliffs, NJ: Prentice-Hall, p 66.

ples and perspectives, deciding on the best course of action, implementing the decisions, and evaluating the results of the actions taken.

Nurses in leadership positions may not see the relevance of this type of bioethics to their managerial responsibilities. Bioethics, for the most part, has focused on concerns of a clinical nature that take place at patient bedsides. Management and leadership ethics reside both in the world of bedside ethics and organizational/managerial/policy ethics. Where might nurse leaders look for assistance in clarifying, discussing, and solving their moral conflicts, especially as they face the growing managed care environment?

Codes of Ethics

One avenue of assistance to all nurses is their professional code of ethics. The American Nurses' Association Code for Nurses (1976/1985) (Table 15–2) provides guidelines for ethical practice. The addition in 1985 of interpretive statements to the code has added to its usefulness. The code stresses nurses' obligations to respect human dignity no matter what the circumstances of the patient might be. Through the code, nurses' traditional responsibilities to their individual patients are highlighted. The code also speaks to the obligation of nurses to maintain their own competency as well as their responsibility for their own practice.

Familiarizing themselves with the code will give broad guidance to nurses in how to uphold the cherished values of their profession. However, just as ethical theories are meant as guides to structuring discussion and not specific answers concerning ethics and moral conflict, the code of ethics does not delineate specific answers to questions that arise in the daily work world. For example, Plank 3 of the code stresses that nurses act in a manner that will safeguard the health of patients from incompetent practice (ANA, 1976/1985). This plank provides a firm foundation for Jane Miller's strong belief that a high ratio of unlicensed personnel will not assure her of the safety of the patients on her unit. The code does not, however, give Jane a plan of action for how she might enact this provision of the code and go about protecting the safety of her patients.

The code for nurses does not take a strong position on the responsibilities of nurses to their em-

Table 15–2.

American Nurses' Association Code for Nurses

1. The nurse provides services with respect for human dignity and the uniqueness of the client, unrestricted by considerations of social or economic status, personal attributes, or the nature of health problems.
2. The nurse safeguards the client's right to privacy by judiciously protecting information of a confidential nature.
3. The nurse acts to safeguard the client and the public when health care and safety are affected by the incompetent, unethical, or illegal practice of any person.
4. The nurse assumes responsibility and accountability for individual nursing judgments and actions.
5. The nurse maintains competence in nursing.
6. The nurse exercises informed judgment and uses individual competence and qualifications as criteria in seeking consultation, accepting responsibilities, and delegating nursing activities to others.
7. The nurse participates in activities that contribute to the ongoing development of the profession's body of knowledge.
8. The nurse participates in the profession's efforts to implement and improve standards of nursing.
9. The nurse participates in the profession's efforts to establish and maintain conditions of employment conducive to high-quality nursing care.
10. The nurse participates in the profession's effort to protect the public from misinformation and misrepresentation and to maintain the integrity of nursing.
11. The nurse collaborates with members of the health professions and other citizens in promoting community and national efforts to meet the health needs of the public.

From American Nurses' Association (1976/1985). Code for nurses with interpretive statements. Kansas City: Author.

ploying organization. Plank 9 speaks to nursing's concern for the establishment and maintenance of conducive conditions for the practice of nursing, but does not address the possible common or differing goals and objectives of nursing and health care administration. Nor does it give guidance to those nurses who may be in an administrative position in a for-profit HMO and feel conflicting obligations between the needs of the patients and those of the stockholders. The code is currently being reassessed and revisions may address more managerial issues of nursing leadership (Scanlon, 1996).

Nurses in management positions may also find assistance from the code of The American College of Healthcare Executives (1995) (Table 15–3). This code emphasizes health care executives' strong commitment to their profession and the patient. It also brings to the forefront the concept that managers are strongly committed to the organization and its employees. The code discusses the standards of ethical conduct for health care organizations in the community, in patient care, and organizational conduct. As with the Code for Nurses, however, the health care executives' code only provides a platform for the discussion of broad ethical conduct. In looking to this code, Jane Miller would not find delineated the parameters of good moral behavior by management personnel. The code would help her to search her own value system for her beliefs about her current problem. Her own values then would help her weigh between conflicting beliefs on what she would consider the right action to take. Discussion with others could then identify for her how best to implement her plan of action.

Nursing and Interdisciplinary Ethics Committees

Maryland is currently the only state that mandates that all health care organizations have an ethics committee. However, Joint Commission on Accreditation of Healthcare Organizations (JCAHO) regulations also state that hospitals must have some way of addressing ethical issues in an interdisciplinary manner. Until recently, this has meant clinical care questions directly involving patients and staff. However, expectations now are that hospitals begin to include overall organizational ethics in their focus.

Some hospitals are also finding value in administrative and unit-based managerial ethical rounds similar to the more familiar clinical ethical rounds (Reiser, 1994). In these administrative/managerial ethical rounds, matters concerning the functioning of the leadership are discussed, the effectiveness of future polices or those already enacted, and whether a commitment is being maintained to the ethical standards of the institution. For instance, health maintenance organizations have set certain criteria for discharge of newborns and their mothers. An organizational ethics forum would discuss this policy and its fit with the mission statement of the maternity department. If the policy is not

Table 15–3.
Code of Ethics: The American College of
Healthcare Executives

Preamble

The purpose of the *Code of Ethics* of the American College of Healthcare Executives is to serve as a guide to conduct for members. It contains standards of ethical behavior for health care executives in their professional relationships. These relationships include members of the health care executive's organization and other organizations. Also included are patients or others served, colleagues, the community, and society as a whole. The *Code of Ethics* also incorporates standards of ethical behavior governing personal behavior, particularly when that conduct directly relates to the role and identity of the health care executive.

The fundamental objectives of the health care management profession are to enhance overall quality of life, dignity and well-being of every individual needing health care services; and to create a more equitable, accessible, effective, and efficient health care system.

Health care executives have an obligation to act in ways that will merit the trust, confidence, and respect of health care professionals and the general public. Therefore, health care executives must lead lives that embody an exemplary system of values and ethics.

In fulfilling their commitments and obligations to patients or others served, health care executives function as moral advocates. Since every management decision affects the health and well-being of both individuals and communities, health care executives must carefully evaluate the possible outcomes of their decisions. In organizations that deliver health care services, they must work to safeguard and foster the rights, interests, and prerogatives of patients or others served. The role of moral advocate requires that health care executives speak out and take actions necessary to promote such rights, interests, and prerogatives if they are threatened.

From The American College of Healthcare Executives (1995). *Code of Ethics.* Chicago, IL: Author.

---

congruent with their standard for postpartum care, then the board and administration would address a course of action to modify either the standard of care or the discharge policy. This type of discussion might not take place without the attention paid by a forum for ethical discussion of organizational values. Jane Miller might find such an ethics forum of assistance as she works through to a decision regarding her own ethical dilemma. By taking her dilemma to an administrative ethics forum she would be able to alert administration to consider the ethical ramifications of this proposed policy. Unit-based ethics rounds could also be expanded to include issues other than questions of patient decision-making. For Jane Miller, this might provide a forum for brainstorming solutions to the licensed-to-unlicensed ratio and for identifying her nurses' values in regard to staffing issues.

Nurses are relatively new to the interdisciplinary ethics arena. Nursing has a great deal to offer to interdisciplinary ethics committees from both its clinical and leadership practice. At first, the new nurse member may feel uncomfortable in speaking up or participating in the ongoing discussion and give and take of ethical consulting, policy review, and educational programs—typical functions of ethics committees. A more comfortable arena to start from would be a nursing bioethics council or committee (Edwards & Hadaad, 1988; Zink & Titus, 1994). A nursing bioethics committee provides a forum for nurses to discuss and learn about ethical nursing practice. Nurses have ethical concerns that do not always fit in the parameters of most interdisciplinary ethics committees, such as communication with patients, working conditions, and relationships with coworkers. A nursing bioethics committee can address these issues and concerns and assist nurses in gaining the needed education and confidence to effectively intervene in ethical matters at both the clinical and the managerial level of nursing practice. If Jane Miller's hospital does not have a nursing bioethics committee, she could be instrumental in starting such a forum for nurses. In this committee, she could bring forth moral practice issues that concern all nurses, such as the use of unlicensed personnel.

Continuing Ethical Education

Ethics and the teaching of ethical decision-making is receiving more emphasis in nursing education programs (Frisch, 1987). However, a recent survey by the American Nurses' Association (Scanlon, 1994) noted that 59% of nurses do not feel adequately prepared for dealing with the ethical dilemmas they face in their nursing practice. Hospitals, home care agencies, ambulatory care centers, managed care facilities, and nursing associations must provide continuing education for nurses to increase their knowledge and confidence when faced with the innumerable ethical dilemmas that arise in practice (O'Neil, 1991). Jane Miller could be instrumental in bringing into her unit a nurse ethicist to provide inservice education for her staff nurses.

Nursing education for nursing leadership must include an ethics component to familiarize nurse executives with the realms of business/organizational ethics and nursing ethics. Practice is needed in examining ethical dilemmas and the resulting moral conflict that may arise for a leader in nursing. The use of decision-making frameworks, case studies, mock ethics rounds, and other simulation exercises is valuable to nursing managers. Jane Miller as a new nurse manager will need to expand her own ethics education to include more management-oriented ethics. This will assist her in bringing into congruence her value system developed as a staff nurse and her new responsibilities.

Creating an Ethical Environment

Nursing leaders are not only responsible for their own ethical behavior, but must work to create an ethical environment for those who work for and with them (Levine-Ariff & Groh, 1990). They must be cognizant of the role-modeling they provide of ethical nurse leadership. Nurses are taking leadership positions in traditional areas such as hospitals, home care agencies, and nursing homes. In these organizations, nurses are also finding new spheres of interest open to them that go beyond traditional nursing departments and responsibilities, such as quality assurance and risk management. Nurses are also moving into leadership in such nontraditional venues as health maintenance organizations, insurance companies, legislative offices (former-Senator

Dole's chief legislative aide was a nurse), social policy agencies, and the legal profession. To all of these venues nursing must bring its established concern for quality patient care and professional nursing practice.

Creating an ethical environment means taking risks, thinking clearly, looking at the possibilities open to nursing, acting professionally, not being afraid to challenge, and having confidence in one's self (Wise, 1991). A sense of humor is also advisable in stressful situations such as the current health care climate. In a time of down-sizing, re-engineering, and bottom-line management, it may seem impossible to achieve a milieu that fosters these behaviors, but if nursing does not accept this challenge, the profession will be among the driven rather than the drivers of the inevitable changes in health care.

Aroskar (1994) notes that to create an ethical environment, nursing leaders must be cognizant of the dynamics of power and politics in any organization. Only then will they be able to effectively work to maintain the moral integrity of their nursing staff and other employees and the profession of nursing. Power and politics are involved in deciding who gets what of the moneys associated with health care benefits. The ethical implications of these questions and answers are of importance to the kind of environment nursing leadership desires to create.

Distributive Justice and Ethics

Many of the issues that cause concerns for the nurse in a leadership position revolve around justice issues. Distributive justice refers to how a society fairly, equally, and appropriately distributes its available goods. Distributive justice issues become of particular concern during times of scarcity. For example, some 20 years ago, gasoline was a scarce commodity and issues of access and rationing were of concern to motorists. In the past the United States has not recognized the scarcity of health care "goods," whether they were money, supplies, technology, or personnel. An underlying assumption of society was a belief in the unlimited potential of the society, its citizens, and its resources.

The philosopher Rawls put forth a theory of justice that held as an ideal that equals should be treated equally and that those of unequal status (through no fault of their own) should be compensated for the disadvantages of their handicaps (Beauchamp & Childress, 1994). This ideal, of the obligation of society to care for the less fortunate, is being questioned. Is government the proper place for this responsibility? If so, what are society's obligations? Should health care professionals and the organizations they work for be guided solely by altruistic concerns? Is it ethical for health care organizations, such as for-profit managed care organizations, to exist simply as profit-making businesses? Within the last few years, these questions have become of major ethical concern to all involved in providing or receiving health care. At this time, there is no overall agreement on these distributive justice questions, much less consistent policies to guide health care providers. However, questions are being asked, and this is a first step to resolving issues of this importance.

Global questions are being asked regarding how much money is appropriate for a nation to spend on health care needs, whether universal access to health care should be the moral norm, whether more health care assets should go toward hemodialysis or toward well-baby check-ups, and whether educational efforts and funds should go toward supplying more advanced-practice nurses or baccalaureate nurses. For the nurse entrepreneur, ethical questions may be directed toward how many medically indigent clients a home health agency can serve at once. The unit manager may ask whether it is better to shift critically ill ICU patients to a step-down unit or to refuse new admissions.

All these are questions of distributive justice. How we arrive at answers to these questions is reflective of the ethical theories discussed earlier in this chapter: What is our duty to fulfill societal needs for health care? What answers and policies will prove the most beneficial to the most members of society? What is the character of the people entrusted to find answers and set policies in motion? Again, reflection on the answers to these and similar questions will more than likely involve a blending of theories to explore as fully as possible all ramifications of justice issues. It is important that nursing leaders be cognizant of the different theoretical perspectives from which other health care leaders' thoughts are arising. Certainly, creating and maintaining an ethical environment in times of scarcity can be challenging.

AN ETHICAL FRAMEWORK FOR NURSE LEADERS

The ethical frameworks for decision-making in individual patient care situations do not easily translate to the broader policy and managerial concerns of nurses in leadership positions. All nurses are in a position to express their opinions on national, state, and local health issues. In addition, nurses in management positions are in a position to be proactive as policies are developed for and by, for example, their nursing unit, home health agency, or state board of nursing. But how are they to address their ethical concerns for developing policy at the organizational level? Kelman and Warwick (1978) have described a process of evaluating the social interventions put forth in planning for change in organizational units, whether small nursing units, hospitals, HMOs, states, nations, or international organizations. They outline four key areas to be examined and questions to be answered by all involved: (1) The choice of goals, (2) defining the target of change, (3) the choice of means used to implement interventions, and (4) assessment of the consequences (Table 15–4).

First, the nurse leader needs to have a clear understanding of the goals of any planned organizational change. She or he needs to assess the goals and reflect on the fit of the projected goal with the mission statement of the organization and her or his own personal and professional value system. Only then will the nursing leader be able to engage in effective dialogue with others on the appropriateness of the goal and the planning of strategies for implementation or revision of the stated goal. For example, is the overall goal of a specific plan for health care reform geared toward providing citizens full access to desired health care or is the goal one of maintaining a minimal level of services for all citizens? Is the goal clearly stated? If the underlying implicit or explicit goal is the maintenance of minimal services, does this goal fit with the traditional goals of this society?

Second, it must be made clear exactly who is being asked to change and how the change will affect their lives. For example, in the case of Jane Miller and the unlicensed personnel, not only is Jane involved, but also affected are the working conditions of the staff nurses on her unit, the physi-

Table 15–4.
Framework for Ethical Policy Decision-Making

I. WHAT IS OUR GOAL?
   A. Is this a morally good goal?
   B. How do we know it is?
   C. Who disagrees and why?

II. WHO WILL BE AFFECTED BY OUR GOAL?
   A. Who is being asked to change?
   B. Are they represented in the planning for this change?

III. WHAT MEANS WILL WE USE TO REACH OUR GOAL?
   A. What alternative means are possible?
   B. Are the means coercive?
   C. Do the means chosen allow for respecting individual autonomy?

IV. WHAT DO WE EXPECT TO BE THE CONSEQUENCES OF ACHIEVING OUR GOAL?
   A. What will be the benefits/harms to society?
   B. What will be the benefits/harms to the affected groups?

From Kelman HC, Warwick DP (1978). The ethics of social intervention: Goals, means, and consequences. In Bermant G, Kelman HC, Warwick DP (eds). *The Ethics of Social Intervention.* New York: John Wiley & Sons, p 3. Reproduced with permission. All rights reserved.

cians who admit patients to the unit, and the patients themselves. All are being asked to change and accept a significantly different level of patient care. Including representation from the unit staff, community members, and physicians would allow for a fuller exploration of the effect of the proposed change as well as generating a broader range of means to implement the change.

Third, a full presentation of exactly how a change is to be carried out will display the moral rightness of the means. In the current efforts to contain costs in the Medicare program, members are being given the "choice" of joining an HMO. A full discussion of how members are being offered a choice of providers would reveal whether they are actually given freedom of choice or are being coerced into joining HMOs. Promoting this discussion then allows for a fuller discussion of the goals of the proposed change.

Last, assessing the consequences of proposed change allows for a re-evaluation of exactly which values of a society or organization are to be given priority at this time. Both the long-term and short-term benefits and harms need to be assessed as well as the direct and indirect consequences of any change. In assessing the consequences of the use of more unlicensed personnel, Jane Miller might find that their use prevents the short-term direct harm of closure of cardiac services at her hospital. However, the long-term indirect harm to the community might be an overall lowering of the standards of care for cardiac patients.

It is this type of airing of the ethical issues involved that allows for a fuller exploration of the moral concerns of importance both to nursing and to all health care providers. If nurses are being asked to be risk-takers in ethical dialogue and discernment (Wise, 1991) they must forthrightly address these ethical demands in the broader arenas of health care. As health care reform moves forward it is imperative that any changes have a solid ethical base of justification and that nurses' voices be heard on these issues.

WORKING TOGETHER FOR AN ETHICAL SOLUTION

The framework of organizational ethical decision-making can assist nurses to be part of the interdisciplinary environment of the current leadership involved in solving health care problems. Along with their problem-solving skills, gained through professional education and experiences, the nurse leader is in an excellent position to influence the moral debate about management and policies of the organization in which they work.

Working Together for Change

When discussing either the ethics of individual patient care decisions or broader organizational policies and decisions, each member of a committee, task force, board, or agency brings his or her own professional viewpoint to the discussion. The hospital administrator brings a concern for management and economics. The risk management department represents concerns for safety and institutional liability. Physicians are concerned with their ability to cure the patients under their care and the organization's ability to fulfill its role of patient care.

Nursing concerns center around the relationship between the nurse and the patient. As Plank 3 of the Code for Nurses (ANA, 1976/1985, p 6) states, "The nurse acts to safeguard the client and the public when health care and safety are affected by incompetent, unethical, or illegal practice by any person." It is through their own personal and professional integrity that nurses acting as patient advocates, as noted in the interpretative statements accompanying this plank, can assist interdisciplinary bodies to maintain a focus on the human element of all decision-making in health care management and reform. This strong connection with the individual patient has made nurse leaders concerned about balancing the needs for group compromise with the needs of individual patients or specific groups of patients. How is this focus maintained when working in interdisciplinary groups? Compromise of traditional nursing focuses may be required (Winslow & Winslow, 1991).

It is through group problem-solving that reasonable compromise arises instead of a decision that upholds traditional ideal values of one profession or group. For example, the hospital administrator may find that his or her value in fiscal soundness must still allow for a certain level of free services to the homeless population of the community. This value in "charity" services is stated in the mission statement of the religious organization that owns the hospital. Physicians may find that a home health agency must join a cooperative purchasing group to cut costs. Physicians using the services of the home health agency must then compromise on their desire for a specific brand of equipment.

Nurses, in turn, participating in deciding the future of health care services, will find that cherished values centered on relationships and the needs of individual patients may have to be re-evaluated in terms of the current health care environment. Yarling and McElmurry (1986) conclude that in today's health care agencies, nurses are not able to act as free moral agents because of the constraints placed on their professional autonomy by the practice environment. Bishop and Scudder (1987) view nurses as placed in an in-between position able to mediate between administration, physician, and patient needs. More and more, all parties to discussion and organizational decision-making are in a position in between competing demands for time and moneys. Just as nurses may feel constrained by competing demands, physicians also feel pulled between high standards of medical care and the demands placed on them by third-party payers.

Winslow and Winslow (1991) assert that it is possible for nurses to take part in the compromises inherent in managerial and policy planning and still maintain their professional integrity. Compromise that preserves the integrity of all can be a morally worthy and realistic goal of dialogue and decision-making in health care. Even within nursing services, conflicts arise over the priority of one professional value over another. Trade-offs are expected between the needs of one patient on a nursing unit and the overall needs of all patients. Similarly, compromise in organizational ethics requires trade-offs that will leave some or all participants less than satisfied with the results of the authorized actions, but understanding the impossibility of fulfilling the totality of desired values of all those affected by the decisions. For instance, in accessing the use of licensed and unlicensed personnel on her unit, Jane Miller may find in the administrative ethics forum that all share her concerns for maintaining patient care standards. Jane may also value the primary care nursing model over the team nursing model for patient care. Compromise could be reached by changing to a modified primary care–team nursing model incorporating the best points of both models. This model may then allow for a certain degree of the use of well-trained unlicensed personnel.

Winslow and Winslow (1991) cite four elements that are needed to allow for the maintenance of individual and organizational integrity in compromise situations (Table 15–5).

Sharing a basic moral language requires those engaged in dialogue to focus their discussion on the commonalities they share rather than the differences that separate them. For example, a discussion regarding what is perceived as inadequate funding for an inner-city clinic may require both clinic staff and city administrators to speak of and agree on less than optimal goals for the clinic. The clinic staff may value universal access to care for all in the community, and the administration may value lowering the burden of debt they carry. To maintain services for those needs identified as having a top priority in this particular community, both staff and administration must be able to talk about what they

Table 15–5.
Compromise with Integrity

1. Integrity-preserving moral compromise requires sharing some basic moral language.
2. Integrity-preserving compromise requires a context of mutual respect.
3. Integrity-preserving compromise is facilitated by the honest acknowledgment of moral perplexity.
4. Integrity-preserving compromise must admit legitimate limits to compromise.

From Winslow BJ, Winslow GR (1991). Integrity and compromise in nursing ethics. *Journal of Medicine and Philosophy* 16:307. With kind permission from Kluwer Academic Publishers.

agree on as having value, so that they can set realistic goals for the clinic.

In all discussions, participants must approach one another with an underlying inherent respect, a respect that requires listening and a dedication to not using coercive methods of obtaining agreement on contested issues. Compromise is what is desired, not capitulation. This is an issue of particular importance to nurses, who have long felt that their professional views have not been given due respect. At this time, nurses may be particularly concerned that expressing their own moral values may be a threat to continued employment.

An acknowledgment by all involved of their own moral perplexity and the moral complexity of situations health care now faces is essential. Humility is needed by all who sit around the conference table. If the issues were not complex and did not give rise to moral conflict, decisions on action plans would be simple. It is because these are not simple, easily reached decisions that they call for a depth of exploration unknown in the past.

At some point, however, there may be limits to the compromise allowed on any given issue. Moral integrity may require the nurse leader to take a stand, to be a risk-taker, against morally repugnant decisions. Winslow and Winslow (1991, p 320) note that "personal integrity is always a quest of the self in conversation with others." When a point of certainty is reached, each nurse leader will need to decide whether her or his own integrity is preserved or threatened and must act accordingly. For instance, Jane Miller believes strongly that the mix of licensed and unlicensed personnel on her unit

should not exceed 60/40. In discussion with others, she will need to then explore whether a moral compromise is possible and decide what she is willing to risk to maintain her own moral integrity. Does she see any room for compromise on this belief? If not, what is she willing to do to uphold her belief?

Role of Ethical Theories and Principles

At this point, a few words need to be added as to how the ethical theories discussed at the beginning of this chapter could assist Jane Miller, Bob Littleton, and John Vargas in defining and resolving their moral conflicts. Ethical theories, according to Jonsen (1991), are the "big picture" surrounding ethical decision-making. Theories proposed by philosophers such as Plato, Aristotle, Hobbes, Spinoza, Kant, Mill, and Rawls try to incorporate all the questions and answers of importance in the overarching question of how humans may and should lead a good life. The problem now is how to take these broad and diverse visions of the good life and apply them to the everyday problems and moral conflicts of nursing and nursing leadership.

There is a need for ethical theory just as there is a need for nursing theory. Theory allows for stepping back and approaching issues from a wider vision without having to answer the practical questions of implementation. It allows for the nurse to look at the totality; for example, to approach a question of scarce resources from a view of the good of a society as a whole without focusing on the good of one vulnerable person. Theory provides space and time for deeper reflection on the ethical issues of today. When nurses and other health care professionals consider what type of access to health care they desire for the population of a given community, they turn to ethical theory to justify their belief in the value of all patients having equal access to services. However, as Jonsen (1991) notes, the logical clarity that seems so evident in abstract theory comes into conflict with other equally logically clear theories. There is no "right" theory or absolute guidance. The "real" world intrudes and asks, "But what are we to do about this vulnerable human standing here right now?"

In the same manner, the principles of respect for autonomy, beneficence, nonmaleficence, and justice can provide a forum to discuss individual situations but cannot provide specific actions for specific cases. Principles set parameters and how "to keep going straight" (Jonsen, 1991, p 16). They provide a ruler for leaders and others to gauge how well they are upholding the values they cherish. Ethical theories can prove especially helpful as society and individuals must address new ethical issues where no precedent is present, such as the rights of genetic versus gestational parents or the genome mapping projects. A broad theoretical discussion is necessary for reaching long-term societal vision and goals.

In the ordinary day-to-day discussions that nurse administrators, clinical nurse specialists, and nursing case managers take part in, however, practical judgment is needed and moves more readily on a case-to-case historical basis than on broad ethical theories. Jane Miller might summarize her own reflections on the increased use of unlicensed personnel by reflecting on previous instances when a nursing *shortage* occurred because of low nursing school enrollment and expanding demands. She could ask what parameters were established for providing nursing care in previous times when licensed personnel were in short supply. What services were deemed essential to good patient care and what were judged desirable but able to be discontinued or provided by a lower level of skill? Did the implementation of these adjustments to care cause irreparable harm to overall patient care? If so, what might be done to minimize harms in this present situation? Jane's values and the theoretical basis for her ethical practice will guide her and warn her when practical judgment will not effectively resolve the current situation. It is at this point that she must decide whether to be the risk taker, able to provide a plan of action that focuses on patient well-being rather than simply an economic solution. Both ethical theory and previous practice will guide her in deciding on what actions are called for in her present moral conflict.

Similarly, it would prove helpful to Bob Littleton, in assessing whether to accept the assignment to the pediatric unit, to have knowledge of theories surrounding his obligations as a nurse and to be able to think clearly as to the benefits and harms that might occur from his actions. John Vargas, in evaluating whether to assign nurses and aides to his ventilator-dependent patients, would find it useful to balance his knowledge of his obligations to care for patients and his clinical knowledge of each of his patients' parameters of needs. With knowledge gained from ethical theories and their own caring practice, nurses will be better able to discuss and analyze the ethical issues of the present and future.

CURRENT ETHICAL ISSUES FOR THE NURSE LEADER

Health care has changed immensely in the last 10 years. One of the most important changes has been the issue of change itself. Health care professionals now realize that change is not a short-term period of adjustment to a new situation or policy, but an unending process of constant reviewing and reconceptualization of the provision of health care in the United States. For the nurse leader, this means that a continual re-evaluation of current ethical issues and future trends is imperative. Home health case managers, hospital unit managers, clinical nurse specialists, and nurse practitioners all must become comfortable with the ambiguity between what society desires of health care providers and what it is possible to provide (Cammuñas, 1994). What are some of the issues that nurse leaders must address?

Health Care Reform

Although the Clinton administration's reform initiatives of the early 1990s have passed into history, health care reform is still a national priority. The impetus for change is now coming from insurance companies, managed care organizations, other third-party payers, and the consumer. Nursing leadership is caught in the middle once again.

The nursing profession has articulated a commitment to universal access to basic health care services. As noted, nursing's strong commitment to quality patient care is being sorely tested. How can nurse administrators and policy planners maintain their commitments and participate in down-sizing efforts and limitation of patient services? Using the framework delineated by Kelman and Warwick (1978), nurse leaders can begin to outline courses of action that will enable them to be morally proactive in securing services for patients as well as facing and dealing with the realities of the current state of cost-containment efforts.

Rise of Managed Care

One of the most noticeable elements of the current cost-containment efforts in health care has been the switch from fee-for-services insurance plans to capitated payment plans and the use of managed care organizations to provide services. Many of the same ethical questions arise in this type of third-party payer arrangement as in any other service area, but for the nurse manager, additional concerns may arise that he or she may not have dealt with in more traditional settings.

Ethical concerns arise out of the relationship contracted between the HMO and the care providers. Not all, but some, HMO contracts require that physicians and nurses provide information only on the specific treatment options available as stated in the contract of the HMO. These options may not always include cutting-edge therapies such as organ transplants or more experimental treatment regimes. The nurse in such a situation is caught in the middle between respecting the patient's autonomy and right to knowledge of all treatment options and the stated policy of the HMO that forbids sharing information on options they will not pay for. How is the nursing leader in this situation to counsel nurse practitioners or case managers who may be restricted from referring patients for evaluative testing that until now has been considered to be the standard of care? How is an ethical environment to be created when physicians and other care providers receive bonuses for not referring patients to specialists? Once again, nurses and nurse managers may find themselves in moral conflict between their obligations to patients, the organization, and their own professional and personal values.

Issues of justice and the totality of society's needs may indeed necessitate restrictions on the type and amount of health care available to members of our society. However, at this time there is no considered approach as to how to achieve just distribution of available resources.

From Nursing Shortage to Down-Sizing Nursing

In the past, nurse managers had to deal with efforts to provide quality patient care in times of nurse shortages. They asked the same hard questions be-

ing addressed today: How can I continue to meet the needs of patients of this home health agency or this ambulatory care facility when I can not afford to hire enough (or must lay off) qualified nurses? What are my moral obligations to my present staff? How can I meet the needs of the patients and not exhaust my nurses who must deal with added overtime, increasing patient loads, and fewer support services? Nurse managers today must consider how they are to reduce their workforce in an ethical manner. Both respect for human dignity and concepts of justice must be of concern when addressing reduction in staff. Weber (1994) suggests that all options other than layoffs must be evaluated first to confirm the need for workforce reduction. If no other means of reduction are identified, the reasons for layoffs and the criteria for selection of those to be laid off must be considered carefully and logically and these criteria clearly communicated to employees. In respect of the dignity of the affected employees, they must be informed in advance and given time to adjust to their termination. Notifying employees on the day of termination and asking them to immediately clear out their desks, workstations, or lockers characterizes an organization that does not respect its employees. Managers find notifying employees of termination to be one of the most troubling aspects of their jobs. All managers should receive instruction on how to handle this distressing responsibility. Ethically responsible nurse leaders will reflect on their own core values of respect for human dignity and commit themselves to a workforce reduction that is committed to maintaining this value.

Role of Unlicensed Health Care Workers

The American Nurses' Association Code for Nurses (1976/1985, pp 10–11) is direct in stating that:

The nurse should not delegate to any member of the nursing team a function for which that person is not prepared or qualified. Employer policies or directives do not relieve the nurse of accountability for making judgments about delegation of nursing care activities.

Jane Miller, in our case example, is keenly aware of the moral conflict she is facing between her duty to provide nursing care in a cost-effective manner and care that maintains a standard of quality inherent in the obligations of professional nursing. Not only must she re-evaluate the desirable ratio of unlicensed to licensed personnel, but she must also carefully evaluate which services can be provided by each group. Many nurses currently employed have been schooled in nursing practice that emphasizes primary nursing concepts. The concept of team nursing, with the professional nurse as case manager, is more in line with the needs of cost containment and the use of unlicensed personnel. The moral conflict for the nurse manager may not be between using or not using unlicensed personnel; the conflict may be more in regard to what tasks and services are appropriate to delegate to unlicensed personnel. The establishment of administrative ethics rounds, as suggested by Reiser (1994), can be helpful in highlighting and determining acceptable ethical resolutions.

Nursing Home and Home Care Services

As cost containment issues in the acute care setting necessitate earlier and earlier discharge from the hospital, the use of the nursing home and home care options has increased. More and more, nurses are employed in these areas. Nursing has taken the lead in management of both nursing homes and home care agencies. The ethical challenges nurses find in these practice areas have certain aspects in common with the acute care setting: standards of service, the use of unlicensed personnel, nurse-physician relationships, and patient privacy and confidentiality. However, the resources available to the nurse manager to deal with the ethical dimensions of these issues may be minimal or nonexistent.

In a large hospital organization, colleagues are available to serve as a sounding board and to assist in analyzing difficult ethical issues (Burger et al, 1992). Working for a home health agency, nurses find themselves alone in homes with only the patients and their caregivers available to reason through difficult situations. Nurses in the home care setting do not spend 10 to 12 hours a day with their patients. They may visit their patient three or four times a week and have only a 40- to 60-minute period of time to assess the situation and implement a plan of action. More and more, hospitals have ethicists and ethics committees available to assist

practitioners with moral conflict. Such services are a rarity in nursing home and home care settings.

Nurse managers in such situations must ensure that they and their staff are comfortable working with an ethical decision-making process. Inservice presentations by a consulting ethicist are important. Counselors and clergy may also be of assistance in consulting with staff and offering support as families and staff make care decisions. The nurses within an agency or nursing home can be encouraged to form support groups or journal clubs to help them reflect on the ethical dimensions of their practice. Another way the nurse manager may create an ethical environment is to begin to form an interagency ethics committee or bioethics network. Most home health agencies in and of themselves are too small to support the diversity and commitment necessary to the establishment of an in-house committee, but an interagency home health ethics committee could prove to be a valuable resource for a community as well as individual agencies. Similarly, nursing homes might benefit from community-wide or regional ethics committees to address the moral conflicts common to all nursing homes. As the use of nursing home and home health services continues to increase, the ethics committee forum within an individual agency may prove more feasible. All of these avenues to improve ethical decision-making will support the nurse leaders' creation of an ethical work environment as much as in the acute care situation (Burger et al, 1992).

Sexual Harassment

Sexual harassment is not new to the world of nursing. Male health care professionals and male patients by their words and actions have frequently shown a lack of respect for female nurses. With the rise in the number of male nurses the same potential for sexual harassment exists between female health care professionals and female patients and the male nurse. What is new since the Anita Hill–Clarence Thomas hearings is the awareness by nurses that they need not put up with unwanted advances by colleagues, supervisors, or patients either in their professional or personal lives (Libbus & Bowman, 1994). It is up to the leadership of all health care workplaces to see that an environment is created in which sexual harassment is not tolerated, an environment in which *all* staff feel comfortable and supported when bringing concerns to their supervisors. The nurse alone in the home is especially vulnerable to sexual advances from patients. The young nurse in the acute care situation may feel vulnerable to the advances of senior nursing and medical staff. Nurses in both these situations may be morally unsure of how to handle such situations. Nurses must feel secure in the knowledge that their immediate supervisor is a supportive presence. The ethically responsible nurse manager will be sure that all staff are knowledgeable regarding their legal rights in regards to sexual harassment. Inservice programs must be ongoing to ensure that all new staff members know how to recognize sexual harassment when it occurs, how to report it, and how to be proactive in preventing sexual harassment (Thobaben, 1993).

Although most sexual harassment is directed toward female staff, as more men enter nursing, the nurse leader must also be cognizant of the potential for the harassment of male staff. Male nurses may perceive their work assignments as unduly heavy or that advancement is blocked by female nurse leaders (King, 1995). No matter where the potential for sexual harassment arises, it is nursing leadership that must set an example for the resolution of any and all morally reprehensible behavior.

SUMMARY

Where is Jane Miller now? Has she been able to resolve her ethical dilemma in a manner that has preserved her moral integrity? Has she been able to find help from colleagues in working through her dilemma? Has a resolution come about that satisfactorily allows for continued excellent patient care by the licensed and unlicensed staff? And, most importantly, have lessons been learned that will assist Jane and the organization to address future moral issues in health care in an ethical manner?

The nursing profession demands that its leaders maintain the highest of ethical standards. The challenges facing all nurses as we approach the 21st century require leadership that will assist nurses to understand and deal with the increasing ethical complexity of their practice. In this chapter, the

exploration of ethical issues that nurses in managerial positions must face has been initiated. The underpinnings of ethical decision-making both at the bedside and in the administrative and policy arenas was described. The responsibilities of leadership to create a healthy ethical environment in the hospital, home health agency, nursing home, and managed care were discussed. It is important that all nurses continue their education regarding ethical decision-making and ethical nursing practice.

■ DISCUSSION QUESTIONS ■

1. What environments or factors have influenced your own moral development? Identify three values that are important to you personally and analyze why they receive priority over others.
2. Discuss how various health care disciplines can work together to establish guidelines for ethical patient care in a community-based practice setting.
3. Discuss why ethical issues are more complex at the end of the 20th century than at the end of the 19th century. How have the factors contributing to this change affected nursing practice?

■ LEARNING ACTIVITIES ■

1. Write a short description of an ethical dilemma you believe is of concern to nurse leaders and use it in the next activities.
2. Review the Kelman and Warwick framework described in An Ethical Framework for Nurse Leaders. Write a brief description of where you believe conflict might arise between individuals brought together to decide on a plan of action to deal with this problem.
3. Begin a discussion with a small group of nurses concerning your dilemma. Try to decide what ethical theory nurses are using to address resolution of the dilemma (duty, outcome, relationship, character). Do different ethical theories enhance or hinder discussion? In what way? Do the discussion participants stay with or switch theories as the discussion proceeds?
4. Use the Kelman and Warwick framework with the group of nurses and decide on a course of action to resolve the ethical dilemma.
5. Briefly describe roadblocks that might occur if

you were in the position of implementing your plan of action.

■ BIBLIOGRAPHY ■

American Nurses' Association (1976/1985). *A Code of Ethics with Interpretive Statements*. Kansas City: Author.

Aroskar MA (1994). The challenge of ethical leadership in nursing. *Journal of Professional Nursing* 10:270.

Beauchamp TL, Childress JF (1979). *Principles of Biomedical Ethics*. New York: Oxford University Press.

Beauchamp TL, Childress JF (1994). *Principles of Biomedical Ethics*, 4th ed. New York: Oxford University Press.

Benner P, Wrubel J (1989). *The Primacy of Caring: Stress and Coping in Health and Illness*. Reading, MA: Addison-Wesley.

Bishop AH, Scudder JR (1987). Nursing ethics in an age of controversy. *Advances in Nursing Science* 9(3):34.

Burger AM, Erlen JA, Tesone L (1992). Factors influencing ethical decision making in the home setting. *Home Healthcare Nurse* 10(2):16.

Cammuñas C (1994). Ethical dilemmas of nurse executives, Part 2. *Journal of Nursing Administration* 24(8):45.

Carse AL (1991). The 'voice of care': Implications for bioethical education. *Journal of Medicine and Philosophy* 16:5.

Edwards BJ, Hadaad AM (1988). Establishing a nursing bioethics committee. *Journal of Nursing Administration* 18(3):30.

Frisch NC (1987). Value analysis: A method for teaching nursing ethics and promoting the moral development of students. *Journal of Nursing Education* 26:328.

Fry ST (1994). *Ethics in Nursing Practice*. Geneva, Switzerland: International Council of Nurses.

Gilligan C (1982). In a different voice. Cambridge, MA: Harvard University Press.

Jameton A (1984). *Nursing Practice: The Ethical Issues*. Englewood Cliffs, NJ: Prentice-Hall.

Jonsen AR (1991). Of balloons and bicycles or the relationship between ethical theory and practical judgment. *Hastings Center Report* 21(5):14.

Jonsen A, Toulmin S (1988). *The Abuse of Casuistry: A History of Moral Reasoning*. Berkeley, CA: University of California Press.

Kelman HC, Warwick DP (1978). The ethics of social intervention: Goals, means, and consequences. In Bermant G, Kelman HC, Warwick DP (eds): *The Ethics of Social Intervention*. New York: John Wiley & Sons, p 3.

King CS (1995). Ending the silent conspiracy: Sexual harassment in nursing. *Nursing Administration Quarterly* 19(2):48.

Leininger M (1981). The phenomenon of caring: Important research questions and theoretical considerations. In Leininger M (ed): *Caring: An Essential Human Need*. Thorofare, NJ: Charles B. Slack.

Levine-Ariff J, Groh DH (1990). Creating an ethical environment. Baltimore: Williams & Wilkins.

Libbus MK, Bowman KG (1994). Sexual harassment of female registered nurses in hospitals. *Journal of Nursing Administration* 24(6):26.

National Commission for the Protection of Human Subjects of Biomedical and Behavioral Research (1978): *The Belmont Report*. Washington, DC: DHEW Publication OS 78-0012.

Noddings N (1984). *Caring: A Feminine Approach to Ethics and Moral Education*. Berkeley, CA: University of California Press.

O'Neil JA (1991). Teaching basic ethical concepts and decision-making: A staff development application. *Journal of Continuing Education in Nursing* 22(5):1.

President's Commission for the Study of Ethical Problems in Medicine and Biomedical and Behavioral Research (1982). *Making Health Care Decisions*. Washington, DC: US Government Printing Office.

Reiser SJ (1994). The ethical life of health care organizations. *Hastings Center Report* 24(6):28.

Scanlon C (1996). Revisiting the code for nurses with interpretive statements. *American Nurses' Association Center for Ethics and Human Rights Communique* 4(3):9.

Scanlon C (1994). Survey yields significant results. *American Nurses' Association Center for Ethics and Human Rights Communique* 3(3):1.

Sharpe VA (1992). Justice and care: The implications of the Kohlberg-Gilligan debate for medical ethics. *Theoretical Medicine* 13:295.

The American College of Healthcare Executives (1995). *Code of Ethics*. Chicago, IL: The American College of Healthcare Executives.

Thobaben M (1993). Sexual harassment. *Home Healthcare Nurse* 11(6):66.

Warren VL (1992). Feminist directions in medical ethics. *HEC Forum* 4(1):19.

Watson J, Ray MA (1988). *The Ethics of Care and the Ethics of Cure: Synthesis in Chronicity*. New York: NLN.

Weber LJ (1994). Ethical downsizing: Managers must focus on justice and human dignity. *Health Progress* July/August:24.

Winslow BJ, Winslow GR (1991). Integrity and compromise in nursing ethics. *Journal of Medicine and Philosophy* 16:307.

Wise PSY (1991). Creating the leadership ethic. *Journal of Continuing Education in Nursing* 22:183.

Yarling RR, McElmurry BJ (1986). The moral foundation of nursing. *Advances in Nursing Science* 8(2):63.

Zink MR, Titus L (1994). Nursing ethics committees: Where are they? *Nursing Management* 25(6):70.

16

Quality Management

Jacqueline A. Dienemann, PhD, RN, CNAA, FAAN,
and Dorothy M. Nyberg, MS, RN

. . . .

LEARNING OBJECTIVES

This chapter will enable the learner to:

1. Explore the scientific and historical bases for quality management.
2. Describe the performance improvement process as it relates to nursing.
3. Illustrate how quality management tools and methods can be applied in nursing.
4. Differentiate risk management and performance improvement.

. . . .

INTRODUCTION

Quality is important to nurses, managers, patients, physicians, and other groups involved in health care. At the extremes, all agree on whether quality is present or absent, but the standard for "good enough" varies widely by person and group because quality judgments are based on personal values, experience, and expectations. This becomes problematic when deciding how to measure quality care. When asked by Congress to design a quality review and assurance program for Medicare in 1986, The Institute of Medicine defined quality of health care as "the degree to which health services for individuals and populations increase the likelihood of desired outcomes and are consistent with current professional standards" (Lohr, 1990, p 1).

This definition is useful but does not go far

enough. It fails to acknowledge that quality is not wholly objective. Dennis O'Leary, president of the Joint Commission on Accreditation of Healthcare Organizations (JCAHO), observed that "quality of care is a judgment shaped by the interests of the individual or group making the judgment" (O'Leary, 1993, p 219). Nurses, physicians, managers, patients, families, and others involved in health care have an interest and point of view regarding quality of care. Each group defines quality differently using its own perspective. These multiple views only partially overlap. When a person receives health care, his impression of the quality of that care is influenced by his expectations and the total experience. This experience is never separate from the technical quality of what was done. For instance, a person experiencing treatment for an injury in an urgent care clinic judges the quality of her care based on the outcome of the injury and her experience in the clinic. The experience includes the decor of the clinic, courtesy of the staff, cost, waiting time, pain she experienced while there, and whether a pay telephone or snacks were available while she waited.

Quality of care is a complex concept that is perceived differently by involved individuals and groups; in fact, the perceptions of these individual and group stakeholders may even conflict regarding desired outcomes. The solution for JCAHO and other accrediting agencies has been to change their focus from *quality assurance* to *performance improvement*. Health care organizations are required to demonstrate how they have improved care between accreditation visits.

Performance data must include information on objective facts about how well the organization is carrying out its important health care functions as well as subjective perceptions about quality by stakeholders such as patients, families, nurses, physicians, and managers. All data must include analysis of improvement using standards and repeated measures over time.

STAKEHOLDERS AS CUSTOMERS

Each group with a professional, personal, or financial interest in health care has a particular definition of quality care. The primary groups with a stake in health care outcomes are patients, families, physicians, nurses, other health care professionals, insurers, and provider organizations. Leaders in quality improvement point out the value of viewing each stakeholder as a customer. Viewing patients and coworkers as customers has sensitized providers to the importance of patient satisfaction and teamwork in providing quality care.

Quality improvement stresses that by defining and understanding the needs and expectations of the customers and suppliers, the quality of work processes can be improved. This way of reframing health care work has dramatically changed the focus on how to improve health care.

Patients and Families

Historically, lay persons, including patients and families, were considered to be recipients of health care who were unable to measure quality of care because of lack of technical expertise. Now it is recognized that patient expectations and satisfaction with the care and service provided have a direct impact on patient health outcomes. Expectations and health practices vary widely among patients based on personal differences in health care goals and previous experiences. However, as customers of health care, patients and families generally agree that they desire competent care, respect, reasonable comfort, caring attitudes, information about their condition, consent regarding choices and treatment, and continuity in care.

Health Care Professionals

Expectations of nurses, physicians, and other professional providers about the quality of health care

Research Box 16–1
Patient Satisfaction

Patient satisfaction information assists health care providers in remaining patient-focused and identifying areas for improvement. One hospital developed a survey form using patient interviews about their experiences and having patients critique a current patient satisfaction form. Simultaneously, each department was asked to submit objective measures of patient satisfaction with their services. For instance, waiting time was suggested for the imaging department. A draft that incorporated both patient and professional suggestions was developed and piloted using a five-point Likert type scale and interviews concerning the meaning of each question. Revisions were made for clarity. The survey is given to each patient on discharge with a stamped return envelope. The return rate is 23%. Monthly reports are sent to each department with the percent of responses as either very negative (highly disagree) or very positive (strongly agree) for department-related questions as well as an overall agency report. The returns have been useful for targeting performance improvement projects, measuring impact of changes over time, and providing positive feedback to employees. The initial 6-month overall percent of "strongly agree" responses was 56%. This slowly rose to 66% within 1 year.

Davis S, Adams-Greenly M (1994). Integrating patient satisfaction with a quality improvement program. *Journal of Nursing Administration* 24(12):28–31.

also vary, owing to differences in socialization and treatment functions as well as personal values and beliefs. However, the common goal of these suppliers of health care is to provide excellent care in a professional manner. There also is agreement that technical competence and ethical respect of patients are highly valued and constitute a personal, professional responsibility. Agreement on the efficacy of different treatment alternatives has been limited by insufficient health services research. Professional associations and the federal Agency for Health Care Policy and Research (AHCPR) developed and published practice guidelines based on research, legal regulations, consensus conferences, and expert testimony compiled by multidisciplinary expert panels. For instance, the AHCPR panel on low back pain included nurses, physicians, physical therapists, and chiropractors (Deyo, 1995). These practice guidelines provide assistance to health care professionals in defining standards of care.

Payers

Insurers of health care include the government, managed care organizations, and private insurance companies. Their interest in quality of care focuses on receiving value for their money. They want data that compare cost per case with others with similar outcomes. Such financial data assist them with calculating their return on investment for specific prevention and treatment interventions. Their goal is to pay for minimum safe, appropriate care at the lowest cost that results in desired outcomes.

Provider Organizations

The final important customers who define and monitor the quality of health care services are the organizations that provide health care. They insist that measurements include data on efficiency of effective care that can be used to compare their performance with that of their competition. This is referred to as *benchmarking*. Their goals are a yearly surplus of revenues over expenses and a competitive advantage over their competitors.

NURSING PERFORMANCE IMPROVEMENT

Nursing management, in partnership with nurses in an agency, is responsible for defining and measuring quality of nursing care for that setting. Priorities are mutually established to measure certain patient care outcomes or aspects of a process of care that can potentially identify performance issues. For example, a hospital may track the number and type of medication errors that occur over time; a home care agency could measure the effectiveness of patient teaching; an ambulatory clinic may measure patient adherence to self-medication regimens; or a mental health facility may measure the number of episodes per week in which leather restraints were used. When performance rates in these areas show sig-

nificant variation or do not achieve pre-established targets, more focused measurement can be initiated to provide the data necessary to reveal the root cause of the problem and help target interventions for improvement.

Performance improvement activities may be carried out by nurses at the point of care or may be conducted at the organizational level. Performance improvement may focus on processes of care that apply to a specific group of patients, such as orthopedic or pediatric patients, or generically to the care of all patients, such as the patient care planning process.

Performance improvement is a problem-solving process, similar to the nursing process. The same identification, tracking, and intervening processes are also conducted by physicians, pharmacists, and other professional providers of health services. Traditionally, these separate activities made up the entire quality assurance program.

Performance improvement programs emphasize that performance of the entire system is more than simply the sum of these separate, although vitally important, parts. Assumptions have changed from "poor quality is due to performance of an individual" to "poor quality is due to an organizational failure." Staff nurses are involved in both nursing and agency-wide health care performance improvement activities.

QUALITY STANDARDS

Quality may be defined by a profession or through legal law and regulation such as laws for safety standards. Traditionally, society accepted the expertise of professions to set internal standards and self-regulate member performance. Quality standards set by professional bodies delineate the scope of practice and the minimal qualifications required for general and specialized practice. Quality standards are promulgated through codes of ethics, standards of care, standards of performance, and practice guidelines published by professional associations. These standards are monitored and sanctions applied through accreditation agencies, peer review, and certification processes (American Nurses' Association, 1990). The responsibility for enforcing the standards is shared with state boards of nursing under each state's nurse practice act. To the degree a society views a profession as effective in setting its own standards to protect the public and regulating its practice to maintain quality, it is less likely that additional laws for government regulation will be passed (Tilbury, 1992).

Within nursing, multiple associations have developed standards for different purposes, using different criteria, scopes, and formats. Until recently, this led to confusion in the health care industry and lack of acceptance by external bodies. Joint efforts among the nursing specialty organizations—American Organization of Nurse Executives, American Association of Colleges of Nursing, National League for Nursing, and American Nurses' Association—have resulted in closer coordination and standardization in formats, criteria, and purposes of both certification and practice standards. One outcome was the publication in 1991 of *Standards of Clinical Nursing Practice* by the American Nurses' Association, which describes the basic competencies for any registered nurse in two areas, utilization of the nursing process in the provision of patient care and professional performance in areas such as collegiality, peer review, and governance. The standards also state that all nurses are expected to engage in professional role activities appropriate to their level of education, position, and practice setting.

Standards of care established by national organizations are supplemented by specialty standards, practice guidelines, and internal agency standards of care, policies, procedures, and protocols. However, even with these resources for guidance, the individual nurse must exercise judgment in determining what is appropriate, pertinent, and realistic in a particular patient situation.

QUALITY ASSURANCE

The concept of systematic evaluation of health care can be traced back to the mid-1800s. Florence Nightingale was a pioneer in the assessment and assurance of quality health care. She kept statistics on the mortality of British solders during the Crimean War and demonstrated, after 6 months of improvement in hospital conditions, a decrease in mortality rates from 32% to 2%. In 1860, she established what are considered to be the first standards for nursing practice (Bull, 1992).

Another pioneer in the assessment of health care quality was Ernest Codman, a physician at Massachusetts General Hospital. In 1914, he advocated the routine collection and publication of patient outcome data as a basis for assessment and improvement of patient care. Although his specific proposals were not accepted, they did influence the initial hospital accreditation standards. In 1918, the minimum standard of the American College of Surgeons' Hospital Standardization Program stated that the medical staff should review and evaluate the quality of care provided to hospitalized patients on a regular basis (JCAHO, 1994). Patterns from this program were later adopted by the Joint Commission on Accreditation of Hospitals (Bull, 1992), and the activities now known as quality assurance were derived from this requirement in the minimum standard.

Quality Assurance in Health Care Provider Agencies

The term *quality assurance* was adopted by JCAHO (then the Joint Commission on Accreditation of Hospitals) (1992b) in the 1970s to refer to health care quality efforts. It was commonly used until the late 1980s, when health care began to adopt new concepts in quality management from the business sector. JCAHO defined quality assurance as a process of objectively and systematically monitoring and evaluating the quality and appropriateness of patient care to identify opportunities to improve care and resolve problems (Katz & Green, 1992). The purpose of quality assurance was to identify when individual providers were noncompliant with standards of care.

In 1975, the first JCAHO standards required every hospital to have a plan for QA using explicit, measurable criteria that could be used in retrospective, time-limited audits of care documented in the medical record. Hospitals complied by collecting voluminous data, which unfortunately were seldom put to use in a systematic effort to improve care (JCAHO, 1991). Reviews for JCAHO accreditation focused on the capability of the organization to provide quality care based on the structures and procedures in place to provide care, not an actual outcome of care.

Medical Peer Review

Unlike Dr. Codman, most physicians and hospital administrators firmly believed that outcomes of care were primarily related to the acuity of the patient's condition and the training, experience, and expertise of the physician. Thus, internal quality assurance efforts centered on peer review of physicians, not patient outcomes. The review processes were informal, subjective individual case reviews done by physicians to identify questionable practices. Recommendations for sanctions of specific physicians were based on the reviewer's knowledge and experience.

Nursing Quality Assurance

In 1976, the American Nurses' Association published its *Model for Quality: Implementation of Standards.* Its purpose was to assist nurses to implement a program of ensuring quality nursing care. This document defined quality assurance as a process of systematic evaluation to ensure excellence in health care. The goal was to *improve patient care* (American Nurses' Association, 1976). This was a shift from physician peer review of care to compliance with standards as a method to ensure quality. The quality model was open and circular, indicating that the components of the implementation process cycle proceed ad infinitum. Each cycle of the process begins with identification of values, followed by the establishment of structure, process, and outcome standards and criteria to reflect the values held, collection of data to determine to what degree standards and criteria were met, interpretations about the strengths and weaknesses, identification of potential courses of action, choice of a course of action, and the introduction of changes to improve care (American Nurses' Association, 1976). The process then begins again with the assessment of values reflected in the changes and continues through the cycle.

Integrating Medical and Nursing Quality Assurance

In 1979, JCAHO standards were written that emphasized a coordinated, organization-wide program that included both medical and nursing quality assurance. These standards emphasized that quality assurance activities should focus on problems whose solution would have a significant effect on patient care outcomes. However, many hospitals had difficulty designing and implementing organization-wide programs. First, nursing care and medical care, although complementary, had very different emphases and responsibilities. Second, the management systems in place to set standards, conduct reviews, and apply sanctions for nurse and physician misconduct were totally separate because nurses were usually hospital employees and physicians were usually community-based individuals with admitting privileges. A third major difficulty involved designing data collection methods that were realistic and effective in assessing and improving the quality of care. Patient problems were increasingly recognized as complex and affected by the patient's personal factors as well as by the actions of multiple caregivers.

Monitoring and Evaluation

In 1985, the JCAHO standards replaced the broad problem-based approach with a narrower, systematic *monitoring and evaluation* of important aspects of patient care in response to the difficulties experienced with previous approaches. The standards focused primarily on specific departments or services, with each department or service conducting its own systematic monitoring and evaluation. Monitoring and evaluation were to be carried out by *concurrent audits of both medical records and patient care processes* whenever possible, so problems could be resolved while the patient was still receiving care. Again, health care organizations requested assistance with methodologies. As a result, the Joint Commission formulated a detailed monitoring and evaluation process, known as the 10-step process, to guide health care providers with assessing, measuring, and improving the quality of care (JCAHO, 1991). Table 16–1 presents an overview of the 10 steps.

Over the 30-year history of quality assurance, several difficulties with this process became apparent. First, it was recognized that *quality was an elusive concept,* and providers were having difficulty defining and measuring it. Second, the notion of

Table 16–1.
Ten-Step Monitoring and Evaluation Process

1. Assign responsibility.
2. Delineate scope of care and service.
3. Identify important aspects of care and service.
4. Identify indicators.
5. Establish a means to trigger evaluation.
6. Collect and organize data.
7. Initiate evaluation.
8. Take actions to improve care and service.
9. Assess the effectiveness of actions taken and ensure improvement is maintained.
10. Communicate results to relevant individuals and groups.

From Joint Commission on Accreditation of Healthcare Organizations (1991). *An Introduction to Quality Improvement in Health Care.* Oakbrook Terrace, IL: Author.

assuring quality was recognized as an unrealistic goal for every patient encounter. Third, it was unclear *which data should be collected* to provide information that would identify opportunities for improvement. Problems were either viewed as obvious, needing no analysis of data to be uncovered, or elusive, with no consensus as to what measures were meaningful indicators of problems and appropriate actions. Fourth, *methods for monitoring, evaluating, and improving care were too subjective.* Data were skewed by the lack of reliability between collectors and could be manipulated to cover up or highlight problems. The use of separate nursing and medical quality assurance departments resulted in a fragmented, uncoordinated approach to the measurement, assessment, and improvement of patient care (JCAHO, 1994a). These difficulties led hospital and nurse leaders to question the value of quality assurance. As a result, in many agencies quality assurance was being done only to placate external regulatory bodies (JCAHO, 1991).

Around this time, other pressures were having an impact on health care that indirectly led to a major shift in quality assurance and its basic assumptions. The pressures of rising health care costs, concerns of third-party payers, burgeoning technological breakthroughs in surgical techniques that shortened hospital lengths of stay, growth in competition, and consumer demands led to an increasing business sophistication in health care. It also led to higher educational standards for health care administrators in business and management that would prepare them to lead efforts to improve productivity and efficiency in health care organizations. As a result, health care administrators began to introduce quality control and quality improvement methods from industry into their organizations. The changes from 1950 to 1995 are summarized in Figure 16–1.

External Peer Review

As part of implementation of Medicare and Medicaid, the federal government established external peer review using peer standard review organiza-

Figure 16–1. Evolution of managing quality in health care. Each step indicates increasing complexity and specificity of the management of quality in health care.

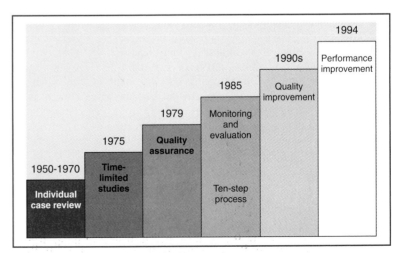

tions (PSROs). They were restructured in 1982 as peer review organizations (PROs) to incorporate current knowledge of monitoring and evaluation using required screening for reasonable, necessary, quality care in appropriate, least-costly settings. In 1992, the Health Care Financing Agency (HCFA), which administers Medicare and Medicaid, again restructured to incorporate quality improvement processes transferred from the business sector with a concomitant upgrading of databases, standardizing of data elements, adoption of practice guidelines, and quality improvement initiatives to work with provider organizations and medical associations to move from quality assurance to performance improvement (Jenks & Wilensky, 1992).

QUALITY CONTROL

For centuries, quality was controlled in business through inspection. Craftspersons inspected their own work as well as the work of their apprentices. With the development of the assembly line, direct inspection was no longer possible. Inspectors were employed to examine the quality of the final products. Statistical methods were used to determine how many samples from a lot should be inspected and to set criteria for when a lot should be rejected due to poor quality of the sample. The cost of inspection and waste from rejecting lots was thought to be justified to ensure that quality was controlled (Berwick et al, 1990).

In the mid-1920s, Walter Shewhart, a physicist at Bell Laboratories, called into question this use of inspection. He advocated that the control of the processes of production was more efficient in ensuring and improving quality than endpoint inspection (Berwick et al, 1990). His emphasis on the need to minimize variation in work processes and to understand the sources of variation led to an extensive theory and set of techniques called *statistical process control* (Aguayo, 1990).

Statistical process control, also known as quality control, is "the application of statistical methods to determine if a process is operating within the established control limits and is producing a product acceptable to the specification requirements" (JCAHO, 1992c, p 8).

Variation is expected to occur in all products manufactured or services delivered. Different conditions, participants, and methods contribute to variation in a process. Two causes of variation are commonly cited. First, *common cause variation*, also known as *random cause*, is due to the sum of all the small causes that combine on a chance basis to produce day-to-day variation. Second, sentinel events due to variation caused by a special event are usually intermittent in nature and attributable to a specific cause (Finison et al, 1993). The goal of statistical process control is to understand and control variation in processes of work (Berwick, 1991).

The adoption of the concept of expecting variation in health care work processes has led to less rigid standards of care. Quality improvement processes in health care define standards for sentinel events in which caregivers should immediately seek the special cause for this variation. Changes in standards for unacceptable common cause variation are achieved by changing the process as a whole.

EMERGENCE OF QUALITY IMPROVEMENT IN HEALTH CARE

Quality Control in Business as Applied to Health Care

One of the outcomes of administrator dissatisfaction with quality assurance was the increasing interest in the business applications of quality control to health care. One of the business practices explored was *total quality management*, an extension of quality control that was initiated in the United States but fully developed and adopted in Japan with the assistance of two US experts in the post–World War II era. Total quality management encompasses continuous quality improvement activities and the management systems that foster such activities as communication, education, and commitment of resources. *Continuous quality improvement* is a more limited term generally used to describe the ongoing monitoring, evaluation, and improvement of processes. The major contributors to the quality improvement field whose ideas seemed applicable to health care include the following:

- W. Edwards Deming introduced three key concepts—organization-wide valuing of quality, employment of methods to empower workers to be more productive, and the use of teams to problem-solve and implement change. These concepts are further explicated in his 14 points (Walton, 1986).

- Joseph Juran introduced the Juran Trilogy of quality planning, quality control, and quality improvement, which are separate, simultaneous, parallel processes directed by top management. He advocated the use of an organization-wide steering committee to choose initiatives with the greatest potential for cost effective improvements (Juran, 1989).

- Philip Crosby introduced the quality maturity grid to direct the introduction and implementation of continuous quality improvement. His primary goal was to change the organizational culture to expect quality (Crosby, 1979).

The National Demonstration Project (NDP) on Quality Improvement in Health Care brought together 100 industrial quality experts who were paired with groups from various health care organizations to address quality issues through the use of quality improvement techniques. The results showed a high rate of success for the projects and indicated that simple industrial-quality control tools could demonstrate processes of care and reveal causes of variation leading to opportunities to improve performance. The overall conclusion was that quality improvement principles and tools can be applied to the health care setting (Berwick et al, 1990).

Based on the results of the NDP, funded by the John A. Hartford Foundation, the Agenda for Change was initiated by JCAHO in 1987. This multi-year project refocused actions to improve quality by incorporating the theories and methodologies of total quality management and continuous quality improvement (JCAHO, 1991, 1994b); this included abandoning the term quality assurance for quality improvement (see Fig. 16–1).

Quality Improvement

Quality improvement is defined as the commitment and approach used to continuously improve processes in the organization with the intent of meeting and exceeding customer expectations and outcomes (Schroeder, 1994). The concepts and principles of quality improvement in health care have been transferred from industry and include (1) a focus on an organization-wide effort to improve the processes of work rather than individuals; (2) the identification of the needs and expectations of the customers, both internal and external, with corresponding organizational changes to meet those needs; and (3) the achievement of greater organizational effectiveness and efficiency through teamwork and innovation. The first tenet of success is a commitment from the leadership to set quality priorities, reorient the organization to a customer focus, define quality for their organization, and incorporate it into the organization's mission statements and planning documents.

This leads to the second tenet that work must be designed to meet the needs and expectations of external and internal customers. Each employee is both a customer, who receives work from others, and a supplier, who sends work to others. In designing quality work processes, all employees need to be involved in defining how to satisfy their coworkers, internal customers, and external customers, described earlier as stakeholders. Proposed work processes are scrutinized for unnecessary repetition, ordering of work, bottlenecks that delay work, and whether communication loops are completed. Work processes are refined as they are implemented based on data and information. This is a change from quality assurance, which depended on refinements based on data and information from quality inspection at the endpoint.

Continuous, systematic assessment and improvement are achieved through formal problem-solving methods that use statistical tools and the scientific method, teamwork, and innovation. The outcome sought is to continuously increase knowledge of and control over both common and special causes of variations in work processes through problem identification, data collection, analysis, and action.

The major change in the shift from quality assurance to quality improvement occurred not in what was done but in the purpose. The goal of quality improvement is the steady improvement of performance based on objective and qualitative information, rather than the goal of quality assurance to provide data indicating the capability of the organization to provide quality care. The distinct differences between quality assurance and quality improvement are summarized in Table 16–2.

Table 16–2.

Differences Between Quality Assurance and
    Quality Improvement

Quality Assurance	Quality Improvement
Focuses on time-limited, clinical problem-solving	Focuses on continuous improvement of performance
Follows organizational structure	Follows patient care
Involves clinical departments	Hospital-wide involvement
Focuses on individuals	Focuses on processes and systems
Correction of special causes (individual, machines)	Correction of common causes (systems)
"Assures" quality	Improves quality
Externally driven	Internally driven
Responsibility of a few	Responsibility of all

PREVENTION OF POOR QUALITY

Over time, quality programs have evolved to include strategies for preventing poor patient outcomes. One concept that contributed to this evolution was *the cost of poor quality.* This was adopted from the business sector as part of the incorporation of total quality management in health care. Manufacturing had always recognized that costs and quality go hand in hand. Costs of poor quality in well-managed organizations are estimated to be approximately 25% of the revenues (Gaucher & Coffey, 1993). Philip Crosby was one of the first individuals to apply prevention strategies to service industries. In his book *Quality Is Free* (1979), Crosby contends that the investment of moneys, usually lost by poor quality, can increase the quality of services "for free." He has estimated that service organizations spend 35% or more of their operating budget on doing things wrong and then doing them over. He contends that most organizations are unaware of poor-quality costs because they do not appear on financial balance sheets.

COST OF POOR QUALITY

When designing a diagnostic testing procedure, clear guidelines on when, where, and how patient education will occur can prevent poor quality. For example, written instructions are not sufficient. A patient may not be able to read and may be unwilling to tell his or her physician. Or a patient may be in a hurry and read the instructions incorrectly. The information given must be appropriate to the patient's understanding, must include an opportunity for confirmation of understanding and questions, and must be reinforced through written instructions and assurance of availability of pretest supplies. Otherwise, insufficient understanding may result in a test having to be rescheduled or given under the wrong conditions, with many ramifications. These consequences may create scheduling problems for the organization and the loss of revenue and time. The patient may lose an extra day of work and suffer anxiety because of the rescheduling and delay in diagnosis. Neither the customer nor the organization is pleased. The worst-case scenario is that the customer will lose confidence in the organization and not return (Marszalek-Gaucher, 1992).

Costs of poor quality are incurred when (1) things are not done correctly the first time, (2) when the right things are not done, or (3) when the wrong things are done. Additional examples are the cost of inspection, customer relations departments to handle complaints or returned goods, loss of market share due to poor reputation, and compensation for rework when work is done incorrectly the first time. Each of these events results in wasted efforts and time, the use of extra supplies, additional labor costs, and decreased productivity. Administrative time is increased in the investigation and follow-up of the problems that occur. In addition, quality failures have a negative impact on the pride and motivation of the employees (Berwick et al, 1990).

Prevention of poor quality is achieved by designing quality into a new service, product, or work process. One example of applying this concept in health care is the training of employees in the use of new technology before implementation, even if the changes are minimal. Misunderstanding of new technology can lead to misuse requiring a procedure to be repeated or even resulting in a patient or employee injury. Another example of prevention is the purchase of safety equipment, such as injection systems without needles to avoid the contamination of individuals by infected blood or body fluids. The expense of these new systems is outweighed by the risk to employees and patients with the normal variation in needle use.

Good quality also has a price. Worker involvement in collaborative teamwork and problem-solving requires nonproductive time away from patient care. Quality improvement is based on data that must be collected and analyzed. The selection of quality indicators should always be within a context of cost awareness of both the costs of collection and analysis and the likelihood that this information will be useful to direct changes. Time must be devoted to understanding work processes and identifying root causes of problems before selecting quality indicators. This reflective time spent describing in detail how processes work is often difficult to justify among coworkers with an action mind-set, yet it may efficiently save time and money otherwise spent on collecting the "wrong" data.

Training and education are often chosen as a strategy to improve quality without determining the root cause of the problem. Careful analysis of data should be used to clarify whether the problem is due to the lack of management attention, ineffective work processes, employees' not valuing a work process, or employees' lack of knowledge before this expensive strategy is implemented.

Quality initiatives should be carefully chosen based on whether the effort is adding value to the customers from cost savings and improved outcomes. The cost of quality initiatives should always be compared with the outcomes.

STRUCTURES FOR PERFORMANCE IMPROVEMENT

With total quality management and continuous quality improvement, it is recognized that the nature and quality of governance and management activities influence patient outcomes. To foster quality, each organization must provide management structures that support local and organization-wide processes of performance improvement. Nurses may work for organizations as small as a free-standing ambulatory surgical center or as complex as a national managed care organization. Regardless of setting, the nurse should be provided with information regarding the quality of her or his performance and how it contributes to patient outcomes. There should also be mechanisms in place to provide the nurse with information on how system processes could be improved and opportunities to participate in change activities.

In organizations with nursing professional practice models, a nurse can contribute to performance improvement through participation in the council or committee assigned to define practice standards and care standards and coordinate nursing quality improvement. Names for these decentralized structures include shared governance, ProAct, professional practice model, and product line manage-

---

Research Box 16–2

Productivity and Work Excitement

A sample of 268 nurses in three hospitals, three ambulatory facilities, and one home care agency was surveyed to identify the relationship between work excitement and a learning environment in the workplace. The Sims Meaningful Work/Work excitement tool was used. This tool had a reliability coefficient of 0.85 to 0.95 and validity had been confirmed through development using grounded theory followed by factor analysis identifying three subscales: interest in work, excitement about work, and frustration with work. Three of the four learning environment variables (availability of learning opportunities; stimulating, motivating, challenging environment; opportunity to work with other professionals) were found to be significantly related to work excitement. The fourth learning environment variable, high technology atmosphere, was not significantly related to work excitement. Other research has shown that learning employees are productive employees; this study confirms that they are also more likely to be excited about their work.

Lickman P, Simms L, Greene C (1993). Learning environment: The catalyst for work excitement. *The Journal of Continuing Education in Nursing* 24(5):211–216.

ment (Hess, 1994). Alternatively, decision-making for nursing may be centralized, and performance improvement may be directed by a specific specialized administrator, such as director of quality improvement, who is assisted by a standing committee of staff and management nurses. Complex organizations may simultaneously use structures that include centralized, advanced practice positions with organization-wide authority, such as case managers, director of quality improvement, or nursing information system experts and decentralized professional practice models for specific divisions. The success of all performance improvement programs is dependent on top management's leadership and commitment to the provision of resources and structures that support implementation of performance improvement at the point of service level.

UNIT-BASED QUALITY IMPROVEMENT

In addition to participation in the organization-wide performance improvement processes, each subunit must identify problems specific to that health service. Unit-based performance improvement must be limited to problems that are within that subunit's control. Nurse leaders need to ask themselves whether this is a problem that involves only nurses or also other disciplines or departments. Is it a local problem that the subunit has authority to resolve? What data support the assessment that this problem is high volume, high risk, problem prone, or costly?

Some tools the staff can use to clarify these answers include *flow charting, Ishikawa cause-and-effect diagrams, interviews and focus groups,* and *pilot data* using *concurrent* or *retrospective audits.* For instance, if assessment data indicate that patient falls are higher for one unit than for others, completing an Ishikawa cause-and-effect diagram and flow-charting the process for managing falls are helpful in determining whether it is a local problem (Figs. 16–2 and 16–3). By using brainstorming to complete the Ishikawa cause-and-effect diagram, which identifies the people, methods, materials and supplies, and facilities and equipment involved in the problem being studied, the factors causing the problem are identified. This diagram is sometimes referred to as a *fishbone* or *whale chart,* which refers to its shape. Flow charts create a picture of

the process of care, both ideal and actual, and help identify how that process can be improved. Review of incident reports and conducting a focus group may help to clarify whether this is a nursing or multidisciplinary problem and identify trends such as degree of injury, location of falls, time of occurrence, or other recurring factors. All groups involved in the process also must be represented on the performance improvement team for any long-term solution to be effective.

Another valuable tool for performance problem-solving is a *story board,* a poster that is displayed to show the process of performance improvement. It serves to assist the team in being systematic in problem-solving, to make staff aware that the problem exists and the investigation is being conducted, and to provide staff with the reason behind changes to resolve the problem, based on analysis of results.

PERFORMANCE ASSESSMENT AND IMPROVEMENT

Performance improvement is a cyclical process that involves the activities of design, measurement, assessment, improvement, and redesign of new or current functions or processes of patient care or services. It is a systematic and scientific approach to improvement of patient care processes, outcomes, and services over time. Improvement efforts may be initiated at any point in this cycle.

Design

Many changes are occurring within health care; as a result, many new services and patient care processes have been designed. In addition, many current processes are being redesigned to be more efficient and provide better patient outcomes. Ideally, quality is one of the factors included in the design of any new service or redesign of a work process. Quality is enhanced by linking the new service or process to (1) the mission of the organization; (2) the needs and expectations of patients, staff members, administration, and payers; and (3) related state-of-the-art practices gleaned from expert knowledge of practitioners, practice guidelines, critical pathways, standards developed by professional organizations, and the professional literature. Planning of the design is

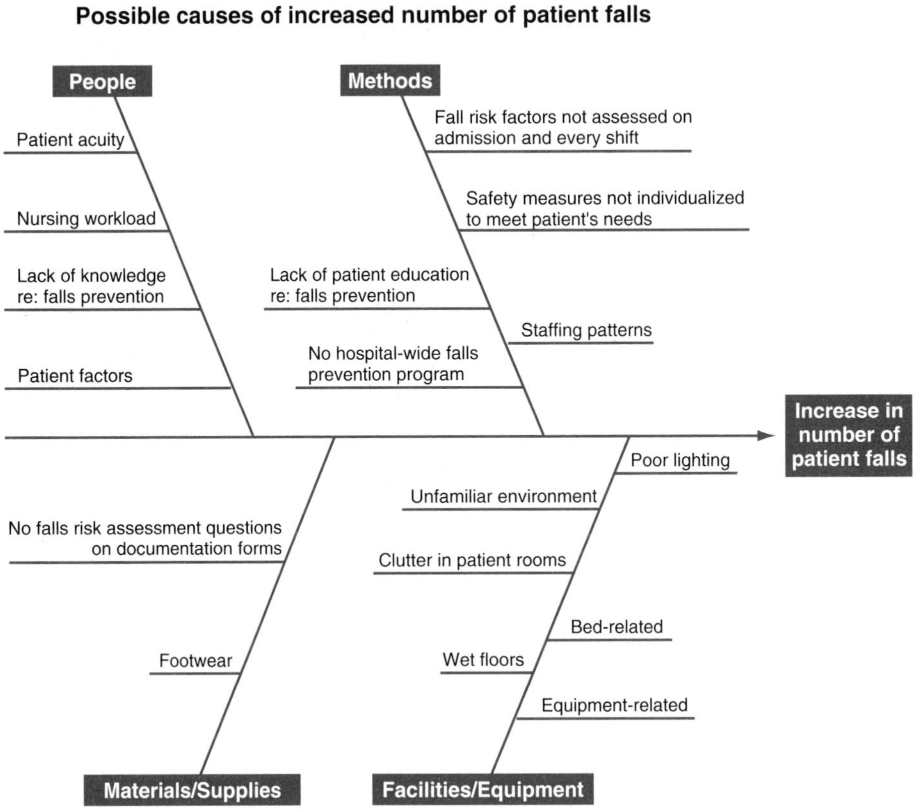

Possible causes of increased number of patient falls

Figure 16–2. Example of an Ishikawa cause-and-effect diagram (fall prevention process).

also directed by the resources of people, facilities, and technology present; level and source of funding for design, people, facilities, and technology needed; and potential revenues to be generated by the service. The coordination and integration of planning and implementation activities between departments and disciplines are crucial to success. Nurses' clinical knowledge, judgment, proximity to the patient, and close cooperation between various disciplines place them in an ideal position to know what new designs or redesigns of problematic processes could help patients and the organization (JCAHO, 1994a).

Measurement

Measurement is the next step in the performance improvement cycle. Measurement is the process of collecting and aggregating data about the perfor-

mance of a new or current process. One purpose of measurement is to provide baseline and evaluation data about a process for which few objective data exist. For example, nurses may want to objectively measure how effectively their patients' pain is being managed or to determine the rate of infections at intravenous line insertion sites. A second purpose of measurement is to systematically gain information about a problematic patient care process, such as skin care as indicated by the development of pressure ulcers during hospitalization. The result of measurement is an organization- or unit-specific performance database that contains information about the structure, processes, and outcomes of a service. Health status and function, satisfaction, cost, and judgments about the quality and value of services are examples of outcomes (JCAHO, 1994a).

Priorities must be established for the service to be measured and assessed. The criteria for choice

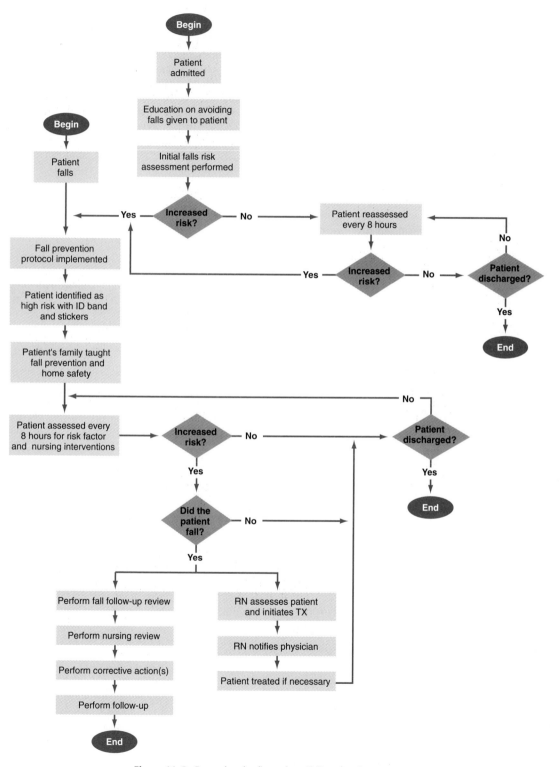

Figure 16–3. Example of a flow chart (fall prevention process).

should be services that involve a high volume of patients or place patients at serious risk if not performed well or not performed at all, are problem prone, or are high in cost.

Indicator is the term used in performance improvement for a measure. An indicator is a valid and reliable quantitative measure that can be used to assess the performance of governance, management, clinical and support structures, and processes that affect patient outcomes. It is not a direct measure of quality but instead directs attention to performance issues that may require more intense review within an organization (JCAHO, 1990). For instance, a structure indicator is the ratio of nurses to patients in a given time period. A process indicator could be the amount of time it takes to triage a patient with traumatic injuries in the emergency department. An outcome indicator could be whether a patient is able to appropriately manage his diabetic diet and insulin injections.

Indicators may be developed for sentinel events or common causes of variation. A *sentinel event indicator* identifies a serious patient care event that requires prompt investigation each and every time it occurs. An example is the administration of incompatible blood. Indicators of common causes of variation are used to monitor structure, processes, or outcomes related to many cases. Table 16–3 presents the core set of nursing quality indicators for acute care settings (American Nurses' Association, 1995). Note that indicators are usually reported one of two ways: rates or occurrences over time. A *rate* typically uses a ratio of those patients with one characteristic experiencing an event to all patients with that characteristic. An example is the percentage of patients who sustained an injury due to a fall compared with the total number of patients who fell during a designated period of time. An occurrence over time is used to monitor a characteristic that can be measured along a continuous scale, such as the precise weight of an individual each day he or she receives total parenteral nutrition (JCAHO, 1994a).

For each service, the relevant dimensions of performance should be identified, and indicators should be designed for measurement. The nine dimensions of performance and their definitions identified by JCAHO (1994b) are shown in Table 16–4; note that *efficacy* and *appropriateness* refer to identifying the right intervention. Availability, effectiveness, timeliness, safety, efficiency, continuity, respect, and caring refer to doing an intervention technically and interpersonally well.

When developing indicators, care should also be taken to use existing data and reliably collect new data in a feasible, cost-effective manner. Data sources may include medical records, incident reports, laboratory reports, direct observations, and surveys or external sources such as third-party payer reports, regulatory agency data, or census data. By using existing data, both time taken from patient care and the cost of collecting new data are saved.

The indicator should be supported by research data where available and the procedures, authority, and responsibilities for data collection should be clearly stated.

Table 16–3.
Core Set of Nursing Quality Indicators for Acute Care Settings

- Mix of registered and licensed practical nurses and unlicensed staff
- Total nursing staff to patients
- Registered nurse education and certification
- Nurse staff turnover
- Use of agency nurses
- Nosocomial infections
- Decubitus ulcers developed during episode
- Medication errors
- Patient injury rate
- Patient satisfaction

From American Nurses' Association (1995). *Nursing Report Card for Acute Care Settings*. Unpublished report. Washington, DC: Author, pp 112–113.

Assessment

Assessment activities include identifying the current levels of performance, interpreting any variations in structures, processes, or outcomes, and drawing conclusions from the data as to whether actions to improve performance are necessary. Assessment uses comparative information to set priorities for improvement.

Initial assessment is ongoing monitoring and evaluation of the data that measure the performance of an important process. Evaluation requires standards that define acceptable levels of variation. When sentinel events or unacceptable variation occurs, a more intensive assessment is conducted to

Table 16–4.
Dimensions of Performance

Doing the Right Thing	
Efficacy	The degree to which the care/intervention for the patient has been shown to accomplish the desired/projected outcome(s)
Appropriateness	The degree to which the care/intervention provided is relevant to the patient's clinical needs, given the current state of knowledge
Doing the Right Thing Well	
Availability	The degree to which appropriate care/intervention is available to meet the patient's needs
Effectiveness	The degree to which the care/intervention is provided in the correct manner, given the current state of knowledge, to achieve the desired/ projected outcome for the patient
Timeliness	The degree to which the care/intervention is provided to the patient at the most beneficial or necessary time
Safety	The degree to which the risk of an intervention and risk in the care environment are reduced for the patient and others, including the health care provider
Efficiency	The ratio of the outcomes (results of care/intervention) for a patient to the resources used to deliver the care
Continuity	The degree to which the care/intervention for the patient is coordinated among practitioners, between organizations, and across time
Respect and caring	The degree to which the patient or designee is involved in his or her own care decisions and that those persons providing services do so with sensitivity and respect for the patient's needs and expectations and individual differences.

From Joint Commission on Accreditation of Healthcare Organizations, *Framework for Improving Performance: From Principles to Practice.* Oakbrook Terrace, IL: Author, p 17. Reprinted with permission.

determine the root cause of the problem and identify actions to resolve the problem.

Continual assessment of common causes of variation uses run charts and control charts. These charts visually display trends. A *run chart* plots points on a line graph to assist in identifying meaningful trends in performance over time. It can help to identify which existing processes need improvement and show whether an action taken to improve performance was successful. A *control chart* adds statistically calculated upper and lower limits of acceptability. An example of a control chart for falls is shown in Figure 16–4. Note the run chart within the control chart showing the number of falls per 10,000 patient-days for each 6-month time period. The differences in control limits between subunits compared with other organizations may indicate opportunities for process improvement.

Intensive assessments are done when trends show either unacceptable variation due to common causes or a special cause. Frequently, intensive assessment is facilitated through the display of data using flow charts, Ishikawa cause-and-effect diagrams, pie charts, and Pareto charts. Flow charts are useful to better understand how a process is actually conducted as opposed to the steps defined in the procedure and policy manual. By documenting the sequence of steps in the process, the steps

Research Box 16–3

Impact of Structure on Quality

A university hospital retrospectively evaluated its four-level, voluntary clinical advancement system over an 8-year period. The goals of the system were (1) to reward nurses as their clinical practice advances, (2) to retain competent nurses in direct patient care positions, and (3) to improve quality of patient care in a cost-effective manner. Measures included qualitative interviews with key administrators and staff, Stamps and Piedmonte's index of work satisfaction, brief scales on intent to leave, promotion opportunities and work rewards, quantitative data on nurse demographics, costs, and turnover. Surveys had a 58% response rate (n = 355), with 152 clinically advanced staff and 203 non-promoted staff.

Although advanced staff had higher job satisfaction, they also reported no statistically significant differences in promotional opportunities or work rewards. Regarding the second goal, turnover was 8.6% lower for advanced staff and intent to leave was much lower (13.3% vs 7.2%), indicating increased retention. The third goal had no objective measure. Comparison of the indirect and direct costs of the program to savings associated with lower turnover found a 0.76:1.0 benefit-to-cost ratio, a total loss of $442,815 over 8 years.

Implications for practice: This evaluation was positive for professional development and retention of nurses but lacked any objective measure of quality patient care and provided no cost savings to the organization. Recommended changes included (1) redesign of the clinical advancement program based on grounded theory with clear differences in competence, (2) clear, distinct job descriptions for each level of nurse, (3) sufficient staffing and preparation of managers so that nurses can fulfill their job descriptions, and (4) development of a database with objective outcome and productivity measures for future evaluations.

Schultz A (1993). Evaluation of a clinical advancement system. *Journal of Nursing Administration* 23(2):13–19.

that cause redundancies, inefficiencies, misunderstandings, waiting times, or confusion can be identified, and actions can be taken to address those problems. An Ishikawa cause-and-effect diagram assists in identifying root causes and the stakeholders involved in a process. It is constructed using the experience and expertise of team members and shows how various parts of the process relate to each other. It identifies conditions that require further attention or might suggest appropriate actions for improvement (see Figs. 16–2 and 16–3).

A *Pareto chart* is a bar chart that arranges the bars representing problems affecting a process being studied in descending order of frequency (Fig. 16–5). This display assists in highlighting priority areas for action that are likely to be the most beneficial. Pie charts display data to show percentages or parts of a whole (Fig. 16–6). Both charts are useful for indicating potential courses of action.

Assessment involves the use of comparative data as a point of reference in determining performance; these data may include (1) historical patterns of performance within that organization or nursing unit, (2) external reference databases from other organizations, (3) practice guidelines or critical paths, or (4) desired performance targets or thresholds.

Improvement

An intensive assessment is part of the focused improvement efforts in which more detailed measurement and analysis of data are done to determine the root cause of the problem and identify actions to resolve the problem.

Design and Redesign

Changes may come about through refinement of existing processes or through innovation and design of new processes. Once a change has been implemented, the cycle of performance improvement begins again.

RISK MANAGEMENT

Rising expectations for health care as a right has been a trend since the early 1980s. This is shown through the demands for universal access through health care reform, the rising numbers of malpractice suits against both agencies and providers, and

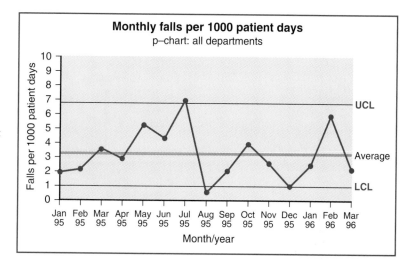

Figure 16–4. Example of a control chart (fall prevention process).

the management and technical innovations to increase quality (Enthoven, 1993). Significant movement has also occurred toward consolidation of health care services under managed care networks and corporations that have resulted in fewer people having a strong relationship with a family physician. These two trends have greatly increased the likelihood that any agency or provider will experience a lawsuit for negligence or malpractice in a given year, regardless of its performance. One outcome of this is an increased interest in risk management among agencies and individuals. Risk management

is defined as activity to promote safety and prevent loss to physical, financial, or intangible assets (Rakich et al, 1992).

At the individual nurse level, the greatest protection from risk is consistent professional practice using accepted standards, thereby preventing harm to patients and others. This requires meeting legal responsibility to (1) be knowledgeable of standards of care and policies of employers, (2) be capable of meeting reasonable expectations for the practice of a nurse with equal credentials and experience, and (3) appropriately provide nursing services using

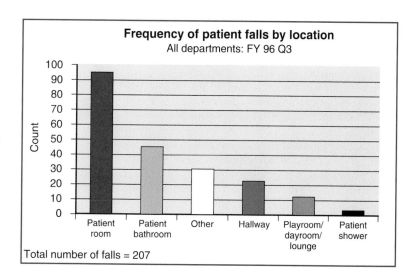

Figure 16–5. Example of a Pareto chart (fall prevention process).

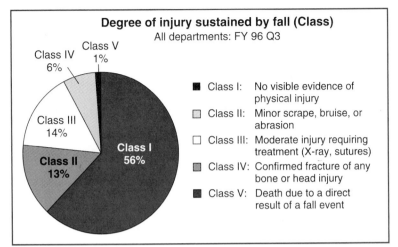

Figure 16–6. Example of a pie chart (fall prevention process).

Note: Classification definitions from "Parameters for Tracking and Trending Patient Falls" by A. Hendrich, 1991, Unit-based Patient Fall Prevention, p. 26–29. Copyright 1991 by A. Hendrich.

clinical judgment and nursing interventions (Hirsh, 1990). This implies an ongoing commitment to professional growth and initiative in seeking out training. Despite his or her best efforts, a nurse may be sued for malpractice.

Each nurse should weigh the purchase of personal malpractice insurance against the risks of loss. Malpractice insurance protects a nurse, within a money and time limit, from losses due to a civil suit that charges him or her with harming a patient by practicing at less than the standard of reasonable expectations for a nurse with equal credentials and experience in the same situation (Hirsh, 1990). On the one hand, it provides peace of mind because it will process and settle all claims regardless of merit. Conversely, insurance premiums are rising, lawsuits do not always name nurses, and attorneys can provide nurses with strategies to protect their assets if they choose to "go bare" without insurance.

Nurses who work in hospitals, home care agencies, nursing homes, ambulatory care centers, or managed care facilities participate in a risk management program with the same elements: identification, analysis, investigation, transfer, retention, education, and prevention (Huber, 1996).

A systematic, continuous *identification* process must include a review of the frequency and severity of all potential threats for losses of physical, financial, or intangible assets. Harm to patients due to

malpractice exposes both the agency and the nurse to loss of the tangible asset of money and the intangible assets of quality nursing practice, image, and reputation.

Analysis of potential risk frequently overlaps with the performance assessment process. Both risk management and performance improvement collect data to assess whether there is sufficient evidence to justify an intervention. With risk management, data are sought regarding potential loss due to asset damage or compensation for harm to patients or others. With performance improvement, data are sought regarding potential threats to meeting a standard of quality. Figure 16–7 shows the overlap of these management processes. Internal sources of

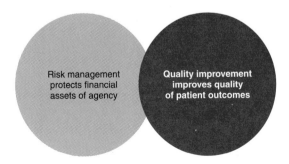

Figure 16–7. The relationship of risk management to quality improvement.

information for both processes include data from performance measures, incident reports, medical records, databases, policies and procedures, critical pathways, and outcomes data. External sources of information include legal laws and regulations, codes of ethics, published reports, clinical practice guidelines, standards of practice and standards of care from professional organizations, benchmarking with comparable organizations, and consultants.

Once a potential risk is identified and a risk incident has occurred, an *investigation* is indicated to identify the likelihood and potential extent of loss. This requires information about (1) the legal duty to the patient, (2) whether a breach of duty occurred, (3) whether the patient was harmed, and (4) whether harm was caused by the breach of duty. Legally, all four must be present, and the patient must file a civil suit against the nurse and/or agency for the nurse to be judged guilty and damages awarded to the patient. The risk manager must also assess the threat of the incident to the organization's intangible assets, such as reputation and image, and take that into account in his or her response. A comprehensive review of tort liability is discussed in Chapter 14.

Handling the risk occurs through *risk transfer* or *risk retention*. Risk transfer occurs through activities that limit risk or finance losses. Examples of limiting risk are use of signed release and consent forms or agreements to share risk between a provider and health insurance agency through guaranteed pricing of a service. Commonly, losses are financed through purchasing insurance or selling a damaged asset, such as a building. Management may decide to retain a risk because the potential cost of transfer, in terms of finances or reputation, is too high. For instance, if a visitor falls, the risk manager may conclude that the agency was prudent and not legally liable but may choose to offer compensation based on protection of agency goodwill and reputation as a responsive, caring health care organization. Risk retention may also be unplanned and costly when there is no awareness of the presence of risk or miscalculation of the magnitude of potential loss.

All risk management programs include strategies to assess risk potential and respond to incidents as well as strategies to reduce and prevent risk. *Education* of all employees, including nurse leaders, is vital in involving employees in the risk management program. Risk management education needs to fo-

Table 16–5.
Nine Leading Malpractice Causes for Nurses

Administration of medications
Assisting in surgical procedures
Patient falls
Patient burns
Patient electric shock
Patient injury due to faulty equipment
Nosocomial infections of patients
Mistaken identity of patients
Misinterpretation of patient signs and symptoms

Data from Poteet G (1983). Risk management and nursing. *Nursing Clinics of North America* 18(3):462.

cus on the (1) legal aspects of nursing negligence and malpractice, (2) policies, procedures, and supporting rationale for responding to risk incidents, (3) expectations regarding standards of practice and standards of care, (4) potential high risk incidents specific to nursing practice that may result in loss (Table 16–5), and (5) the impact of medical records and expert testimony on the outcomes of malpractice suits.

The entire risk management program is an important management strategy to enhance *prevention* of losses. Another important risk management approach is the expectation that employees interact with patients and families with respect and courtesy. A climate of responsive courtesy and attention to comfort promotes positive healing experiences. Patients' expectations and their impressions of staff have as much influence on their satisfaction with care as do outcomes. Satisfied patients rarely resort to legal redress when unexpected or even negative outcomes occur. They are usually willing to work with organizational representatives to resolve their concerns and claims for compensation.

PERFORMANCE IMPROVEMENT AND RE-ENGINEERING

The current stage in the evolution of quality processes is the introduction of re-engineering when

Research Box 16–4
Cooperative Care

New York University's Cooperative Care Unit admits each patient accompanied by a caregiver. Criteria for admission to the unit include the requirement that the patient be independently mobile (may use aids such as wheelchair or walker). Patients assume responsibility for coming to the RN for routine checks, keeping laboratory and radiology appointments, going to meals, and taking medications. Health services include a dietitian at meals to assist in choices and diet applications, a pharmacist to instruct and guide medication administration, and nurses to instruct caregivers and patients in medical and nursing regimens. Outcomes include the achievement of a negotiated level of health care, holistic treatment of patients and families, cost savings of 39.9%, and effective transfer of care from hospital to home.

Smith D (1994). Reducing healthcare costs through co-op care. *Nursing Management* 25(6):44–47.

analysis of a problem indicates the need for revolutionary change. Sometimes analysis reveals that the problem does not lie in poor performance; quality improvement has already produced the maximum benefit from refinement. Additional improvements must answer the questions, Why are these processes used? What is the fundamental business we are in? What totally different alternatives are available to reach this outcome?

Re-engineering is like an earthquake—it changes the basic structure of the organization. To be effective, it must focus totally on the desired outcome and be accompanied by retraining of employees to function within the new structure. Examples include the training of nurses and technicians for multipurpose positions, patient-managed care units, case management of inpatient and outpatient care for one exacerbation of illness, and introduction of critical pathways with hospital information systems.

SUMMARY

Quality in health care links cost and value to management of processes for continuous surveillance and periodic interventions to improve patient outcomes. Nurses are a vital element in quality care and must be involved in improvement processes at all levels for positive patient outcomes to be achieved.

■ DISCUSSION QUESTIONS ■

1. Describe why quality of health care cannot be wholly objective.
2. Identify examples of performance improvement activities at the organizational and nursing unit levels.
3. Compare and contrast, with examples, common and special cause variations.
4. Identify data elements useful in the investigation of a risk incident.

■ LEARNING ACTIVITIES ■

1. Make an Ishikawa cause-and-effect diagram for emergency department waiting times.
2. Ask five people to define quality health care and list the factors they identify.
3. Interview a nurse on how performance improvement is carried out in his or her setting.

■ BIBLIOGRAPHY ■

Aguayo R (1990). *Dr. Deming: The American Who Taught the Japanese about Quality.* New York, NY: Carol Publishing Group.

American Nurses' Association (1976). *Quality Assurance Workbook.* Kansas City, MO: Author.

American Nurses' Association (1991) *Standards for Clinical Nursing Practice.* Kansas City, MO: Author.

American Nurses' Association (1995). *Nursing Report Card for Acute Care Settings.* Unpublished report. Washington, DC: Author.

Bassett SS (1993). Quality assurance/quality improvement. *In* Koch MW, Fairly TM (eds). *Integrated Quality Management: The Key to Improving Nursing Care Quality.* St. Louis, MO: Mosby-Year Book.

Berwick DM (1991). Controlling variation in health care: A consultation from Walter Shewhart. *Medical Care* 29:1212–1225.

Berwick DM, Godfrey AB, Roessner J (1990). *Foundations of Quality Management: Curing Health Care: New Strategies for Quality Improvement.* San Francisco, CA: Jossey-Bass, pp 29–45.

Bull MJ (1992). Quality assurance: Professional accountability via continuous quality improvement. *In* Meisenheimer CG (ed). *Improving Quality: A Guide to Effective Programs*. Gaithersburg, MD: Aspen Publishers, pp 3–20.

Crosby P (1979). *Quality Is Free*. New York, NY: New American Library.

Davis S, Adams-Greenly M (1994). Integrating patient satisfaction with a quality improvement program. *Journal of Nursing Administration* 24:28–31.

Deyo RA, et al (1995). *Acute Low Back Problem in Adults: Clinical Practice Guidelines No. 14*. Rockville, MD: AHCPR publication No. 95-0645.

Donahue MP (1992). Health care values and quality. *In* Johnson M (ed). *The Delivery of Quality Health Care: Series on Nursing Administration*, Vol 3. St. Louis, MO: Mosby-Year Book, pp 3–15.

Enthoven AC (1993). The history and principles of managed competition. *Health Affairs* 12(suppl):24–48.

Finison LJ, Finison KS, Bliersbach CM (1993). The use of control charts to improve health care quality. *Journal for Health Care Quality* 15:9–23.

Fitzpatrick MJ (1994). Performance improvement through quality improvement teamwork. *Journal of Nursing Administration* 24:20–27.

Gardner DL (1992). Measures of quality. *In* Johnson M (ed). *The Delivery of Quality Health Care: Series on Nursing Administration*, Vol 3. St. Louis, MO: Mosby-Year Book, pp 42–58.

Gaucher EJ, Coffey RJ (1993). Why implement total quality management? *In Total Quality in Health Care*. San Francisco, CA: Jossey-Bass, pp 3–25.

Hess RG (1994). Shared governance: Innovation or imitation? *Nursing Economic$* 12:28–33.

Hirsh H (1990). Legal aspects of nursing administration. *In* Dienemann J (ed). *Nursing Administration: Strategic Perspectives and Application*. Norwalk, CT: Appleton Lange.

Huber DL (1996). *Leadership and Nursing Care Management*. Philadelphia, PA: WB Saunders.

Jenks S, Wilensky G (1992). The health care quality improvement initiative. *Journal of the American Medical Association* 268:900–903.

Johnson M, McCloskey JC (1992). Quality in the nineties. *In* Johnson M (ed). *The Delivery of Quality Health Care: Series on Nursing Administration*, Vol 3. St. Louis, MO: Mosby-Year Book, pp 59–67.

Joint Commission on Accreditation of Healthcare Organizations (1991). *An Introduction to Quality Improvement in Health Care*. Oakbrook Terrace, IL: Author.

Joint Commission on Accreditation of Healthcare Organizations (1992a). *Cost of Quality: Exploring Quality Improvement Principles: A Hospital Leader's Guide*. Oakbrook Terrace, IL: Author, pp 100–119.

Joint Commission on Accreditation of Healthcare Organizations (1992b). What is quality improvement? *In Using Quality Improvement Tools in a Health Care Setting*. Oakbrook Terrace, IL: Author, pp 1–10.

Joint Commission on Accreditation of Healthcare Organizations (1992c). The tools and techniques of quality improvement. *In Using Quality Improvement Tools in a Health Care Setting*. Oakbrook Terrace, IL: Author, pp 27–65.

Joint Commission on Accreditation of Healthcare Organizations (1994). *Framework for Improving Performance: From Principles to Practice*. Oakbrook Terrace, IL: Author.

Juran J (1989). *Juran on Leadership for Quality*. New York, NY: The Free Press.

Katz J, Green E (1992). *Managing Quality: A Guide to Monitoring and Evaluating Nursing Services*. St. Louis, MO: Mosby-Year Book.

Lickman P, Simms L, Greene C (1993). Learning environment: The catalyst for work excitement. *The Journal of Continuing Education in Nursing* 5:211–216.

Lohr K (ed) (1990). *Medicare: A Strategy for Quality Assurance: Volume II: Sources and Methods*. Washington, DC: National Academy Press.

Marszalek-Gaucher E (1992). Total quality management in health care. *In* Johnson M (ed). *The Delivery of Quality Health Care: Series on Nursing Administration*, Vol 3. St. Louis, MO: Mosby-Year Book, pp 103–118.

O'Leary D (1993). Defining performance of organizations. *Journal of Quality Improvement* 19:219.

Poteet G (1983). Risk management and nursing. *Nursing Clinics of North America* 18(3):457–465.

Rakish JS, Longest BB Jr, Darr K (1992). *Managing Health Services Organizations*, 3rd ed. Baltimore, MD: Health Professions Press.

Reily P (1992). Quality assurance programs. *In* Johnson M (ed). *The Delivery of Quality Health Care: Series on Nursing Administration*, Vol 3. St. Louis, MO: Mosby-Year Book, pp 71–85.

Schroeder P (1992). Collaboration for quality: The next step in health care. *In* Johnson M (ed). *The Delivery of Quality Health Care: Series on Nursing Administration*, Vol 3. St. Louis, MO: Mosby-Year Book, pp 36–41.

Schroeder P (1994). Improving quality and performance: The concepts. *In* Schroeder P (ed). *Improving Quality and Performance: Concepts, Programs, and Techniques*. St. Louis, MO: Mosby-Year Book, pp 3–11.

Schultz A (1993). Evaluation of a clinical advancement system. *Journal of Nursing Administration* 23:13–19.

Simpson R (1994). How technology enhances total quality improvement. *Nursing Management* 25(6):40–41.

Tilbury MS (1992). From QA to CQI: A retrospective review. *In* Dienemann J (ed). *Continuous Quality Improvement in Nursing*. Washington, DC: American Nurses Publishing, pp 3–13.

Walton M (1990). *Deming Management at Work*. New York, NY: The Putnam Publishing Group.

17

Performance Management

Faye Anderson, MS, RN, CNAA

. . . .

LEARNING OBJECTIVES

This chapter will enable the learner to:

1. Discuss the purposes of performance appraisal.
2. Describe common problems of performance appraisal.
3. List the characteristics of an effective performance appraisal system.
4. Identify five principles for designing a performance appraisal system.
5. Identify sources of performance standards.
6. Describe the purpose and format of job descriptions.
7. List four methods of appraisal and identify the strengths and weaknesses of each.
8. Discuss the benefits of self-appraisal, peer review, subordinate evaluation, and customer evaluation.
9. Identify performance appraisal rater errors and methods to minimize errors.
10. Discuss the benefits of appraiser education.
11. Describe two approaches in determining when and how often to conduct performance appraisals.
12. Identify methods to enhance preparation of the appraisal report.
13. Develop an agenda for an appraisal performance interview.
14. Discuss important aspects of appraising the professional.
15. Describe a legally defensible performance appraisal system.
16. Discuss how performance appraisal can promote empowerment.

. . . .

INTRODUCTION

Changes in reimbursement, rising costs of health care, and a more knowledgeable patient/client are factors increasing the pressure on health care organizations to provide quality care in the most economical manner. Employee performance is critical to this initiative. Promoting effective performance is a management responsibility, and a performance appraisal system that is carefully designed and implemented can aid the manager in this effort.

The purpose of this chapter is to provide the reader with an overview of performance appraisal design and implementation. The purposes and problems of performance appraisal, characteristics of an effective system, and principles of designing a system are discussed. The relationship of performance standards and job descriptions to performance appraisal, and the strengths and weaknesses of various methods of performance appraisal are presented. The section on the appraisal process includes a discussion of who should appraise, how often appraisals should be conducted, preparing the appraisal report, conducting the appraisal interview, and appraising the professional employee. Legal and regulatory considerations are reviewed; and finally, empowerment through performance evaluation is discussed.

HISTORICAL BACKGROUND

Evaluating performance is not a modern management function. Landry (1989) reports that emperors of the Wu dynasty in China in AD 221 to 265 had an imperial rater who evaluated the royal family's performance. In the early 1800s, Robert Owens in

Scotland placed colored blocks at individual workplaces to indicate to workmen how well they had performed the previous day. Different colors were used to designate various levels of performance. Formal appraisals were used in the United States by government agencies in the early 1900s. Although performance appraisal methods that focused on personal traits were used after World War I, integration of work-related qualities into the process did not occur until the 1980s.

Early nursing literature emphasized the need for objective evaluation of personnel. In 1944, Wayland, McManus, and Faddis urged the hospital head nurse to follow the basic management principle of clearly defining the duties of personnel and checking performance. More than 20 years later, Shanks and Kennedy (1965) lamented the lack of valid, reliable instruments to evaluate nursing personnel objectively. They wrote:

The old problem of evaluating personnel performance meaningfully remains. At this point an evaluation of one person by another is nothing more than a judgment. But the quality of the judgment can be improved, if the person making the evaluation collects all the information he can get from all the sources he can find and objectively considers the facts. If sufficient facts are not available, the judgment cannot be made. It is inexcusable to base an evaluation on the findings obtained through the use of an inappropriate instrument of measurement, and it is possible that some evaluators are unable to be objective or lack the sensitivity and understanding necessary to make an evaluation (p. 115).

Court cases and regulatory guidelines developed over the years have reinforced the need for evaluations to focus on job performance and not on personality traits. Legal and regulatory implications will be discussed in a later section of this chapter.

DEFINITION OF PERFORMANCE APPRAISAL

Performance appraisal is a process that determines whether an individual is meeting established objectives or standards (Swansburg, 1990). The activity also includes a plan for improvement. The emphasis in the appraisal process is positive and is directed toward self-awareness, performance, and growth.

PURPOSES OF PERFORMANCE APPRAISAL

Although performance appraisal is often viewed negatively by both managers and employees, appraisal is beneficial to the individual and to the organization. Understanding the purposes and results of appraisal can promote acceptance and proper implementation of the process.

A major objective of performance appraisal is to maintain or improve performance (Gibson et al, 1991). Feedback given to the employee on how he or she is performing and how that performance compares to established standards is useful in identifying additional education or training needs. Training programs and inservice classes can be offered to promote development of the desired knowledge and skills. The individual can use the feedback to identify education courses external to the organization to enhance knowledge and skills required in the present position, or to grow professionally and be able to accept more responsibility.

Reiley (1992) states that performance appraisal is a method of ensuring quality of care because quality is dependent on the competency of those providing care. Performance appraisals assist managers and caregivers in identifying weaknesses that have an impact on the desired quality outcomes.

The appraisal process can be a method to motivate employees to perform the tasks necessary to accomplish the mission of the organization (Gibson et al, 1991; Mohrman et al, 1989). Specific goals can improve performance more than unclear suggestions can, and the employee is motivated by feedback that recognizes and reinforces good performance. Motivation may also occur when appropriate or improved performance results in increased compensation, such as salary increases, bonuses, or promotions.

The appraisal system can provide an opportunity for employees to gain insight and advice on career growth. Objective, accurate evaluation can put strengths and weaknesses into perspective and can assist the person in planning for the future. Energies can be directed toward goals that are valued in the institution.

Organizations routinely use information from the performance appraisal as the basis for a number of personnel decisions (Gibson et al, 1991; Swansburg, 1990). The most common are salary increases, promotions, transfers, demotions, and terminations. As already mentioned, the information can also be used to develop appropriate employee training programs.

Some conflict is inherent when the appraisal is used both for performance improvement and for reward purposes (Gibson et al, 1991; Mohrman et al, 1989). Open, honest discussion of achievements, strengths and weaknesses, and career development should occur when the focus is on improvement and development. The emphasis is not just on the past—what has been accomplished—but is also on what can be accomplished. But when rewards are tied to the appraisal, the focus changes. The employee emphasizes accomplishments and minimizes areas needing development. Thus, the goal of developing the employee and improving performance becomes secondary to achieving monetary rewards.

To minimize the conflict of these very different objectives, one appraisal may be conducted for developmental purposes, and a second at another time for reward purposes (Gibson et al, 1991; Mohrman et al, 1989). The initial discussion focuses on accomplishments and plans for improvement. After decisions are made on salary adjustments, a second meeting is scheduled for the manager to inform the employee of the raise and to reaffirm commitment to the goals previously established.

A final purpose of performance appraisal is to meet accreditation, regulatory, and legal requirements (McConnell, 1993). Disciplinary actions that result in demotions, reduction in pay, or terminations may be challenged. An objective, well-documented appraisal is critical to the defense in a grievance or regulatory hearing or a court case. Health care organizations must also have performance appraisal systems in place to meet accreditation standards by various state agencies and by the Joint Commission on Accreditation of Healthcare Organizations.

PROBLEMS WITH PERFORMANCE APPRAISAL

In spite of the recognized purposes and potentially positive results of performance appraisal, the process is frequently fraught with problems (Meyer, 1991). It may be implemented by less than enthusiastic managers and poorly perceived by uninterested or hostile employees. Mohrman et al (1989) identify the potential negative consequences as the following:

employees leave because of dissatisfaction with how they are treated; data are false; time is wasted; relationships are permanently damaged; motivation is lowered; money is wasted; and lawsuits are filed.

McConnell (1993) describes five problem areas that can compromise or destroy the effectiveness of a performance appraisal system. The first is a lack of managerial support that can originate at the very highest levels. Consider the following comments: "I just dread the month of June. I always have so many personnel evaluations to do." "That evaluation form really doesn't reflect what a nurse does. The whole procedure is just a waste of time." In a study reported by Napier and Latham (1986), managers perceived no consequences, either positive or negative, and no practical value in conducting performance appraisals. If appraisal is seen as an unpleasant task, completed only because it is "required," the process becomes a low priority that is postponed or implemented haphazardly. A negative attitude communicated to the employees can compromise the goal of improving performance. The nurse manager should promote the value and benefits of appraisal to his or her department, even if organization-wide support is minimal. Such efforts may be difficult, but the positive results of performance appraisal might be achieved in at least one department if the manager supports the process.

A second problem is confusion over what is being evaluated. In the past, appraisals focused almost exclusively on personality traits such as attitude or dependability and were evaluated subjectively. The appropriate appraisal focuses on performance, not on personality. Specific standards that reflect the responsibilities and tasks of the job with objective measures should form the basis for the appraisal. Thus the evaluator can be a witness of behavior rather than a judge of character or intentions (Wagner & Hollenbeck, 1992).

Lack of system support contributes to problems in a performance appraisal system. Maintenance of the system is usually the responsibility of the human resource department and involves such activities as notifying managers when evaluations are due, supplying forms, checking on delinquent appraisals, ensuring that appropriate actions are initiated (such as pay increases), and filing completed appraisals. In some health care organizations, a centralized nursing office may be responsible for some of the maintenance tasks.

Failure to provide training in how to implement the performance appraisal can also cause problems. Initial and ongoing training can minimize variations and inappropriate implementation. The reluctance of evaluators to give honest feedback, especially when pay or future career options are affected, can diminish the effectiveness of the appraisal. Training to promote the necessary skills may help overcome the emotional constraints to appraisal. Additionally, when the system has a mechanism to follow up on delinquent appraisals, the reluctant manager will not be able to delay indefinitely.

Finally, McConnell (1993) identifies fear of legal repercussions as a problem. Concern over lawsuits, complaints, or grievances may cause a manager to avoid being totally honest. To minimize negative consequences, the manager should be able to objectively verify all comments. Documentation should be objective with no subjective comments.

Due to current accreditation and legal concerns, performance appraisal must be conducted on a regular basis. Thus, it is important that a performance appraisal system be designed to minimize negative consequences and promote achievement of the primary objective, the improvement of performance.

DESIGNING A PERFORMANCE APPRAISAL SYSTEM

Designing or revising an appraisal system is a project that is usually initiated by senior management. Nurse managers, however, need a basic understanding of how appraisal systems are developed so that they can participate appropriately when the opportunity arises.

Characteristics of Effective Systems

Characteristics of an effective performance appraisal system have been identified (Table 17–1).

Table 17–1.

Characteristics of Effective Performance
  Appraisal Systems

1. The major objective is to improve performance.
   - The focus is on work performed.
   - A variety of formats is used.
2. The system is accepted by managers and employees.
   - The system is seen as fair and is easily understood.
   - Appraisal distinguishes between effective and ineffective behavior.
   - Employees have access to appraisal criteria and receive feedback.
3. Administrative support is present.
   - The system is maintained and kept current.
   - Evaluator training is conducted.
   - The system is evaluated regularly.
4. The appraisal process is continuous.
   - Follow-up occurs on goals and plans for improvement.

Data from Landry (1989), McConnell (1993), and Timmreck (1989).

The focus is on work performance and not on non-performance factors such as personality. Different approaches may be used to meet the needs of different employee groups. A single format may not be adequate in the complex health care organization, with numerous jobs requiring a variety of skills and knowledge.

An effective system has a high level of acceptance from both managers and employees and is perceived as fair and relevant to the work performed. The appraisal distinguishes between effective and ineffective performers and is easily understood and implemented. Employees have access to the criteria and standards prior to evaluation and receive feedback on performance in the appraisal interview. Employee acceptance can be promoted by involving employees in the development and revision of the system as well as through such activities as self-appraisal and goal-setting. Bretz et al (1992) reported that current appraisal systems in use in United States industry were designed primarily by personnel specialists with limited input from managers and almost no input from employees. The current trend, to increase participation at all levels, challenges administrators and human resource personnel to adopt methods that will appropriately involve personnel in the design and revision of performance appraisal systems.

Administrative support is essential in an effective system. Maintaining files, keeping job descriptions and standards current, furnishing forms, and following up on delinquencies are necessary tasks that usually are the responsibility of the human resource department. Evaluator training and retraining is scheduled, and the entire system is evaluated on a regular basis.

Finally, an effective system is one that does not begin and end with the formal appraisal. The process continues over time with both formal and informal follow-up on goals and plans for improvement.

Principles of Design

Mohrman et al (1989) discuss guiding principles for designing a performance appraisal system (Table 17–2). The first principle is to involve the right people and include the managers and the employees who will be affected by the system. Participation promotes acceptance. Experts may assist in development, but input from all levels is essential for support of the final design. The second principle is to recognize that performance appraisal is an integral part of a larger, complex system. The appraisal system will not be successful if it reflects a philosophy or requires support that is not part of the larger system. The third principle is to learn from implementation. The fourth is to be flexible. Some aspects of a system cannot be changed or modified but some can, and modifications should occur when problems are identified. The final principle is to be

Table 17–2.
Mohrman's Principles of Design

1. Involve people who will be affected by the system.
2. Recognize that performance appraisal is part of larger systems.
3. Learn from implementation.
4. Be flexible; modify when problems are identified.
5. Be patient; conduct ongoing evaluation, refinement, and education.

From Mohrman A, Resnick-West S, Lawler E (1989). *Designing Performance Appraisal Systems: Aligning Appraisals and Organizational Realities.* San Francisco: Jossey-Bass Publishers.

patient. Change takes time. A new or revised system will not gain acceptance immediately; ongoing evaluation and refinement and education will enhance acceptance.

Implementing a new or revised performance appraisal system is not easy and requires commitment on the part of the administration, the human resource department, managers, and employees. Outside consultants may be helpful in compiling the necessary data and can assist in developing formats and procedures. If consultants are not an option, a review of the literature combined with the expertise of the human resource department may achieve the desired result. When consultants are involved, they should not be used to the exclusion of involvement by the personnel affected. To repeat, participation promotes acceptance, and participation from all levels is essential to successful implementation (Case Study 17–1).

CASE STUDY ◆ 17–1

DESIGNING A NEW PERFORMANCE EVALUATION SYSTEM

Midtown Hospital is a medium-sized, community-owned, not-for-profit hospital. In the mid-1980s, the organization began to position itself as a regional leader for health care. Major services such as a physical rehabilitation program and cardiac catheterization and open-heart surgery capabilities were added. A shared governance structure in the nursing division was implemented and a clinical advancement program was planned. A complete revision of the performance evaluation system was one outcome of the clinical advancement program.

The design of the program included development of job descriptions, performance standards, appraisal tools, and the appraisal process. A task force composed of staff nurses, unit managers, and representatives from administration worked under the guidance of an external consultant to design the system. The design phase took approximately 2 years. During that time, the task force members would bring information to the nursing units and division committees for review and then bring feedback and suggestions back to the task force. From the outset, the project had the support of both nursing and general hospital administration. The human resources department was consulted as the system began to take shape.

Once the design was completed, members of the task force conducted educational sessions to acquaint nurses with the system and the details of implementation. The system was implemented in 1988.

Questions for Discussion:

1. How did the development of the system at Midtown Hospital reflect Mohrman's principles of design?

2. How could the design process be improved?

PERFORMANCE STANDARDS

The appraisal system will not be effective if personnel do not know what is expected of them and do not know the criteria by which they will be evaluated. Standards are an essential component of an effective performance appraisal system. A *standard* can be defined as the measure by which performance is judged (Gibson et al, 1991). Standards describe quality and quantity of work. They specify what is done, who does it, how much must be done, and when and where it must be done. Standards should be established by an authority, should be based on appropriate knowledge, and should be practical (Swansburg, 1990).

A variety of authoritative sources are available for determining appropriate professional standards; national sources include accreditation and professional associations. *Standards of Clinical Nursing Practice* (1991), developed by the American Nurses' Association, describes a common level of competent professional nursing care and performance and is "authoritative statements by which the nursing profession describes the responsibilities for which its practitioners are accountable" (p. 1). The standards can be used as a basis for job descriptions and performance appraisals.

Job Descriptions

Specific performance standards are derived from the job description (Swansburg, 1990). A job description describes the expectations associated with

a particular job; it is a written document that outlines the general scope, duties, and responsibilities of a job. It usually defines the minimal qualifications of individuals in that position, identifies reporting relationships and limits of authority, and provides the basis for performance evaluation (Table 17–3).

To develop appropriate, comprehensive job descriptions, data must be gathered from a number of sources. Individuals currently in the job can be observed or can keep diaries of duties performed. Interviews and questionnaires can also be used to determine the level of difficulty, the duties and responsibilities, and the skills and abilities required to perform a job.

Organizations usually have standard formats for all job descriptions. Standard information includes title, general summary of the job, required skills and qualifications, physical demands and environmental conditions, and major duties and responsibilities (Table 17–4).

Once a job analysis is completed and the job description developed, care must be taken that the document not become outdated. Regular review and revision are necessary so that the job description remains current and reflective of the work that is to be done and does not serve as an excuse to avoid action (eg, "It's not in my job description.").

It is essential that personnel know, understand, and accept the expected standards of performance. Involving the staff in developing standards can serve two purposes. First, the standards will be more realistic and achievable; and, second, the standards will be more acceptable to all. Fears that the standards will be too low should not be a reason to exclude staff from participating. Employees who are

Table 17–3.
Purposes of Job Descriptions

- Establish basis for salary structure
- Clarify relationships between jobs
- Aid in orientation to a job
- Aid in defining organizational structure
- Evaluate performance
- Assist in hiring, placement, and promotion
- Assign functions and responsibilities
- Maintain continuity of operations

From Swansburg, R (1990). *Management and Leadership for Nurse Managers.* Boston: Jones & Bartlett Publishers.

Table 17–4.
Registered Nurse I: Sample Job Description

JOB CLASSIFICATION: REGISTERED NURSE I
DEPARTMENT: NURSING

I. JOB SUMMARY:

   Performs basic skills independently and seeks collegial consultation from CN II–IV when indicated. RN I is the minimal level of performance for a clinical nurse.

II. POSITIONS SUPERVISED: LPNs; assistive personnel

III. QUALIFICATIONS:

   A. Education/Licensure: Graduation from an accredited, state-approved, school of nursing. Current Mississippi professional nurse license.

   B. Skills/Knowledge: Skill in treating patients with complicated disorders; ability to interpret physician's instructions; skill in equipment and instruments used in patient care. Knowledge of standard nursing principles, practices, and procedures.

IV. OTHER INFORMATION:

   A. Physical Demands: Visual acuity and manual dexterity are required for performance of duties. The ability to speak and hear are required to receive instructions and information and for communication. Must possess sufficient mobility to move freely about the hospital.

   B. Personal Traits: Compassionate, enthusiastic, creative, sincere, willing to accept guidance, interested in self-development.

   C. Post-Hire Training: Kind and length of training: One week of classroom orientation (includes general hospital orientation and CARE Program) plus orientation in the work area under supervision of director or designee. Training and supervision of IV therapy (including required return demonstration). Participates in continuing education.

   D. Working Conditions: Bloodborne pathogen exposure category: Category I (tasks involve exposure to blood, body fluids, or tissues).

   Protective equipment needed: Universal precautions—Equipment is available as needed and includes: gloves, gowns, masks, shields, caps, shoe covers, protective eyewear, space suits, lead shields, scrubs, and fluid barrier clothing.

V. JOB FUNCTIONS:

   A. Nursing Process

   1. ASSESSMENT

      a. Obtains baseline data through completion of systems assessment.

      b. Identifies nursing diagnosis based on information collected.

      c. Projects discharge needs of patient/family.

      d. Assesses patient/family learning needs.

      e. Reassessments of patients completed once per shift.

      f. Completes discharge planning section of admission assessment sheet.

   2. PLANNING

      a. Formulates a plan of care utilizing input from the patient, family, or other health team members.

      b. Identifies a measurable goal for each nursing diagnosis.

      c. Identifies nursing interventions for achieving specified goals and discharge needs.

      d. Develops a plan of care related to the patient/family learning needs.

   3. INTERVENTION

      a. Implements interventions consistent with standards of care.

      b. Employs or initiates environmental measures to promote safe patient care.

      c. Provides patient/family teaching consistent with the plan of care.

Table continued on following page

Table 17–4.

Registered Nurse I: Sample Job Description *Continued*

---

    4. EVALUATION

      a. Documents patient's/family's response to and outcome of the plan of care.

      b. Revises the written plan of care.

      c. Evaluates the effectiveness of the patient/family teaching and capabilities of patient/family to manage continuing care needs after discharge.

B. Professional Development

    1. QUALITY IMPROVEMENT

      a. Attends 75% of QI/staff meetings.

      b. Identifies unit quality issue and completes QI form.

      c. Participates in data collection for unit specific studies.

    2. UNIT ORIENTATION

      a. Assists with basic unit orientation.

      b. Teaches clinical skills to orienting nurse.

    3. EDUCATION

      a. Completes mandatory inservices.

      b. Obtains a minimum of 12 contact hours per year in addition to mandatory and unit certification.

    4. TEACHING PRACTICE (PEERS)

      a. Conducts one inservice per year pertinent to specialty area.

    5. RESEARCH/PUBLICATION

      a. Reads two research articles per year.

    6. MEETINGS

      a. Attends 75% of staff meetings per year.

      b. Attends 75% of committee meetings per year if applicable.

C. Lead RN

    1. Acts as lead RN when needed.

D. Attendance

    1. Meets professional responsibility by reporting to work as scheduled.

    2. Meets professional responsibility by reporting to work on time.

    3. Cooperates with meeting scheduling needs of the unit.

E. Care

    1. Is courteous in all dealings with patients, visitors, and fellow staff members.

    2. Maintains positive attitude toward job and hospital.

    3. Shows respect for fellow employees, supervisors, patients and visitors.

    4. Maintains enthusiasm for job by continually updating skills, knowledge, and desire for growth.

From Memorial Hospital at Gulfport, Gulfport, Mississippi. Used with permission.

committed to the mission of the organization and who are provided information about the purposes and goals of a performance appraisal system can assist in establishing standards that are realistic and achievable yet are also challenging.

Once standards are developed and approved, staff must be educated on the expected performance standards. Everyone should understand that the standards will form the basis for measuring individual performance and achievement.

METHODS OF APPRAISAL

A variety of formats are used for performance appraisal. Some compare employees against one another, either individually or in groups, whereas in other formats, the employee is evaluated against specific standards.

Individual Formats

A number of appraisal methods evaluate employees individually. A *graphic rating scale* is a commonly used format (Gibson et al, 1991). The employee is rated on a specific factor or characteristic on a numerical scale. Specific behavioral statements describe a performance level, and the rater chooses the rating that describes the performance of the employee. Typical factors evaluated on a graphic rating scale include quality and quantity of work, attendance, cooperativeness, dependability, and job knowledge (Table 17–5). The form may include space for comments to justify the rating chosen.

Although the graphic rating scale is easy to implement at a low cost, there are weaknesses in this approach. Different raters may not interpret the scales the same, so a person may be rated very differently by different evaluators. In addition, specific problems may not be identified when an overall positive score is given (McConnell, 1993).

In the *behaviorally anchored rating scale* (BARS), a scale is developed for each major component or task of a position. Descriptions of behavior define levels of performance. The evaluator determines which description best reflects the performance of the employee and notes that scale value. The total evaluation score is determined by combining the

Table 17–5.
Example of Graphic Rating Scale

Instructions: Circle the number corresponding to the value associated with the evaluation of the individual on the defined dimension.

Problem-Solving: Problems are identified and solved in manner consistent with organizational goals; involves personnel affected by the problem; takes action in timely manner in order to minimize delays and escalation of issues.

0	1	2	3
Unsatisfactory	Needs improvement	Satisfactory	Excellent

scale values for all the defined categories (McConnell, 1993) (Table 17–6).

The BARS method places emphasis on job performance rather than on personality traits and is objective. The format also provides specific information to the employee on current levels of performance and identifies the kind of behavior required to improve performance. The dimensions of each job must be identified and statements developed that describe examples of performance, ranging from high to low. The participation of managers and employees in this process promotes understanding and acceptance. The disadvantage of BARS is that it is time-consuming and costly to develop.

Checklists are composed of a number of statements describing behavior related to a job (Gibson et al, 1991). The rater indicates the presence or absence of the behavior (Table 17–7).

In some checklists, a weight may be assigned to each statement. To minimize bias, the actual weights may not be known to the evaluator. The final score is the total of all scores of the items marked. The amount of effort needed to develop and implement checklists can be a disadvantage of the format. In addition, restricting knowledge of the weights may alienate evaluators (McConnell, 1993).

In the *critical incident technique*, specialists prepare statements of effective and ineffective behavior that are organized into specific job categories. A log is kept by the rater of examples of good and poor performance. The log is used to evaluate the employee. This method may be very time-consuming

Table 17–6.

Example of Behaviorally Anchored Rating Scale

Function:	Quality of work:	Documentation	

Standard: Patient care is documented accurately and completely on approved forms. Content reflects patient status and care given.

1	2	3	4
Unsatisfactory performance Care frequently is not documented, documented incorrectly, or documented incompletely.	*Marginal performance* Care is usually documented, but charting frequently lacks all observations or information requested on approved forms.	*Acceptable performance* Care is regularly documented accurately and completely. Charting includes observations of patient progress, implementation of ordered treatments, and patient response to therapy.	*Exceptional performance* Care is consistently documented accurately and completely. Content includes all aspects of #3 with detailed assessments, planning with other health team members, and psychological and physiological problems and responses to care. Content can serve as an example to other employees.

and may not reflect the degree or frequency of a particular behavior (Joiner, 1988).

In an *essay method,* no particular form is used. The evaluator records the strengths and weaknesses of the individual. Educational or training needs may be identified as well as potential for growth and advancement. A guide may or may not be provided to assist the evaluator; thus, this approach may re-

Table 17–7.

Example of Checklist

Function: Patient Care Standards	Rating	
	MET	**NOT MET**
1. Obtains initial nursing history/assessment on newly admitted patients.	_____	_____
2. Develops and/or revises written plan of care based on assessment.	_____	_____
3. Conducts reassessments according to policy.	_____	_____
4. Implements plan of care; performing procedures in accordance with policy and safety standards.	_____	_____

sult in varied and inconsistent appraisals (McConnell, 1993).

A final individual approach to performance appraisal is *management by objectives* (MBO). The process of MBO involves establishing specific objectives and a plan of action, implementing the plan, measuring achievement and taking corrective action if necessary, and establishing new objectives and plans for the next time period. The objectives are established jointly between the employee and the manager; and regular discussions are held to review progress and revise plans if necessary. On the positive side, MBO brings together the needs and interests of the individual and the organization and enables individuals to know in advance how they will be evaluated (Gibson et al, 1991). On the negative side, an MBO system can require considerable time and effort to develop and maintain. In addition, setting reasonable goals is often difficult and may be subject to factors beyond the control of the individual.

Comparison Methods

Appraisal methods that compare employees include ranking, paried comparison, and forced distribution. *Ranking methods* require the evaluator to rate employees from highest to lowest on an overall criterion related to job performance. In the *paried comparison method,* each employee is compared to all others being evaluated. A record is kept of the number of times an individual is preferred over other individuals. A ranking is determined from the results. In the *forced distribution method,* the evaluator must rate employees according to assigned proportions at designated performance levels; for example, 15% are rated in the highest category, 15% in the lowest category, and 70% in the average category (Joiner, 1988).

Joiner (1988) notes that comparison methods are most effective for making decisions related to advancement, especially if more than one rater is involved; otherwise, the comparison method may lead more to evaluation of personality than performance. The method may also be problematic with large groups of employees.

To illustrate a comparison approach, consider how a division director uses ranking to evaluate six nurse managers. Each of the six is compared to all the others, making a total of 15 choices. Ms. Jones is always selected over any other managers, so she is ranked first. Mr. Martin is selected first except when compared to Ms. Jones, so he is ranked second. Ms. Wolf is ranked first three times, Miss Wells, twice, and Ms. Simpson only once. Ms. Lane is never picked over another manager and is ranked last. Even though a ranking is achieved, the differences among the individuals may not be substantial and the performance of all may be acceptable according to established standards. This method of evaluation might be useful if the division director is to select one of the managers to promote. However, this method would not be as helpful for the annual performance appraisal as would a criteria-based format that identifies specific behavior for commendation or improvement.

Whatever format is used, the specific form should be based on the job the person is expected to do and should facilitate the achievement of the objectives of the performance appraisal system, that is, to improve performance, motivate, and provide a basis for personnel action. It is unlikely that one form will meet the needs of all personnel in a complex health care environment. Joiner (1988) states that single measurement systems using formal checklists and ratings should be used only for more routine tasks that have predictable outcomes and are observable. As complexity of tasks and uncertainty of outcomes increases, additional sources of data should be incorporated into the appraisal system. Multiple sources of data should be part of the process if the appraisal has multiple purposes (eg, performance improvement, basis for salary increases, and identification of training needs).

APPRAISAL PROCESS

The performance appraisal process is more than just completing a specific form to be filed in an employee's personnel folder. Once an analysis of the job has been conducted, job descriptions developed, specific standards or criteria established for judging performance, and a format developed, decisions must be made regarding who will do the appraising and how often appraisals will be conducted.

Appraisers

Who appraises performance is an important issue to be decided when establishing the appraisal process. Although the typical appraisal review is conducted by the immediate supervisor, nontraditional sources such as peers, subordinates, and self are valid resources (Bretz et al, 1992). The more people appraising, the greater the chance that biases will be eliminated and that a more accurate picture of the individual will be presented (Mohrman et al, 1989; Reichel & Mehrez, 1994).

Appraisal by the Manager

The manager is usually the rater because it is assumed that the manager has more opportunities to observe behavior and to evaluate it in light of organizational and unit goals (Mohrman et al, 1989). The manager has direct knowledge of and experience with the work being done and has the status and authority to make decisions about performance. Even so, especially with large numbers of personnel to evaluate, input from a variety of sources enhances the evaluation. In a participative or matrix organization, others may actually have more information than the manager, and formal input from multiple appraisers should be incorporated into the process.

Self-Appraisal

Self-appraisal can be a very effective way to promote improved performance and motivation. Meyer (1991) has identified several advantages to self-appraisal. It promotes dignity and self-respect; it places the manager in a role of counselor rather than a judge; it promotes employee acceptance of plans for improvement; and it is likely to be more satisfying than the traditional approach without self-assessment. The individual may complete the same form as the manager or may submit documents and examples of performance. A less structured approach is for the employee just to meet with the manager to compare the self-evaluation with that of the manager, and for the two to develop a joint appraisal. Although self-appraisal is expected in a participative organization, it can be appropriate and helpful in the more traditional organization (Mohrman et al, 1989).

Peer Review

Peer review is examination and evaluation of an employee's practice by associates who are working with and at the same level as the employee. Established standards form the basis of the review (Douglass, 1992). Peer review can promote insight into areas needing improvement and can facilitate growth in both reviewers and employees.

Peer review is promoted among nurses as a component of a professional practice environment. It is supported as a mechanism to maintain nursing's professional accountability, integrity, and self-governance (Waldo et al, 1993).

Mann et al (1990) describe a peer review process that was designed to foster individual accountability for professional development and group accountability for quality practice on the unit. The manager, employee, and a group of two to four peers met at a scheduled time to review accomplishment of previous goals and requirements of the job description. Input from all peers was facilitated by the manager, with the final evaluation incorporating the employee's self-evaluation, the group input, and any areas of supervisory concern. The manager scheduled the appraisal interview with the employee to discuss the final written evaluation. The authors report that the process was viewed positively by managers, and staff interviews validated that the method supported professional accountability and job satisfaction. Managers saw the process as aiding their efforts to be a coach and mentor.

Both self-appraisal and peer review are supported in the ANA "Standards of Professional Performance" (1991). Standard II states "The nurse evaluates his/her own nursing practice in relation to professional practice standards and relevant statutes and regulations" (p. 14). The measurement criteria for the standard require that the nurse seek constructive feedback on practice and participate in peer review as appropriate.

Subordinate Evaluation

The most familiar example of subordinate evaluation of a superior is faculty evaluation by students. Subordinate ratings are helpful in determining how managers are functioning as leaders and as disseminators of information and how staff are functioning as team members. Although input from subordinates may be solicited periodically for developmental reasons, such evaluation on a regular basis is not common (Mohrman, 1989).

Figure 17–1 is an example of a subordinate evaluation of a nurse manager. The form reflects the manager's job description and is completed anonymously by employees at the time of the manager's annual evaluation. The results are used by the nurse manager for self-development and improvement.

Customer Evaluation

Increasingly, data from the customer's perspective are viewed as important in evaluating overall effectiveness. In health care, the patient/client's perception of care and satisfaction with processes are assessed and used in making changes. Although the opinion of the customer is subjective, the information can be very helpful in problem-solving and in improving behavior, especially if negative trends are apparent. Data on individuals or teams can be obtained from surveys, interviews, and letters from patients. A method of tracking responses would be needed to incorporate the input on a consistent basis that would be seen as fair by employees. Use of patient/customer responses in an arbitrary or biased way could undermine the validity of the information and jeopardize any decisions based on it.

Name of person reviewed: _____   **Date:** _____

Objectives	NA	Met	Not met	Exceeds	Comments
1. Participates in the long-range planning for the assigned area(s).					
2. Supports the council structure (Practice, QA, Education, and Nurse Management Council) and utilization of nursing care standards.					
3. Responsible for the operations of the assigned areas to ensure the quality of services on a 24 hour basis.					
4. Initiates and promotes unit activity toward achievement of unit goals and objectives.					
5. Maintains the operations of the department within the fiscal and productivity guideline of the hospital.					
6. Facilitates management of human resources to ensure the operation of the assigned unit(s).					
7. Participates in nursing recruitment activities.					
8. Contributes to the development of Quality Assurance activities.					
9. Conducts on-site rounds a minimum of twice weekly to review the quality of service.					
10. Contributes to and promotes a positive image of the hospital.					
11. Participates in various hospital and department committees.					
12. Demonstrates a commitment to teamwork philosophy within and among departments.					
13. Informs staff of projects and developments in the hospital.					
14. Demonstrates positive problem-solving approach in resolving concerns or issues with: a) Other departments b) Medical staff					
15. Maintains optimal interpersonal relationships with and among: a) Other departments b) Medical staff c) Other departmental employees d) Patients e) Families					
16. Serves as a role model for research activities that will impact quality and delivery of care.					
17. Demonstrates support for research activities that will impact quality and delivery of care.					

Figure 17–1. Example of a director review form. (From Memorial Hospital at Gulfport, Gulfport, Mississippi. Used with permission.)

Rater Errors

A number of appraisal rater errors have been identified (Timmreck, 1989). *Leniency* is rating an employee toward the positive end instead of rating correctly across the scale. When the evaluator rates toward the middle of the scale, the error of *central tendency* occurs. These errors make it difficult to separate those who are performing well from those who are performing poorly. In some cases an individual who performs well (or poorly) in *some* areas is rated high (or low) in *all* areas. This is the *halo effect*. With the *recency effect*, recent events carry more weight than events that occurred early in the evaluation period. In some instances, one negative event weighs heavier than a number of uneventful positive performances. Unfortunately, biases and prejudices of evaluators may also cause errors.

These errors in appraising contribute to a lack of trust in the appraisal system and may undermine the desired goals. Utilizing methods and formats that promote objectivity and minimize subjective comments can help to avoid errors.

Education of Appraisers

The appraiser(s) should have an understanding of the requirements of the job and the standards for acceptable performance and should be knowledgeable of the appraisal system forms and procedures. Adequate training should be conducted with appraisers so that gaps in knowledge do not influence the quality and effectiveness of the process and rater error is minimized. McConnell (1993) lists four specific reasons for appraiser training:

1. To ensure that employees are evaluated correctly and fairly.
2. To ensure consistency of application among employees and departments.
3. To promote full use of the system by managers to improve performance.
4. To ensure that the appraisal is seen as a positive process in the relationship between the employee and the manager.

Training is essential when a new system is implemented or if a current system is revised. In addition, new managers in the organization should receive training in the system procedures prior to evaluating employees. Bretz et al (1992) notes that while most organizations provide training when new systems are introduced, few provide regular ongoing training. Periodic updates are appropriate for all appraisers, especially if implementation problems are identified. Individuals may become lax in following procedures or may lose sight of the primary purpose of improving performance, especially when the evaluation is linked to specific external rewards such as pay increases.

Frequency of Appraisal

When and how often to evaluate is established by the organization as part of the overall appraisal system. Two approaches may be considered. All evaluations may be scheduled for some particular date; or employees may be evaluated on some recurring date, typically the anniversary date if yearly evaluations are conducted. Each approach has advantages and disadvantages (McConnell, 1993). Doing all the evaluations at one time can be overwhelming to the evaluator and may contribute to rater error such as halo or recency effects. The employee may feel that the process is less personalized and relevant. The all-at-once approach does provide a financial advantage when merit pay is directly connected to the appraisal. Funds for merit increase can be allocated and distributed in a more orderly, controlled manner. By conducting all appraisals at one time, overall quality and consistency are improved.

Evaluations done on a recurring basis (such as on an anniversary date) seem more personalized and current to the employee, and managers are able to spread the work over a longer time frame. If comparison evaluations are used, the anniversary approach may make the process more difficult, and merit increases are less predictable. Guidance to managers on distributing merit raises can, however, provide some control (McConnell, 1993).

The second issue related to frequency of appraisal is how often to evaluate. Annual evaluation is the common approach. Another approach is to relate evaluation to a specific task or project and to evaluate at completion. This last option does not lend itself to use in health care organizations, in which activity is ongoing and does not necessarily have a defined completion date (such as end of a semester, or development of a new product that goes to market). Evaluation should not occur before an employee has had an opportunity to demonstrate performance; neither should it be delayed so long that excellent performers lose motivation or it is too late to correct behavior of poor performers (Mohrman et al, 1989).

If performance is to be improved, information related to performance cannot be given just on an annual or semiannual basis. Informal feedback should be ongoing and continuous. Consider the following situation: A football coach notes that an offensive lineman is missing a blocking assignment on running plays. Each time a play is run, the defensive player is able to get through the line and tackle the running back for a loss. After watching the player and analyzing what is happening, the coach realizes the player really does not know his assignment on running plays and blocks the wrong defensive player. Additional training is needed. If the coach just makes a note of the problem with the intent to share this information at evaluation time, chances are the coach will not be back the next year! That is not how performance improvement occurs in sports and should not be the way it occurs anywhere. If the nurse manager or peer identifies problems in performance, positive, corrective feedback and action should occur immediately. Quality of care concerns, risk-management issues, and individual development needs mandate that feedback be continuous and ongoing.

Preparing the Appraisal Report

Conducting the performance appraisal is more than just completing an approved form. Appraisers—whether a supervisor or other individual such as a peer—need to dedicate adequate time and attention to developing the report. Since few people have total recall, most need to develop a system to assist in remembering specifics related to an individual's performance over the period to be evaluated. A system involving *anecdotal note files* has been shown to be effective in promoting recall of specific events (McConnell, 1993). An evaluator should routinely record significant observations that reflect performance. The date and brief notations of the facts can be kept in a file to serve as examples to verify ratings. These incidents should *not* be all negative;

examples of positive and outstanding performance should also be recorded.

When completing the appraisal form, notations should be made to verify ratings. These comments should be concise and objective and be consistent with the rating; subjective, biased personal comments should not be made. All notations should be written as if the record were going to be reviewed in court. If a formal self-appraisal is part of the record, the manager should complete the appraisal prior to reviewing the employee's self-evaluation to minimize bias (McConnell, 1993).

The written appraisal report should not be a surprise to the employee. If positive as well as corrective feedback has been given throughout the appraisal period, then the report will just be a summary of what has already occurred.

McConnell (1993) cautions about appraisal reports that are too lenient and minimalize poor performance. When the appraiser consistently fails to document such behavior, an incorrect message is given to the employee. In addition, if a decision to take corrective action is made, there is no history of unsatisfactory performance in the employee's file. Thus, efforts to improve performance may be very difficult. It cannot be stressed enough that the final report should be accurate and objective, identifying areas of strength and aspects of performance needing improvement.

Appraisal Interview

Although the appraisal interview may be just one part of an overall appraisal system, for the employee, the interview *is* the appraisal. An interview should be scheduled with every employee—excellent, average, and poor performers. The employee who is doing well should not be excluded just because there are no problems; all employees need feedback on how they are performing.

The appraisal interview is the time for assessment and counseling, a time for the appraiser and the employee to discuss how the employee is performing and formulate plans for future development. In many instances, it is also the time for discussion of administrative decisions such as salary changes (McConnell, 1993). The interview is often a major source of stress for the evaluator, especially if the discussion will include negative comments.

Delaying or glossing over the unpleasant aspects should be avoided. By preparing thoroughly before the interview, the evaluator can approach the interview with confidence. Training in interview communication and assertive techniques can also be helpful and can assist the manager in conducting appraisal interviews that are received positively and are more effective in producing the desired outcomes (Mohrman et al, 1989).

Part of preparing for the interview is establishing an agenda or plan for the discussion; without a planned agenda, the meeting may lack focus. If discussion of salary adjustments is part of the interview, this topic must be added to the agenda. Although there is disagreement over whether a discussion of salary or promotion should occur at the same time as the counseling and development discussion, if it is part of the process (and it frequently is), it must be considered when the appraisal interview is being planned.

The appraisal interview should take place in a setting that is quiet and private. The evaluator should make arrangements for the time and place as well as arrange for the meeting to be free of interruptions. One way by which some evaluators try to avoid difficult discussions—especially if the content is unpleasant—is to schedule the meeting at a time when interruptions are expected, such as midmorning on a busy unit when demands on time are great. The employee should never get the impression that the interview has to be rushed or that it is unimportant. The interview is a vital component of the appraisal process, and the setting should underscore that message.

A few minutes of pleasant greeting at the beginning of the meeting can help to establish a positive tone. No matter how well an employee thinks he or she is performing, the interview is stressful. Conveying an interested, supportive attitude can establish an environment for a productive meeting. Caution must be taken, however, to be sure that the attitude is not so casual that the objectives for meeting are minimized; the meeting is not a social occasion. The evaluator should present an attitude of genuine interest and support to encourage participation and promote a positive interaction (McConnell, 1993).

The evaluator can begin by encouraging the employee to present a self-appraisal. If a formal self-appraisal is part of the process, this can be reviewed at this time. If not, the use of open-ended questions and a review of the job description and standards can provide the structure for self appraisal. The evaluator can then review his or her assessment of the employee's performance and focus on areas where the employee's and manager's views are not consistent. Problem areas will need to be explored. It is important that the evaluator avoid making judgmental, subjective comments. Instead of saying "You are prejudiced against teenage mothers," note the source of the problem. "We have received negative feedback on patient satisfaction surveys from teenage mothers. Can you identify a reason for this?" Keep the tone positive and encourage the employee to identify weak areas and ways to achieve improvement.

If specific objectives were established in previous appraisal sessions, a review of achievement should occur. Lack of follow-up on goals and objectives minimizes their effectiveness. The employee may soon realize that setting goals is a paper process and is meaningless in regard to overall performance improvement. The conscientious employee will be frustrated if efforts to achieve objectives are not recognized. The discussion should also focus on satisfactory and exceptional performance, and the evaluator should recognize efforts to improve even if improvement is still necessary. Recognition of achievements and encouragement of continued efforts are just as essential as discussion of problem areas.

The meeting should close with an identification of specific objectives and plans for the next appraisal period. If problem areas have been identified in the review, plans to correct these should be formulated. For the employee performing at an acceptable or exceptional level, objectives may include activities to enhance and challenge his or her capabilities. Any plans should be developed jointly by the appraiser and the employee. The objectives should meet the expected criteria of objectives; that is, they should be specific and measurable. Vague, poorly defined objectives may meet the purpose of "having a plan" but may not result in any perceptible change and may indicate one type of performance to the manager and another to the employee. For example, the manager may interpret the objective "Improve attendance" as less than six unscheduled absences a year; to the employee, it may mean only one a month. The differences in interpretation can result in conflict and frustration rather than an improvement in a problem area.

The interview process is not complete until the results of the interview have been documented. Documentation includes completing the appraisal form with written comments and the agreed-on objectives and plans for improvement or continued growth. The employee should be aware of what is written and in most instances is required to sign the form to ensure that this occurs.

For employees who have major performance problems, consequences of failure to improve should be clearly communicated. Again, if appraisal has been continuous, there should not be any surprises in the formal interview. Documentation of unacceptable performance and proposed corrective action should have already occurred. Failure to comply with standards should be noted and specific consequences outlined if performance does not improve. See Case Study 17–2 for an example of an appraisal interview.

CASE STUDY ◆ 17–2

APPRAISAL INTERVIEW

Ms. Rawlings is a new nurse manager at Smalltown Community Hospital. She is to receive her first annual evaluation from her supervisor. She has not seen the evaluation, but she does have a job description and has attempted to perform her duties in accordance with the job description. Ms. Rawlings expected to have a personal interview with her supervisor to discuss the evaluation. Instead, one day she received the completed evaluation with a message to review it, sign it, and return it to the personnel department. The evaluation was on a standard form and reflected qualities such as cooperation, quality and quantity of work, and leadership. In general, the ratings were positive with minimal comments. Ms. Rawlings was very active in her professional association and had attended a number of meetings during the past year, but she always used personal leave time and did not ask for official time off for these meetings. Her involvement was known to the supervisor when she was hired. The only negative comment on the appraisal was a general statement about too many absences for professional meetings.

Questions for Discussion:

1. What might be Ms. Rawlings' impression of administrative support for the appraisal process?

2. What improvements in Ms. Rawlings' performance might be expected from this appraisal?

3. How can this evaluation process be improved?

Appraising the Professional

Recruitment, retention, and development of professional employees is a challenge for many organizations, as is the case in health care organizations regarding the professional nurse. Von Glinow (1989) reports that the professional must see that the appraisal is reflective of the work and is conducted by a credible source. Thus, peers may be more appropriate as evaluators than a manager who does not possess comparable skills. The appraisal system for the professional employee should be flexible; for example, multiple methods may be used in accordance with the work performed, such as a combination of rating scales and MBO, or the appraisal may be conducted on a less rigid time schedule if special projects are in progress. Appraisal feedback must address relevant issues and be valid. These areas have already been identified as components of an effective appraisal system, but their importance with the highly skilled professional cannot be overemphasized. It is difficult to define and quantify the work of the professional, and sometimes major components may be missing from an appraisal. Von Glinow (1989; p. 201) notes, "If critical aspects of a professional's performance are missing or haphazardly dealt with on the appraisal form, either the appraisal is considered bogus and therefore is discounted or the critical aspects will be overlooked." Since the work of nurses is very complex and difficult to define, appraisals and standards that focus only on more easily defined aspects such as psychomotor skills may be perceived as invalid by the nurses, and the problems identified by Von Glinow may result.

LEGAL AND REGULATORY CONSIDERATIONS

Federal law, Equal Employment Opportunity Commission guidelines, and court cases have established requirements that have an impact on performance appraisal. Title VII of the 1964 Civil Rights Act, amended in 1972 and 1974, makes it illegal in matters of terms, conditions, or privilege of employment to discriminate on the basis of race, color, religion, sex, or national origin. The Age Discrimination in Employment Act of 1967 protects job applicants and employees aged 40 to 70 years from discrimination (Wiatrowski & Palkon, 1987). More recently, the Americans with Disabilities Act requires the fair treatment of qualified individuals with disabilities.

Rulings in court cases underscore the need to have valid appraisal systems that are designed carefully. In *Brito v Zia Company,* the court ruled that the performance appraisal used for layoffs did not have established validity and that ratings were made by supervisors who did not have sufficient information to judge performance (Gibson et al, 1991). In *Griggs v Duke Power Company,* the Supreme Court ruled that testing procedures for specific jobs must relate to the tasks of the job. When performance appraisals are used for selection, transfer, or promotions, the rulings of this court case apply (Joiner, 1988).

In a legally defensible appraisal system, the content of the appraisal is developed from a job analysis and is behavior oriented, not trait related. Appraisers are trained in the process; employees are aware of performance criteria and standards; and the results are reviewed by the employee (Gibson et al, 1991).

A further consideration is to establish an appeals process (Balkin, 1994; Mohrman et al, 1989). No individual evaluator or system is perfect; errors are made and biases are present. An appeals process can promote employee acceptance of the appraisal system and provide additional incentive for the evaluator to present a fair, unbiased evaluation.

In addition to legal concerns, accreditation agencies have established guidelines for performance appraisal. For a number of years, the Joint Commission on Accreditation of Healthcare Organizations has required the use of performance evaluations that are criteria based and related to the job description (JCAHO, 1995).

EMPOWERMENT VIA PERFORMANCE EVALUATION

In today's health care environment, competent, productive employees are a valuable asset. Developing individuals and teams and empowering them to act in accordance with an organization's mission are critical to long-term organizational survival and success. The philosophy that the manager is in complete control and has all the pertinent information while the employee just follows orders is obsolete and ineffective. The pace of change, the escalating body of knowledge, the expansion of technology coupled with a more highly educated technical/professional staff require a management approach that recognizes the expertise of skilled workers and empowers them to do their job. Nurses bring specialized knowledge and skills to the health care setting and must be allowed to function without encumbering rules and policies.

Empowered nurse managers are facilitators and coaches who assist the nurse to do the job and to obtain additional training as knowledge and expectations change. Empowered employees understand the mission of the organization and receive regular feedback related to achievement of organizational objectives. They understand their role in achieving the mission and receive education to increase skills. Performance appraisal systems with the primary objective of improving performance can assist in an organization's efforts to empower staff. Clear descriptions of roles and responsibilities eliminate questions and confusion. Employees can be given authority and responsibility for defined activities and then can be trusted by management to execute that authority without having to check and gain approval for each activity (Dveirin & Adams, 1993). Explicit expectations (standards) that are known by the employee promote coordination of efforts and achievement of goals.

Meaningful feedback given to empowered employees includes appraisal of their performance and how well they are meeting goals. Halamandaris (1992) supports self-evaluation as empowering and proposes establishing categories of raises that would enable staff to suggest their own raises. An example of this approach is shown in Table 17–8.

The benefits of involving the staff at all levels when developing and implementing a performance appraisal system have already been identified. Such participation also promotes empowerment. When roles, responsibilities, working relationships, and standards are established with input from the employees, overall understanding and support are en-

Table 17–8.
Sample Criteria for Above-Standard Performance: Staff Registered Nurse

Instructions for Performance Criteria/Validations
Performance criteria reflect expectations for the RN to provide safe, efficient, and therapeutically effective patient care through assessment, planning, implementation, and evaluation, and expectations for professional development.
To be eligible for a 4% merit raise, the RN must meet 100% of the performance criteria. To be eligible for a 6% merit raise, the RN must meet 100% of the performance criteria plus 80% (four of the five criteria) of the performance criteria for "above-standard performance."

PERFORMANCE CRITERIA	VALIDATION
1. Completes one special project specific to unit needs as mutually agreed upon by staff member and director prior to evaluation.	1. Submits evidence of completed project.
2. Holds membership in nursing organization and attends 50% of meetings per year.	2. Submits copy of membership card and evidence of attendance at meetings.
3. Achieves 100% of nursing process criteria for present level on four additional charts.	3. Random concurrent review of four charts by a peer shows evidence of meeting Assessment, Planning, Intervention, and Evaluation Criteria. Peer will be mutually agreed upon by nurse being evaluated and director.
4. Obtains 10 additional contact hours beyond hospital/unit's mandatory hours, and beyond contact hours required for standard performance.	4. Shows evidence of 10 additional contact hours beyond hospital/unit's mandatory hours and beyond contact hours required for standard performance.
5. Reads an additional research article, summarizes, and presents pertinent information at a staff meeting.	5. Unit meeting minutes reflect presentation of article summary.

From Memorial Hospital at Gulfport, Gulfport, Mississippi. Used with permission.

hanced, and efforts are directed toward desired goals.

SUMMARY

What is the future of performance appraisals? Although much information is available for developing and implementing effective systems, Bretz et al (1992) conclude that organizations continue to undermine effectiveness. Training is lacking, the role of the employee is ignored, and sources of information, such as peers and self, are overlooked. The demands for increased efficiency and quality may, however, result in a greater emphasis on designing and implementing appraisal systems that can assist in improving performance. New formats may be developed and extensive training of both evaluators and evaluatees may be instituted. Redesign of health care organizations may also result in a totally different approach to appraisal. Emphasis on teams

and work groups is changing the focus to productivity of teams rather than the individual. Outcomes, continuous quality improvement, and customer satisfaction are areas receiving more attention. Perhaps in the future, individual appraisals will not be conducted; instead appraisal may be of the work team and the team's achievement of goals and objectives. Whatever the approach, an appraisal system that is fair, focuses on performance, is implemented by knowledgeable evaluators, and is designed to improve performance can be a valuable component of the organization of today and tomorrow.

■ DISCUSSION QUESTIONS ■

1. Discuss the purposes of performance appraisal.
2. Identify common problems associated with performance appraisal.
3. Discuss the strengths and weaknesses of four different individual performance appraisal formats.

4. Describe a situation in which a comparison method of appraisal is more appropriate.
5. Discuss the benefit of including information from a variety of sources in the performance appraisal review.
6. Identify common errors made by evaluators. How can they be minimized?
7. Discuss the components of a successful performance appraisal interview.
8. Identify requirements of a legally defensible appraisal system.

■ LEARNING ACTIVITIES ■

1. As the manager of a medical unit, you are to chair a committee to review and revise the staff nurse job description, which has not been revised in 5 years. Develop a plan of action identifying potential members of the committee, sources of standards, and specific tasks.
2. As a new nurse manager just promoted from a staff nurse position, you are very aware of the dissatisfaction of the staff with the performance appraisal system. You would like the system to be revised to include input from peers. Describe how you would promote a peer review component to your supervisor.
3. As a manager in a home health agency, you are part of a team developing the job description and self-appraisal for the new position of case manager. How would you proceed with the assignment?
4. You are the nurse manager of an outpatient surgery unit. A nurse employed 8 weeks earlier is obviously having problems getting to work on time. Her lateness is causing unrest with the rest of the staff. She is due to receive her 3-month probation evaluation in 1 month. How should you handle this situation?

■ BIBLIOGRAPHY ■

Alexander Hamilton Institute, Inc (1989). *Performance Appraisals*, 2nd ed. Maywood, NJ: Modern Business Reports.

American Nurses' Association (1991). *Standards of Clinical Nursing Practice*. Washington, DC: Author.

Balkin D (1994). Comment: Managing the inherent bias in personnel evaluation. *Journal of Management and Inquiry* 3(1): 96–97.

Bowen DE, Lawler EE (1992). Total quality oriented human resources management. *Organizational Dynamics* Spring: 29–41.

Bretz RD, Milkovich GT, Read W (1992). The current state of performance appraisal research and practice: Concerns, directions, and implications. *Journal of Management* 18(2): 321–352.

Douglass A (1992). *The Effective Nurse: Leader and manager.* St. Louis: Mosby-Year Book.

Dveirin G, Adams K (1993). Empowering health care improvement: An operational model. *Journal of Quality Improvement* 19(7):222–232.

Gibson J, Ivancevich J, Donnelly J (1991). *Organizations: Behavior, Structure, Processes,* 7th ed. Homewood, IL: Irwin, Inc.

Halamandaris VJ (1992). Empowering people: Key to the future. *Caring Magazine* Sept:36–41.

Houston S, Luquire R (1991). Measuring success: CNS performance appraisal. *Clinical Nurse Specialist* 5(4):204–309.

Joiner CL (1988). Performance appraisal. In Fottler M, Hernandez SR, Joiner CL (eds). *Strategic Management of Human Resources in Health Services Organizations.* New York: John Wiley & Sons, pp 319–346.

Landry JA (1989). Performance management systems. In *Productivity and Performance Management in Health Care Institutions.* Chicago: American Hospital Publishing.

Mann L, Barton C, Presti M, Hirsch J (1990). Peer review in performance appraisal. *Nursing Administration Quarterly* 14(4):9–14.

McConnell CR (1993). *The Health Care Manager's Guide to Performance Appraisal.* Gaithersburg, MD: Aspen Publishers.

Meyer HH (1991). A solution to the performance appraisal feedback enigma. *Academy of Management Executives* 5(1): 68–76.

Mohrman A, Resnick-West S, Lawler E (1989). *Designing Performance Appraisal Systems: Aligning Appraisals and Organizational Realities.* San Francisco: Jossey-Bass Publishers.

Napier N, Latham G (1986). Outcome expectancies of people who conduct performance appraisals. *Personnel Psychology* 39:827–837.

Nathan BR, Cascio WF (1986). Introduction. Technical and Legal Standards. In Berk RA (ed). *Performance Assessment: Methods and Applications.* Baltimore: Johns Hopkins University Press, pp 1–50.

Peglow DM, Klatt-Ellis T, Stelton S, et al (1992). Evaluation of clinical nurse specialist practice. *Clinical Nurse Specialist* 6(1):28–35.

Plachy RJ (1988). *Performance Management: Getting Results from Your Performance Planning and Appraisal System.* New York: AMACOM.

Reichel A, Mehrez A (1994). Employee selection and performance evaluation biases and organizational efficiency: A mathematical modeling attempt. *Journal of Management and Inquiry* 3(1):85–95.

Reiley P (1992). Quality assurance programs. In Johnson M (ed).

The Delivery of Quality Health Care: Series on Nursing Administration, Vol 3. St. Louis: Mosby-Year Book, pp 71–85.

Roland HS, Roland BL (1985). *Nursing Administration Handbook*. Rockville, MD: Aspen Publications.

Shanks M, Kennedy D (1965). *The Theory and Practice of Nursing Service Administration*. New York: McGraw-Hill.

Staff (1993). Performance evaluations: Making them meaningful. *Personnel Manager's Letter.* July 10:1–3.

Swansburg RC (1990). *Management and Leadership for Nurse Managers*. Boston: Jones & Bartlett Publishers.

The Joint Commission (1995). *1996 Accreditation Manual for Hospitals*. Oakbrook Terrace, IL: Author.

Timmreck T (1989). Performance appraisal systems in rural western hospitals. *Health Care Management Review* 14(2):31–43.

Von Glinow MA (1989). Appraising the performance of professional employees. In Mohrman A Jr, Resnick-West S, Lawler E. *Designing Performance Appraisal Systems: Aligning Appraisals and Organizational Realities.* San Francisco: Jossey-Bass Publishers, pp. 196–203.

Wagner JA, Hollenbeck JR (1992). *Management of Organizational Behavior.* Englewood Cliffs, NJ: Prentice-Hall.

Waldo JM, Hofschulte L, Mango L, Colleran M (1993). Peer review for nurse managers. *Nursing Management* 24(5):58–59.

Wayland M, McManus RL, Faddis M (1944). *The Hospital Head Nurse.* I. Stewart (ed). New York: MacMillan Co.

Wiatrowski MD, Palkon DS (1987). Performance appraisal systems in health care administration. *Health Care Management Review* 12(1):71–80.

Young L, Hayne A (1988). *Nursing Administration: From Concepts to Practice.* Philadelphia: WB Saunders.

2

Index

Note: Page numbers in *italics* refer to illustrations; page numbers followed by t refer to tables.